The China Gadabouts

The China Gadabouts

New Frontiers of Humanitarian Nursing, 1941–51

Susan Armstrong-Reid

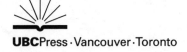

UBCPress · Vancouver · Toronto

27 26 25 24 23 22 21 20 19 18   5 4 3 2 1

Printed in Canada on FSC-certified ancient-forest-free paper (100% post-consumer recycled) that is processed chlorine- and acid-free.

Library and Archives Canada Cataloguing in Publication

Armstrong-Reid, Susan, author
 China gadabouts : new frontiers of humanitarian nursing, 1941-51 / Susan Armstrong-Reid.

Includes bibliographical references and index.
Issued in print and electronic formats.
ISBN 978-0-7748-3592-3 (hardcover). – ISBN 978-0-7748-3594-7 (PDF)
ISBN 978-0-7748-3595-4 (EPUB) – ISBN 978-0-7748-3596-1 (Kindle)

 1. Nursing – China – History – 20th century. 2. Nurses – China – History – 20th century. 3. Humanitarian assistance – China – History – 20th century. 4. Missions, Medical – China – History – 20th century. 5. Sino-Japanese War, 1937–1945 – Health aspects – China. 6. Friends Ambulance Unit – History – 20th century. I. Title.

RT13.C6A76 2018   610.73095109'044   C2017-905969-6
                                                    C2017-905970-X

Canadä

UBC Press gratefully acknowledges the financial support for our publishing program of the Government of Canada (through the Canada Book Fund), the Canada Council for the Arts, and the British Columbia Arts Council.

Printed and bound in Canada by Friesens
Set in Museo and Warnock by Artegraphica Design Co. Ltd.
Copy editor: Francis Chow
Proofreader: Carmen Tiampo
Indexer: Noeline Bridge
Cover designer: George Kirkpatrick
Cartographer: Marie Puddister

UBC Press
The University of British Columbia
2029 West Mall
Vancouver, BC V6T 1Z2
www.ubcpress.ca

To   **DR. GLENNIS ZILM** and **JANE ZAVITZ-BOND,**
whose encouragement and enthusiasm for
their respective fields, nursing history and
the Peace Testimony, inspired this book

Contents

PART 3: Unwelcome Visitors: Negotiating Access with the Communists, 1947–51

Maps

Acknowledgments

Recovering the stories from the field of the Quaker-sponsored relief organization commonly known as the China Convoy, from 1941 to 1951, took many unexpected turns in the six years from its conception to completion. It is based upon a diverse range of materials from public archival and private papers held in Canada, the United States, Great Britain, and New Zealand. Archivists at Canadian Quaker Yearly Meeting Archives (CQYMA) (Pickering, Ontario); the American Friends Service Committee Archives (AFSCA) and Haverford College (Philadelphia); Friends House London (the Library of the Religious Society of Friends) and the Imperial War Museum (London); the Woodbrooke Quaker Study Centre (Birmingham); and the National Library and the Alexander Turnbull Library (Welland, New Zealand) made my research trips both more profitable and pleasurable. Don Davis at the AFSCA and Jane Zavitz-Bond at the CQYMA merit special thanks for encouraging and tolerating me during this project.

The study's direction, however, was refined as a rich trove of untapped private sources informed its critical engagement with the scholarly conversations on humanitarian nursing's contested place within the wider global context. My family will attest that the process of unearthing new sources held by Convoy members or their families became somewhat addictive. What set this project apart was the generosity and trust exhibited by Convoy members and their descendants. They not only consented to be interviewed or to share private letters, diaries, and photos but also opened their homes to me on my research trips, or made connections with other Convoy members' descendants. There was a need to be attentive to the subjectivity of Convoy members in selecting what to record or how they reconstructed their involvement, as well as my own relationship with them; nonetheless, their diaries, memoirs, and letters and my own interviews enlivened, confirmed, or, at other times, corrected the portrait of events painted by official documents. They led to a deeper appreciation of how race, profession, gender, nation, culture, and place figured quite differently in shaping members' intensely personal odysseys, sometimes within the same medical team. From this perspective, I am particularly indebted to Edwin Abbott, Joe Awmack, Harriet Brown Alexander, Douglas Clifford, and Graham Milne, as well as the families of Connie Bull and Ron Condick, Lindsay Crozier, Jack Dodds, Al Dobson, Shirley Elliott Gage, Kathleen Green Savan, Gordon Keith, Frank Miles, Mark and Mardy Shaw, Francis Starr, Margaret Stanley Tesdell, Rita Dangerfield White, and Joan Kennedy Woodrow. Craig Shaw and Rebecca Stanley Tesdell offered constant encouragement as the work progressed. Collectively, these private papers and archival sources revealed a far more contested and complex portrait of the China Convoy's humanitarian endeavours on the ground than would have been possible otherwise.

While researching this book, I had the good fortune to connect with a lively group of scholars engaged in unpacking the stories of individual members of the China Convoy. Conversations with David Brough, Caitriona Cameron, Cathy Miles Grant, Andrew Hicks, and Thomas Socknat provided different vantage points that enhanced my understanding of the interplay of personalities and pacifist views that imbricated the Convoy's humanitarian work. Caitriona Cameron graciously granted access to the oral interviews that she had conducted while writing her study of New Zealanders' contribution to the China Convoy. Andrew Hicks, David Brough, Sacha Denton White, and several descendants of other China Convoy members meet annually and work to keep the memory of the Convoy's relief effort alive. Their passion for uncovering, preserving, and sharing Convoy stories was contagious.

Over time, as we exchanged information, China Convoy members and their families became friends. An invitation to travel with Cathy Miles, her brother Dan, and his wife, Shelly Stickel-Miles, to China in the spring of 2016 stands out among my cherished memories of this project. Their father, Frank Miles, served on medical team 19 (MT19) in Yan'an, on MT21 in Zhongmou, and then as chairman of the China Convoy.

Capturing the many moving moments that I experienced as the enduring personal connections and national commemoration of this Quaker relief organization's legacy unfolded in surprising ways over those three weeks is difficult to do. Obtaining a visa to travel to China is fraught with bureaucratic challenges and requires being sponsored by a Chinese citizen. Our sponsor was Wang Yunying, whose father had worked closely with Cathy's father. Frank Miles, Douglas Clifford, and Jack Dodds were instrumental in arranging for the Chinese Student Foundation of Ontario to sponsor

Yunying's studies at the University of Toronto from 1985 to 1987. The connection strengthened during the years that Dan and his family lived in China and on Yunying's visits to the Miles family home. Yunying's translation skills were surpassed only by her hospitality and continued geniality as she deftly orchestrated all of our travel arrangements and presentations with 8th Route Army Office museum officials in Xi'an and Yan'an and the modern Henan hospital that traced its roots to 1947 in a humble Quonset hut.

As we were feted and swept away on private tours where tourists seldom venture, the legacy of the Convoy's desire to foster global friendship was clearly discernible. During each visit, our hosts attempted to share the few surviving Chinese sources; in turn, we were able to present digital pictures and film footage of the China Convoy's work that documented the agency of its Chinese staff. In 2014, the 8th Route Army Museum, together with Xi'an Municipal Administration and David Brough, who acted as liaison with Friends Ambulance Unit (FAU) members and their descendants, had opened an exhibition called "Our Common Memories" of the FAU China Convoy, in Xi'an, Shaanxi Province. Our desire to share the historically important photographic record of Douglas Clifford, Margaret Stanley, and Frank Miles was crucial as new exhibitions depicting the Convoy's humanitarian work were being planned. During our visit to Xi'an in April 2016, we met Li Gang, son of Li Xingpei, who had worked in Yan'an with MT19. At our hotel later that evening, we were delighted to be presented with photos of MT19's 1978 visit to Yan'an.

I am especially grateful for the friendship and support of colleagues within the dynamic transnational network of scholars re-evaluating the history of global nursing. During the formative stage of this book, I was particularly fortunate to receive funding as the 2012 Lillian Sholtis Brunner fellow from the Barbara Bates Center for the Study of the History of Nursing at the University of Pennsylvania. The fellowship not only funded my research at the America Friends Service Committee Archives but also provided the opportunity for thought-provoking conversations with centre scholars Barbara Mann Wall and Julie Fairman. Our conversations probed the project's scope, foundational analytical frames, and contribution to the scholarly debates swirling around the contested concept of "humanitarian nursing." Later I had the opportunity to contribute a chapter, "Two China 'Gadabouts': Guerrilla Nursing with the Friends Ambulance Unit, 1946–48," in *Colonial Caring: A History of Colonial and Post-colonial Nursing* (Manchester University Press, 2015), edited by Helen Sweet and Sue Hawkins, whose insight and expertise proved invaluable for situating this work within the global scholarly conversations. Equally, I gratefully acknowledge my Canadian colleagues, Jane Elliott, Cynthia Toman, Wendy Mitchinson, Jamie Snell, and Glennis Zilm. Their careful reading of and comments on individual chapters, offered from different perspectives, improved the final manuscript.

At every stage of this publishing journey, I also benefited from sage editorial direction. While preparing the manuscript for submission, Ian Mackenzie, a veteran editor and Canadian "mish kid" born in Henan, consistently offered both excellent technical and structural advice, often within tight timelines. The professionalism of UBC Press's editorial staff, Darcy Cullen, Nadine Pedersen, Megan Brand, and Francis Chow, was surpassed only by their approachability and enthusiastic support for this project. Marie Puddister, a very talented cartographer at the University of Guelph, created the maps that will enable my readers to visualize where the teams worked, especially as many of the village names are not easily locatable.

Ultimately, my greatest debt is to my husband, Richard, the "senior" historian in the family. Despite his teasing that "family vacations" somehow always involved the China Convoy, or that writing diminished my culinary skills, he was an ardent supporter and an exceptional in-house editor, even when it meant setting aside his own manuscript.

The China Gadabouts

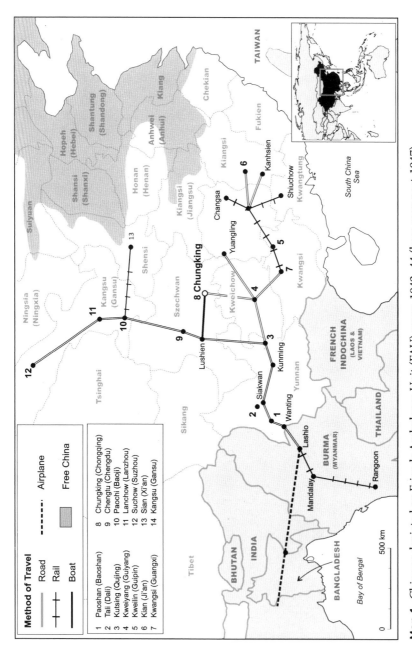

Map 1 China as depicted on Friends Ambulance Unit (FAU) maps, 1942–44 (base map post-1947)

Method of Travel

Road
Rail
Boat
Airplane

Free China

1 Paoshan (Baoshan)
2 Tali (Dali)
3 Kutsing (Qujing)
4 Kweiyang (Guiyang)
5 Kweilin (Guipin)
6 Kian (Ji'an)
7 Kwangsi (Guangxi)
8 Chungking (Chongqing)
9 Chengtu (Chengdu)
10 Paochi (Baoji)
11 Lanchow (Lanzhou)
12 Suchow (Suzhou)
13 Sian (Xi'an)
14 Kangsu (Gansu)

Introduction

[The Friends Ambulance Unit] was an agency through which members of the Society of Friends and like-minded persons carry into action their deepest religious convictions and insights ... Through relief service we are able to express our sense of responsibility for and unity with our fellow human beings. We feel we need to bring food, clothing, and shelter to those in distress, but far more important than even such vital material assistance is the opportunity to share the burden of suffering of another, to help restore his sense of self-respect and integrity, and to restore his faith in love and good-will through a practical demonstration of human sympathy and brotherhood. Convinced of the error of the way of violence, Friends seek to make love the basis of their relationships with others.

– FAU SERVICE CONTRACT

On 18 April 2014, the Chinese government opened an exhibition at the 8th Route Army Museum in the city of Xi'an, Shaanxi Province, to commemorate humanitarian work performed over seventy years earlier by the Society of Friends Ambulance Unit (FAU) and its successor after 1947, the Friends Service Unit (FSU).[1] It was a surprising overture, considering the passage of time and the small size of the FAU's China section, commonly known as the China Convoy. The opening remarks of Zheng Yulin, director of the Xi'an Municipal Administration for Cultural Heritage, explained the exhibit's purpose:

We would like to share these stories with all the people whose lives and happiness today were made possible by the sacrifices of the China Convoy and their colleagues. Through these precious and moving images, we can commemorate [their] brave deeds ... in rescuing Chinese wounded soldiers and civilians in those terrible times, and feel the scars made by brutal war and the healing through the humanitarian activities and the perseverance and kindness of these individuals. The history is passed, but showing what happened is to commemorate the hard-earned peace and to enlighten thinking about history and the present, war, peace, life and its purpose.[2]

This was the first time the Chinese public had been made aware of the Convoy's humanitarian activities. More remarkably, other exhibits have continued to spread the stories of their shared cultural heritage; the next held in Yan'an, the cradle of Revolutionary China, is currently scheduled for the fall of 2017.

Going to China as a conscientious objector in the 1940s was not for the faint-hearted. The dangerous transport job and arduous medical work claimed the lives of seven idealistic young men. This book considers the confluence of two separate yet intertwined stories. It is the history of the China Convoy's humanitarian endeavours at a pivotal moment in China's social and structural revolutions and today's humanitarianism. Understanding how Convoy members framed their humanitarian action and, in turn, were profoundly changed by their experience deepens our understanding of the continuing ethical dilemmas of acting humanely, impartially, and neutrally across borders and cultures to ensure basic human security.

Mining archival collections, untapped diaries, letters, interviews, memoirs, private and official photo collections, and film footage, this book selected nurses' experiences to shed new light on the Convoy's pacifist principles, culture, and struggles to realize its transnational pacifist vision. The lived experiences of nurses provide a window into the tangled professional and political relationships that underpinned the Convoy's humanitarian actions. Nurses witnessed every aspect of the cultural shift to reconcile the Convoy's pacifist beliefs and medical work with the gruesome reality of war-ravaged China, yet historical accounts privilege the narrative of the Convoy men in traditionally gendered roles as conscientious objectors, leaders, physicians, medical mechanics, and truck drivers.[3]

Despite the constraints that class, gender, place, and race imposed on their life choice, nurses exercised agency to advance their lives personally and professionally. This book examines how humanitarian work gave meaning to women's lives as nurses and as private individuals, and how they carved out personal and professional space despite a chaotic, unfamiliar, and sometimes hostile environment, to create a sense of home and belonging. The history of the Convoy nurses is not only the history of the nurses themselves and, by association, humanitarian nursing as a contested concept. It is about women's historically constructed place in the historiography of global society that marginalizes their contributions and power. This volume is the first comprehensive study that critically interrogates the multi-faceted and contested agency exercised by Western and Chinese nurses in the China Convoy's humanitarian efforts from 1941 to 1951.

Physicians' stories and accounts provide an important counterpoint throughout the book, however. Although their experiences were intertwined, nurses were subject to different biases, discriminations, and challenges. Male physicians' narratives reveal nurses' gendered and sometimes racialized place within this Western humanitarian organization. Those of female physicians expose women's gendered experiences across professional lines. I have attempted to find nurses' voices as women, alongside and in relation to the Convoy men, to understand how gender and professionalism defined and shaped the Convoy's history. Physicians' accounts spotlight the tensions across cultural and professional boundaries that nurses were expected to manage, many of which extended well beyond bedside matters. In addition, the historical narratives of nurses, especially those of Chinese nurses, were often refracted or embedded in accounts written by men for family members or for the Convoy's newsletters. While these must be read with the intended audiences in mind, they evidence the agency, professional identity, and nation-building role of Chinese nurses.

This book raises questions of why a small group of Westerners were chosen by the Chinese government in 2014 to be captured in China's cultural memory. Members viewed the Convoy as distinctive from larger Western groups, especially missionary groups with a longer history of working in China. Their humanitarianism, Convoy members claimed, was driven by compassion and their desire to help relieve human suffering, regardless of race, nation, or religion. Subscribing to the Quaker Peace Testimony, their goal was to model global fraternity rather than impose their religious beliefs on others. They maintained that their practice of impartiality and their indomitable faith in the victory of the human spirit over violence could provide the basis for peace. That view, foregrounding the China Convoy's compassion and neutrality, was reflected in Zheng Yulin's opening remarks at the 8th Route Army Museum quoted above. Moreover, in recognition of their long tradition of providing neutral and impartial assistance, the China Convoy's sponsors, the American Friends Service Committee (AFSC) and the British Friends Service Council

(BFSC), were jointly awarded the 1947 Nobel Peace Prize. During the Peace Prize presentation ceremonies, the attributes singled out and praised were the same ones pointed to by Convoy members to distinguish their work in war relief and postwar reconstruction.[4]

The China Convoy was born of a spirit of adventure and youthful soul-searching in the hope that it might foster international fellowship and reconciliation in a world at war. Pacifism, the glue that bonded the independent-spirited Convoy members, was their rejoinder to war. Just as war brought them together, "so China was the challenge that kept [them] together."[5] China captured their hearts and minds and cemented their enduring ties to each other and to China. The China Convoy has therefore long been regarded within and beyond Quaker circles as a positive example of Quaker humanitarian practice. The perception that it was not just the work but also the ethical way in which it was done gained currency within the Convoy's ranks[6] and in A. Tegla Davies's 1947 official history of the FAU: "One does not come to appreciate China in a day nor to realize that the whole world must not be judged by Western standards. But once the corner was turned, there was no other section of the Friends Ambulance Unit that attained so much character and coherence, so much sympathy and integration with the life of the country in which it served."[7] This legacy, however, was forged within the grim reality of the unimaginable suffering, social dislocation, and loss endured by the Chinese people in a country where war never abated.

In this challenging environment, negotiating a distinctly Quaker approach to humanitarian action, premised on a depoliticized model of humanitarian relief, took many turns. Recently historians have produced a more nuanced assessment of the Quakers' record of impartial global humanitarianism, and at times generated lively debate about inconsistencies in Quaker humanitarian practice.[8] This book joins these scholarly conversations to better understand the complex politics that enmeshed the China Convoy's humanitarian efforts. Deepening our comprehension of the Convoy's humanitarian action sheds light on the contours of and cracks within the nascent modern humanitarian system.

Until recently, moreover, nursing's voice has also been marginalized in the scholarly literature on the development of the humanitarian system, which prioritizes diplomacy orchestrated by politicians and international bureaucrats. Revisionist scholars challenge, or at least complicate, earlier interpretations of the role of nursing as imperialist cultural aggression.[9] This book moves beyond merely recovering nurses' stories as unsung heroes on the periphery of the history of humanitarianism. Since the emergence of the humanitarian system at the time of the Geneva Convention of 1863, nursing has provided crucial and enduring service in wars and natural disasters, yet the concept of humanitarian nursing is poorly understood. The notion of the humanitarian nurse is a multi-faceted and contentious concept.[10] The origins of humanitarianism are entrenched in the West's colonial and imperial past, especially in faith-based organizations. Nursing has been traditionally cast as part of the wider process of making imperialism more palatable; others ascribe to it a more sinister role as an "agent of empire," imposing Western cultural standards or institutions while undermining local ones.[11] This book critically examines how nurses navigated the cultural schism and the mesh of ethical dilemmas, professional challenges, and opportunities presented by humanitarian nursing within a Western-based relief organization.

Nurses' life narratives elucidate the uncertainties and complexities encountered by the Convoy's multinational staff, who were brought together by their pledge to relieve China's suffering. For Connie Bull, as for many other nurses, her China years led her to question her role and contribution within a Western-based humanitarian organization that presumed a "right" way for communities to ensure their survival and that of their members. As she remarked:

> I think this is a good place to come to if you ever had any young ideas about changing the world and helping mankind towards a better life. You realize that if there is a God, then in His eyes you and the dirtiest Chinese beggar stand equal, that the coolie and the old woman tottering on bound feet, intent on their own lives, are living out more fully than we [do] the life [that is] ordained for them. By our restless striving towards the ideal, or our unceasing consciousness that we are not seeking the ideal, we so divide ourselves that we can do nothing wholeheartedly.[12]

Recovering Convoy nurses' stories from the field also unsettles accepted interpretations and suggests that a more complex historical portrait of humanitarian nursing is warranted. Their letters, diaries, photos, official reports, and rare published materials offer new perspectives on their identity formation as humanitarian nurses in the intimate contact zone of patient care during wartime. This tantalizing trove provides fresh perspectives on the intersections of power with faith, gender, class, race, and nation that shaped their work and life in the field. Their testimonies illuminate the extraordinary

diversity of Convoy nurses' humanitarian work as it was imagined and practised in war-devastated China. The experiences of Western and Chinese
nurses therefore provide a litmus test for humanitarian nursing and, by association, for the iconization of FAU members' cross-cultural humanitarian
exchanges in the field as distinct from those of other aid organizations.

At a turning point in Chinese history, the views of Convoy nurses offer a
different means of examining the relationship between women and war, and
women's political commitment and attitudes towards pacifism and communism. Some nurses witnessed the realignment of power during global
war that set the stage for the birth of modern China. Later, others witnessed
China's emergence from both sides of the conflict. For some Western nurses,
their involvement in China reflected a broader interest in and advocacy of
social justice. While nation building was often the path taken by Chinese
nurses to achieve that goal, for Western nurses it meant promoting international peace and reconciliation, and sharing their nursing knowledge to
relieve human suffering.

In sum, this book explores the historical meaning and development of
humanitarian nursing, its current relevance to the profession, and the vibrant
global discourse swirling around the perceived failure of contemporary humanitarianism. It illustrates how the politics of impartiality shaped the development of the modern humanitarian system; it is still necessary but is an
inadequate foundation of the modern humanitarian system to ensure human
security. It raises questions about the fine line between international humanitarian actions as legitimate humanitarian intervention, and a newer
cultural or economic imperialism that raises the spectre of a continued
militarization of humanitarianism. Beyond these contributions, this book
offers implications for the direction of future research on humanitarian nursing across disciplines.

Before exploring how the China Convoy personnel conceived of their
work in China, it is useful to start with who they were and what brought them
to China. With the outbreak of the Second World War, the British Society of
Friends, with assistance from the American Friends Service Committee,
reconvened the Friends Ambulance Unit. Former members of the FAU of the
First World War had continued to hold reunions; at one such gathering in
1938, plans began to be formulated to launch a new FAU to meet the growing

world crisis.[13] As in the First World War, it provided conscientious objectors with a state-sanctioned opportunity for humanitarian service as an alternative to military service. Between 1939 and 1946, more than 1,300 FAUers served as unpaid volunteers in Britain, France, Finland, Norway, Egypt, Greece, Syria, Ethiopia, India, and China. FAU membership was never restricted to Quakers, however.[14] The Unit welcomed anyone who adhered to the Quaker Peace Testimony, as exemplified in the principle "Go anywhere, do anything," or GADA, to relieve suffering, regardless of race, religion, or politics – hence the nickname the "Gadabouts." When it became clear that substantial funding could not be obtained in England, which was already overwhelmed by demands for relief for victims of the Axis air raids, the American Friends were approached. Since the British and American Quakers had cooperated in the First World War, and intermittently since then, it was natural to rekindle that connection. Like its British counterpart, the AFSC had been formed in 1917 to meet the needs of American conscientious objectors, and then expanded its humanitarian mandate during the interwar era to include peace education and relief activities conducted worldwide on the basis of depoliticized impartiality. As the prospect of a Second World War loomed closer, the AFSC sought safe and meaningful options for alternative service that helped conscientious objectors transcend their feeling of social ostracism.[15] It became an increasingly important source of funds and personnel for the China Convoy and eventually assumed administrative responsibility for its successor, the Friends Service Unit in 1947.

The China section was formed in 1941 after a year of multilateral negotiations between London, Philadelphia, and China.[16] The China Convoy was unique. It was the only section to undertake transport work – hence its name, the China Convoy. Begun as a British operation, it became the most international section in its composition and funding. Over time, Canadians, New Zealanders, Americans, and Chinese, both volunteers and paid staff, swelled its ranks, and their governments and private donors contributed to its coffers. Drawn from all walks of life, with a variety of reasons for joining and a diverse set of beliefs and commitments, they found common refuge in pacifism. The China Convoy "was a great leveller of social distinctions and backgrounds." Everyone was "in the same boat. They were all expected to perform the same duties and to learn the same skills. Faced with the challenges of hospital and relief work, of driving and motor mechanics, practical skills and gumption were more significant than qualifications or vocabulary."[17] Women were recruited later and came with a similar mix of motives and aspirations. Some sought adventure or a new beginning, whereas others sought more meaningful wartime work.

Quaker principles remained embedded in its organizational culture until the China Convoy closed its doors in 1951, but getting the Convoy members' diverse ideals aligned in China was another matter. Renowned as a fiercely democratic, self-critical, and idealistic risk taker, the Convoy always operated at arm's length from its Quaker sponsoring organizations and remained vigilant in preserving its administrative autonomy in the field. The fledgling Convoy soon discovered "what a tough nut we have to crack" in a country riddled with political intrigue and suspicion.[18] While many of its members were eager to share the dangers and work on the front lines during the global war, they were unwilling to sacrifice the Convoy's pacifist principles and financial independence or subsume its distinctive identity.[19] Working with military authorities, the International Relief Committee,[20] the Chinese National Health Administration (NHA), or British civilian aid bodies proved fraught with tension. Moreover, building relationships and finding adequate funding in Great Britain, the United States, and eventually Canada would be crucial to its survival. Grumblings about the lack of consultation and honest differences of opinion with those in command back in London and Philadelphia fuelled discontent within the rank and file.

Tensions were rife within the Convoy and beyond; the maverick "China Boys" marched to the beat of their own drum. They blatantly disregarded the authority of London or Philadelphia or of their own leaders more than once. Almost immediately, the rank and file disputed the choice of a Canadian medical missionary, Dr. Robert McClure, to direct its medical and relief work. In 1937, McClure had been seconded from the United Church Mission in Henan to the International Red Cross as field director for Central China. At first glance, the appointment of a missionary seemed out of character for a Quaker organization. Clearly, McClure's extensive knowledge of China and its culture and language, and his impressive political network in China and abroad, took precedence over strict fidelity to Quaker principles. His lifelong attitude that the "wrong decision is better than the right decision too late" proved problematic.[21] As we shall see, his maverick leadership style would be disputed, but his guiding hand remained evident until 1946. His successors, chosen from the rank and file, learned the job on the ground.

The Convoy's humanitarian endeavours spanned an era in which the Chinese experienced regional war, then global war, then the final stages of a civil war that culminated in the establishment of the People's Republic of China in 1949. China's wars were nested within each other, like Russian matryoshka dolls, embedded within global conflicts or containing other sub-intrastate conflicts among warlords.

By 1940, the Sino-Japanese War (1937–45) had had a devastating impact on China. War fractured the social fabric. The fighting in the latter half of 1937 triggered massive civilian evacuations and the flight of millions into exile. The Japanese occupied the seaboard provinces of the east and south, while the Chinese Communists controlled the northern provinces. The remaining parts of western and southern China that were not occupied by the Japanese, commonly referred to as "Free China," were landlocked, with restricted supply routes. Braving bandits, disease, and dangerous roads, the transport division of the FAU delivered almost all medical supplies for civilians and famine relief in Free China. Meanwhile, FAU medical personnel on the front lines struggled, often in primitive conditions with makeshift facilities, to carve out a humanitarian enclave as the first Western aid group to work under the Chinese Red Cross and alongside the Chinese army.

The nuclear bombing of Hiroshima and Nagasaki in August 1945 brought a sudden end to the war, and Japan's surrender marked a watershed in the China Convoy's history. The Convoy now shifted its focus from emergency work to undertake a long-term agricultural, industrial, and medical rehabilitation program centred primarily in Henan. Could the FAU and the FSU, its successor after 1947, reinvent the Convoy's mandate in line with its pacifist principles in a very different humanitarian landscape? For eight years the Chinese people had lived in terror and endured unimaginable hardships as their nation was torn apart. Long before the war ended, it was widely recognized that a massive humanitarian relief and rehabilitation task lay ahead. Allied plans were well under way to establish the United Nations Relief and Rehabilitation Administration (UNRRA) as a bridge to peace that would allow the liberal economic order and democracies to flourish.[22] Returning missionary societies and new international aid agencies flooded into China, further complicating the Convoy's humanitarian negotiations.

The formation of the FSU in 1947 coincided with a turning point in the Chinese civil war. Its work was increasingly held hostage by events beyond its control. As the civil war intensified, the Convoy struggled to maintain its integrity and to honour the primacy of the humanitarian imperative to receive and give humanitarian relief. The tenuous wartime truce between the Guomindang led by Chiang Kai-shek and the Communist Party of China led by Mao Zedong was short-lived. On 1 October 1949, Mao proclaimed the creation of the People's Republic of China.[23] As China entered the final chapter of a vicious civil war, foreign aid workers became increasingly unwelcome. The dictates of the Cold War after 1946 shifted Western aid priorities from multilateral programs under UNRRA's umbrella to "help people to help themselves" to bilateral aid to contain communism. When the FSU could no longer obtain funding and replacement personnel, it reluctantly closed its doors in 1951.

Before interrogating the specifics of the China Convoy's humanitarian endeavours, it is useful to situate it within the tradition of Quaker humanitarianism. What did it mean to give aid in a "Quakerly fashion"? How did Quaker ethics shape the Gadabouts' collective memory of being unique among Western aid groups? What tensions within Convoy ranks resulted from the diversity of opinions on the Quaker Peace Testimony in practice?

Quakers have long been an authoritative force for peace and justice. Over the years, the China Convoy remained open to admitting non-Quakers who shared the Quaker belief in non-violence and peacemaking rooted deep in Quaker convictions about the dignity and worth of all persons. The "inner light" or "inward light," a distinctive theme underpinning their belief that God can be seen in each person, meant that Quakers believed all men were equal and therefore had the right to reach their full human potential. It meant that they did not have enemies and therefore could not kill. This was the essence of the Peace Testimony. It was not a passive peace but one that had to be built on a daily basis on all levels: in the family, in the community, in the nation, and in the world. Quaker beliefs are related to the belief that the direct awareness of God enables each person to discover God's will for him or her. The Quaker ideals of resolving conflict through individual witness and of demonstrating love as a prerequisite for solving human conflicts therefore informed FAU and FSU humanitarianism. It should be kept clearly in mind, however, that while the Convoy as a whole maintained its absolute pacifist position, members were at liberty to act as the "inward light" directed them to in wartime.

Convinced that there were alternatives to war, Quakers – or Friends, as they refer to themselves – had long felt the need to provide a practical demonstration of human sympathy and global fraternity through relief services. The humanitarian imperative that impelled Quakers to alleviate suffering wherever it was found was designed "to protect life and health and to ensure respect for the human being." It also promoted "understanding, friendship, co-operation and lasting peace amongst all peoples."[24] Working for pacifism and belief in the human capacity for goodness were central to Quakers' humanitarian action. This human capacity for goodness, Quakers believed, had to be fostered through interpersonal action, not proselytization.[25] Most Convoy members took a pragmatic approach and distanced their humanitarian endeavours from the work of other, evangelistic missionary groups working in China. In sum, peace for them never meant merely the absence of war but a positive peace predicated on justice and human reconciliation.

Since the ethics of method was as important as the ethics of outcome, members constantly reflected on whether the China Convoy's humanitarian aid was being delivered in a Quakerly fashion. The Convoy always had to measure its desire to protect its operational space against the imperative to provide impartial aid on the basis of need. By defining their objective as the relief of the individual rather than of the nation, members believed that the China Convoy's organizational identity as a neutral and impartial pacifist organization could be insulated from the politics of humanitarianism.

For several reasons, humanitarian negotiations were more difficult than the idealistic Convoy volunteers first realized. Other aspects of what is now commonly referred to as "humanitarian space" – broadly understood as the agency's ability to operate freely and meet humanitarian needs in accordance with the principles of humanitarian action – became evident. The fluidity of their operating environment, particularly the security conditions and the inability of the most vulnerable to reach life-saving aid, constrained their humanitarian negotiations, determining where and how they worked.[26] China's humanitarian terrain was a crowded and contested space, occupied by institutions and actors with competing agendas.

Stories from the field offer perspectives on the ability of relief organizations to provide aid, rehabilitation, and resettlement assistance where humanitarian aid often becomes strangled by bureaucratic red tape, conflicting agendas, and modern warfare. Unit members came to understand that Quaker principles provided a framework for negotiating access to those in need of assistance across political divides but could not ensure the outcome. The China Convoy's humanitarian ethics, this book argues, proved situational. Ultimately it would be the FAU's or FSU's persuasion and relevance in particular locations and times that mattered in the end. This raises two larger questions. First, when allied to the practice of Quaker ideals, can humanitarian nursing – and, by association, medical humanitarian aid – remain neutral only to a limited degree? Second, was there ever a "golden age" of humanitarian action when independence, neutrality, and autonomy were respected? In so doing, this book challenges the now dominant narrative of a "shrinking humanitarian space,"[27] which defines and defends the contemporary humanitarian system more as an interventionist stance to protect human rights and security without the prior consent of a country's government.

This book also critically examines the tensions, clashes, and compromises between the converging cultures that coloured all the China Gadabouts' humanitarian exchanges at all levels of the Convoy's operations. Nurses' experiences offer an appraisal of what it means to be thrust into chaotic settings armed only with limited professional experience. Humanitarian nursing quickly took all Convoy nurses outside their normal scope of practice. Many found their work frustrating but rewarding as they battled administrative inefficiency, indifference, racism, political intrigue, and sheer pettiness beyond their control. Humanitarian nursing involved negotiating personal and professional space and resolving ethical dilemmas. For some, it was the most powerful experience of their lives; for others, it was a time best forgotten. Hence the coping strategies that the Convoy nurses developed to navigate unfamiliar professional terrain form a thread throughout the narrative that connects their individual, and often very different, stories within the same teams.

Both Western and Chinese nurses discovered that humanitarian relief work was contentious, perilous, and sometimes life-changing. Both were expected to be diplomats, cultural brokers, and purveyors of expert Western nursing services, all without losing sight of the Convoy's pacifist ethos. Hence, the cross-cultural brokerage role of both Western and Chinese nurses is also a central theme of this book, as is an examination of the way in which both legitimized their work. Did the Western Convoy nurses embody and uphold Western standards of nursing, and how did they vary over time and place? Did they prioritize the China Convoy's interests over those of the Chinese people? Or was theirs a far more complicated and contested story? Examining the agency, assimilation, and accommodation of Chinese nurses exposes the complexity of the China Convoy's humanitarian exchanges. Why did Chinese nurses join a Western relief group, and what did they expect in return? How did they perceive their wartime role as modern Chinese women? Why were some nurses more effective cross-cultural brokers than others?

Accordingly, unpacking the China Convoy nurses' collective narratives pushes scholars to re-evaluate nursing's historic role within the Convoy and, by association, its contested contribution in Western-driven humanitarian diplomacy.[28]

For both Western and Chinese women, joining the China Convoy made it possible to recreate their lives inside and outside of nursing. This book probes how gender as a constructed concept shaped nurses' sense of identity and their work within the Convoy. Gender as an analytical construct, as used in this study, is viewed as socially constructed and embraces men's and women's gendered experiences as humanitarian workers. Even though women had a long history of nursing on the front lines, their place within the Convoy sparked heated debates. Gender identities, especially for Chinese nurses, were sometimes more contested as they straddled traditional Chinese feminine norms and Western professional modernity. This book also pays attention to the gendered experience of men providing nursing services. Until the China Convoy closed its doors, it was taken for granted that men, frequently trained on the spot, would fill key nursing roles. As pacifists, the Convoy men already challenged hegemonic masculinity and "were often constructed as irresponsible and sexually suspect anti-citizens."[29] Nursing, as a caring profession, was considered women's work. How were male nurses' experiences in the China Convoy reconciled with prevailing notions of manhood?

Understanding nursing's historic global involvement in health promotion and humanitarian assistance demands a transnational perspective open to engagement across disciplines that no longer privileges the nation state or its predominantly male representatives as a historical paradigm for understanding nursing's past. As the international relations discipline conventionally constructed state identities and citizens' responsibilities, most women's lived experiences were excluded. Recovering nurses' stories challenges the gendered nature of international relations scholarship that relegated women to the sidelines of humanitarian action, and of foreign policy more generally. Collectively, for some feminist historians, their gendered world as humanitarian workers exposes the ragged intellectual edges of our scholarship, mandating more radical revision of how we think and write about global history. I argue that good global nursing history should expose the lacunae in analytical constructs that frame our historical inquiry into humanitarian nursing's historic global presence, suggest new directions for research, and inform the role of nursing in policy formation.

New analyses and theoretical approaches are required to examine the historical work and worth of nursing globally.[30] Nurses are often key cultural conduits between Western medicine and traditional medical practitioners. The history of nursing offers an alternative perspective for interrogating how Western-based humanitarian organizations insinuated their culture into the lives of indigenous people. Accordingly, my examination of humanitarian nursing's textured past requires a multidisciplinary approach incorporating cutting-edge trends across disciplines that situate race, class, gender, ethnicity, place, nation, and postcolonialism in a transnational framework. It engages with revisionist investigations, across disciplines, into the contested humanitarian exchanges between privileged Western health workers and their counterparts in conflict-ridden or emergent nations with different political or cultural traditions.[31] Recently, feminist international relations scholars have argued that nurses were not always agents of cultural imperialism but could be "authentic knowers" who develop cultural sensitivity once in the field.[32] Works by cultural anthropologists illuminate the tensions that FAU nurses experienced as cross-cultural brokers[33] and the reasons why some proved more effective humanitarian diplomats than others.[34]

This book explores the movement beyond a state-centric approach that privileges the nation state and security. Instead, it alters the concept of power to admit nurses' agency and activism in global humanitarian diplomacy. The China Convoy nurses' narratives of their humanitarian work offer fresh perspectives that refocus the boundaries of international relations studies from the causes and cost of war to the drastic consequences the Chinese people suffered due to militarism and oppression. Building on my previous work, I am attracted to the work of international relations scholars that, by distinguishing between "power over" and "power with," questions whether women exercise power differently in global society.[35] This enables me to treat seriously nurses' contribution to global civil society, war, and nation building – an area that has been addressed only recently by historians of global nursing and remains invisible in mainstream international relations studies.

Centring human security – commonly understood as freedom from violence to ensure basic food, shelter, health protection, and human rights – instead of national security within a transnational analytical frame better contextualizes the Gadabouts' experience and the enduring trends, ethical ambiguities, and challenges of the modern humanitarian landscape. These transnational frames instead scrutinize how nursing has addressed the opportunities and challenges of disseminating Western-based medical knowledge, ethics, and resources globally through a wide range of transnational non-state actors. These frames focus scholarly attention on the resilience, cultural awareness, and innovative leadership required for anyone contemplating humanitarian nursing in conflict zones or complex humanitarian crises. They suggest a far more contested and complicated picture of humanitarian nursing, and indicate that, in general, women's role within the global humanitarian landscape has been undervalued.

Good global history reveals the enduring themes, trends, and ethical ambiguities in humanitarianism. A retrospective of the China Convoy's humanitarian endeavours during this transformational era, when what it meant to be a humanitarian was not fully settled, provides important perspectives on the implications of humanitarian neutrality. The adoption of two key documents are watershed moments in the development of humanitarian law. The Geneva Conventions of 1949 updated the regulation of the conduct of armed conflict and sought to limit its effects, and the Universal Declaration of Human Rights by the United Nations General Assembly in 1948 reinforced the idea that humanitarian action should be based on rights rather than needs. Humanitarian relief implies short-term rather than long-term action. In the period after the Second World War, however, what was intended to prevent imminent harm became transformed into attempts to promote social and economic development and protect citizens. Promotion of economic and social development and peacekeeping appeared to follow provision of humanitarian relief, with the distinction between them becoming increasingly blurred.[36]

As Baroness Amos, the UN's Under-Secretary-General for Humanitarian Affairs and Emergency Relief Coordinator from 2010 to 2015, contended: "To shape our future, we must understand our past."[37] A review of the Convoy's humanitarian endeavours as the new world order was being formulated offers valuable insights for conversations among scholars and practitioners today.[38] A stronger engagement with the history of humanitarianism's origins and identity establishes a sounder vantage point from which to engage with those who were shaped by different sets of circumstances.[39] Central to the debate on global governance is the militarization that accompanies the "new humanitarianism" predicated on moral and human rights; it means an a priori departure from the basic humanitarian principle of supplying aid on the sole basis of need with prior state consent for any given humanitarian action. As the UN's adoption of the Responsibility to Protect (R2P) concept in 2005 attests,[39] the global debate increasingly focused on agreement that the international community has a right, and even a duty, to alleviate distress, and whether acceptable means include forcible intervention to end suffering and protect human rights when a state fails to do so.[40] The Gadabouts' humanitarian ethics as practised in China contribute to scholarly debate on the overlap between the development of human rights and humanitarianism.[41]

The Second World War signalled a change in humanitarianism with the development of new structures and organizations to administer relief and rehabilitation. During their China years, new players entered the "contested humanitarian marketplace."[42] Long before the term "nurses/doctors without borders" was coined, the China Convoy attempted to reconcile its humanitarian imperative with the changing face of modern warfare. It also foreshadowed the meteoric rise of international non-governmental organizations (INGOs) and other non-state actors worldwide, which complicated post-1945 global humanitarian governance.[43] This book spotlights an understudied area of global nursing – its role within INGOs, now more active than ever in global health care.

Taking a transnational perspective on global nursing unsettles our parochial assumptions about the invisibility and powerlessness of nursing within the gendered and Western-derived global humanitarian community. Giving voice to nursing's historic contribution to humanitarianism issues a challenge for nurses to be more critically engaged in the global health community today. The stories of humanitarian nursing in China may seem far removed from the concerns of contemporary nursing leaders, but I was struck otherwise in writing this book. Issues that China Convoy nurses confronted remain relevant today: the struggle to build healthcare facilities that are sustainable and tailored to local needs; the battle against agendas driven by political or economic rather than healthcare needs; the dogged leadership and personal resilience required to provide compassionate care and high standards of nursing service in difficult and dangerous circumstances; and the recognition that health and human security are inextricably interwoven. However, if today's nurses are to move beyond a clinical perspective on global health to become human rights advocates and engaged citizens for health for all, our historical inquiry should support them by providing a sound historical understanding of nursing's complex role in global health diplomacy and the socio-economic structural issues that underpin and connect health and social justice. This book takes a modest step in this direction.

Historians face many challenges in trying to understand and write global nursing history. They are sensitive to the ethical and methodological challenges of conducting transnational research.[44] They have long since abandoned the idea that sources enable us to mirror an objective representation of the totality of nurses' life experiences. They have, for the most part, embraced subjectivity, including their own selection and interpretation of those sources. Quaker accounts written for family and friends may have prioritized different issues than those written by conscientious objectors of other denominations. Memory has become an inescapable feature of the historical landscape.[45] Scholars must display sensitivity to both the advantages and disadvantages of using private recollections or published "redemptive narratives" that paint a positive portrait of wartime humanitarian nursing.[46] With one significant exception, the photographic record and the official publicity film footage that create historical memory of the Convoy's humanitarian work were taken and preserved by Convoy men. Moreover, women's contributions, especially those of the Chinese nurses, are often embedded in male narratives. These sources nonetheless reveal societal norms as Convoy men depict nurses' life stories. Fortunately, nurses' private diaries, poetry, letters, and reports written at the time, accompanied by two redemptive narratives, provide a counterpoint to male accounts of Convoy life in the field. These sources reveal their authors' attempts to preserve recollections or rationalize their presence as the events evolved. Despite these limitations, they bring to life the voices and vastly different experiences of nurses seldom evoked in official records or caught in the colourful Convoy newsletters portraying and celebrating life in China. Taken together, they provide a window to interrogate how Quakers perceived their social interaction in wartime China as being distinct from that of Christian missionaries or other international aid agencies. Oral interviews conducted afterwards, vetted against other primary sources, can shed light on the complexity of larger events or themes, revealing far greater contours or nuances in their agency or presence than previously realized. They are essential for situating individual nurses' perspectives within the organization for which they worked and within the global political context.[47] Incorporating oral and personal testimonies into historical writing enables me to convey the major ethical and personal challenges of humanitarian nursing in a more relatable manner for scholars, practitioners, and others interested in the relationships between peace, global health, social justice, and human security.[48] Paraphrasing Naomi Rogers, I also recognize my own work "as part of the process of memory working, as an additional layer to [the Convoy nurses'] stories."[49]

The nurses presented in this study do not constitute an exhaustive examination of the Convoy's humanitarian work in China. Moreover, the stories of some of the Chinese nurses have been obliterated by time and the lack of identifiable personal records. They do, however, represent the human drama and professional vagaries encountered during three periods of the Convoy's history: the transition from regional to global war from 1941 to 1944; the transition to civilian work in 1945 until the Friends Service Unit took over in 1947; and the FSU's humanitarian endeavours under the new Communist regime until 1951. The voices of the China Convoy continue to resonate today.

PART 1

From Regional War to Global War, 1941–45

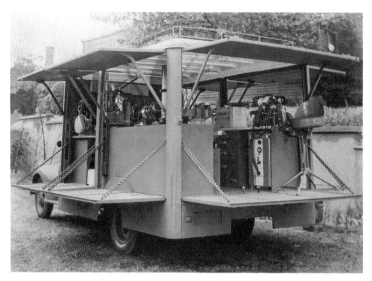

A Friends Ambulance Unit surgical truck proved ill-suited to battlefront conditions on the Salween front during the Sino-Japanese War. *Source:* American Friends Service Committee Archives

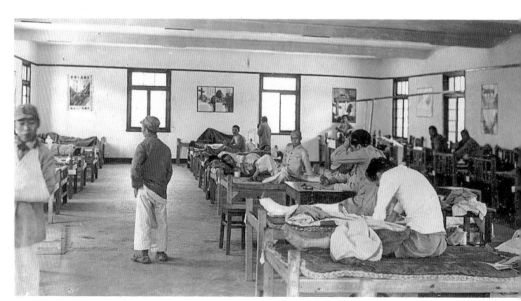

Medical Surgical Team 2 (MST2) at Baoshan. *Source:* American Friends Service Committee Archives

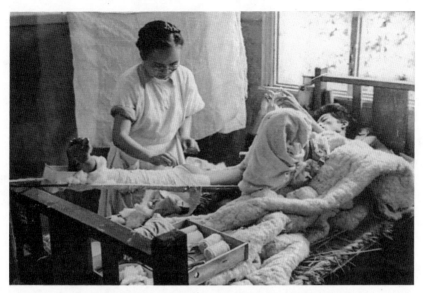

Chinese New Life Movement nurses serving with Medical Team 3 (MT3).
Source: American Friends Service Committee Archives

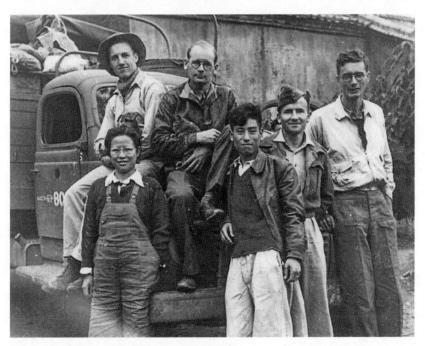

MT6 leaving Mohei. Edwin Abbott sitting on truck (back); Jane Wong standing
in front. *Source:* Edwin Abbott Private Papers

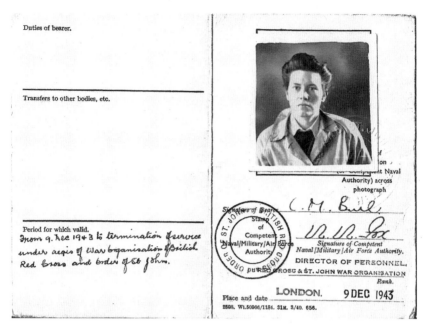

British nurse Connie Bull Condick. *Source:* Connie and Ron Condick Collection

British nurse E. "Rita" Dangerfield White. *Source:* E. Dangerfield White Collection

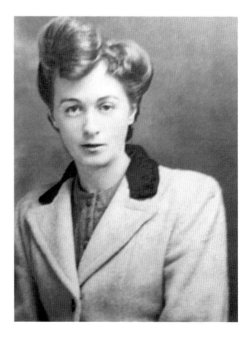

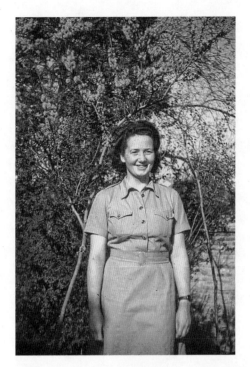

British nurse Margaret Briggs Matheson. *Source:* Margaret Stanley Tesdell Collection

Harriet Brown Alexander and the second Canadian contingent at Pendle Hill, completing their field orientation in the winter. *Source:* American Friends Service Committee Archives

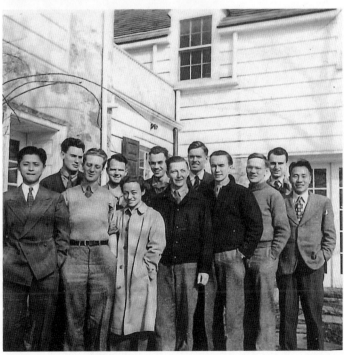

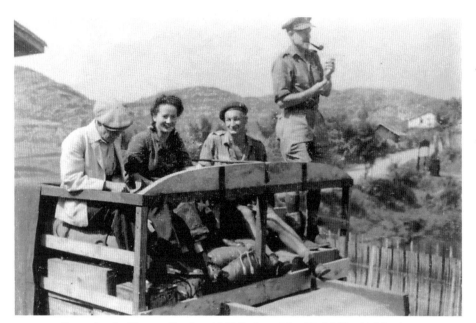

Departing for Henan, October 1945. Left to right: J.B. McHattie (North China Mission), Margaret Briggs, Neil Johnson, Dr. Robert McClure. *Source:* George Lindsay Crozier Collection

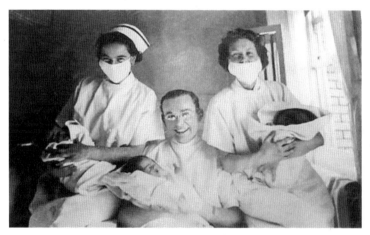

Dr. Arthur Barr and FAU Chinese nursing staff holding babies. *Source:* Arthur Barr Collection

In the late summer of 1940, with opportunities for further work in Europe cut off,[1] the Friends Ambulance Unit (FAU), headquartered in Gordon Square, London, explored opportunities to work in China. In the meantime, the American Friends Service Committee (AFSC), established in 1917 to provide conscientious objectors with opportunities for alternative war service, had redefined its wartime mandate in the intervening decades to include a broader humanitarian mission that set the stage for its later involvement in China.[2] Throughout the interwar period, the AFSC, headquartered in Philadelphia, had explored opportunities in China for a distinct project that would not replicate the mission boards' work. It now appeared that such an opportunity might open up. More immediately, the haphazard formation of FAU's China section, commonly known as the China Convoy, laid the basis for future schisms between London and Philadelphia over its pacifist purpose, leadership, administrative structure, and financial backing. But the character of its volunteers and the vagaries of war that produced modern China would fundamentally shape the China Convoy's humanitarian endeavours and its relations with British and American Friends.

By late 1940, the devastating impact of the Sino-Japanese War on the civilian population was well known in British and American Quaker circles. Both had long and complex missionary ties in China dating back to the late 1880s. Following Japan's invasion of China in 1937, the American Friends Board of Foreign Missions agreed to work with British Friends to establish the Friends Centre in Shanghai. These missionaries "established a network of relationships that allowed Quakers, and more specifically the AFSC, more of an influence than their otherwise small numbers would suggest possible."[3]

American and British Friends held both combatant nations culpable for the atrocities that the Chinese populace endured. In December 1937, in the Rape of Nanking (Nanjing), one of the worst atrocities during the Second World War, the Japanese Imperial Army murdered half of the 600,000 civilians and soldiers in the city. The Nationalist Chinese government's decision in June 1938 to break the dikes on the Yellow River to deter the impending Japanese capture of Wuhan had equally tragic consequences. Nearly 4 million Chinese civilians in three flooded provinces became refugees.[4] In the expanding theatre of battle, the escalation of the Second Sino-Japanese War (1937–45) ushered in a nationwide catastrophe. Between 1937 and 1945, more than 95 million Chinese became refugees.[5]

Given the need for humanitarian assistance, a Joint China Committee, chaired by an Old China Hand, Dr. H. Gordon Thompson, the secretary of the British Fund for the Relief of Distress, was established to coordinate the FAU work with the fund and the British Relief Unit that was already assisting the International Red Cross Committee for Central China. Right from the start, funding the China Convoy caused friction between London and Philadelphia. The limited British relief funds available to the FAU were primarily directed to the relief of civilian suffering caused by air raids. Consequently, Christopher Sharman, who was responsible for the FAU's work overseas, was dispatched to the United States to raise the necessary funds. The United China Relief (UCR) funds coursed through the AFSC were the China Convoy's chief source of income.[6] The UCR's insistence that the AFSC be fully responsible for the administration of its funds placed the AFSC in "an awkward position."[7] The solution was to send more American personnel to lead what would continue to be an essentially British organization until 1945. Meanwhile, the British Foreign Office's grant-in-aid to the British Fund for the Relief of Distress in China caused uneasiness in Philadelphia.[8] First, the AFSC worried that the British grant would mean British government control. It remained adamant that the FAU was "not going to China to pull any gov't's chestnuts out of the fire but that the venture was an expression of our Christian pacifism."[9] Second, grant-in-aid was earmarked primarily for work involving military medical services with the Chinese army. At the time, the AFSC was very civilian-minded and viewed this proposal as tantamount to making an important contribution to the war effort.[10] While a satisfactory agreement was eventually reached for accepting help from the British government, tensions persisted as to whether the Convoy should focus on military or civilian casualties.

The decision of the British Joint China Committee (BJCC) in early May 1941 to parachute Dr. Robert McClure in to lead the Convoy as a fait accompli was surprising and in some ways unwelcome. The charismatic McClure would be the commandant; the incumbent, Peter Tennant, "very much the old school tie sort of fellow, a bit stiff,"[11] was now relegated to second seat. The BJCC wanted a proven Old China Hand to direct the fledgling organization's field operations. Seconded in 1937 by the United Church of Canada's mission in Henan to the International Red Cross as field director for central China during the Sino-Japanese conflict, McClure had a wealth of medical experience, "spoke Chinese like a native," and knew China "like the palm of his hand."[12] His perfunctory appointment and maverick personality, however, affronted the rank and file's esprit de corps and tainted his leadership.[13]

The Quakers' unique process of decision making collided with Robert McClure's individualistic leadership style. The decision-making process is a matter of spiritual discernment that takes place within a specially convened meeting for worship, a "Religious Meeting for Business." Historian A. Paul Hare explains:

> For over 300 years the members of the Society of Friends (Quakers) have been making group decisions without voting. Their method is to find a "sense of the meeting," which represents a consensus of those involved. Ideally this consensus is not simply "unanimity," or an opinion on which all members happen to agree, but a "unity": a higher truth, which grows from the consideration of divergent opinions and unites them all.[14]

The intent of a Quaker business meeting is not to find what most people want to do but to discern the will of God for the body that is meeting. The Quakers' core belief that there "is but one Truth, [and that] its Spirit, if followed, will produce unity" provides a central principle of corporate guidance. Quakers seek to discern that as a body they are called in a particular direction based upon their individual sense of the transcendental being rather than personal preferences, prejudices, or convenience. Quaker business practice is premised upon the belief that every human being can perceive God's will and that, consequently, all who genuinely seek the will of God can find unity in what it is referred to as the "Sense of the Meeting." Communal silence "plays an active role in decision making through a process understood to take precedence over its outcome."[15] In the context of Quaker "Meetings for Business," silence prepares those present to take part in the decision-making process as participants wait and listen for guidance. Decisions are made together through worshipful attention to the "Spirit" and deep listening to one another to discern the "higher truth," the "Sense of the Meeting." The clerk of the meeting is responsible for stating when a "Sense of the Meeting" appears to have been reached. If the meeting decides to approve this "Sense of the Meeting," members "not being in unity" with the decision can request to have their concerns recorded. When no "Sense of the Meeting" can be agreed upon, divisive matters are held over. Managing this process in wartime China among widely scattered groups, not all of whom were Quakers but were independently minded conscientious objectors, would be a challenging process. This decision-making process operated at the Yearly Meeting called to determine the Unit's overall direction and within each section or team responsible for field operations. The process proved a better fit with the philosophy of non-violence, in accordance with which individuals strove for an understanding of the heart and motivation of their opponents rather than for the rapid, unified decision making needed in China's fluid wartime conditions. As we shall see, individual Unit sections or teams, guided by the dictates of their own conscience, would frequently feel compelled to veer from the course of action set by the Yearly Meeting or Unit leadership.

McClure was astute enough to realize that leading American and British Friends questioned his leadership, especially after he established increasingly close working arrangements with the Chinese military authorities and abandoned the Convoy's intended ambulance work. His carefully crafted letters and reports heralded the China Convoy's fitness to serve as a cultural bridge between the British and Chinese in providing for China's wounded.[16] His letters offered reassurance "that the religious life and spiritual tone of [the] group and ... members who are joining us is very high indeed ... and is a credit to the name of Friends in China." Closing with the promise "to do all in my power to keep it that way," McClure expressed his confidence "that the Friends in America will stick with us in this job."[17] But McClure's conciliatory gestures did little to alleviate the AFSC's concern throughout the war that the work had developed along lines that ran "counter to basic Quaker principles" and that the "major emphasis should be on civilian work."[18]

Moreover, budget allocations remained a bottleneck for the next five years. "More energy was probably expended in letters and cables and meetings and visits to straighten out the China section's finances than on any other piece of Unit administration, particularly when, later on, the spiral of inflation made budgeting ahead a matter of little more than guesswork."[19] Although the China section craved operational control, it would have to dance to the tune of its financial backers.

Peter Tennant whittled down over 150 applicants to join the China Convoy's first contingent to 40. The "holy forty," as these Convoy boys became known, were purportedly selected on the basis of their concern for China rather than a desire to travel abroad. Equally, China offered an opportunity for more manly alternative service. An association between military service and male citizenship and virility shaped British culture. As conscientious objectors, the applicants faced pressure to prove their bravery and loyalty, and to defend their pacifist ideals. Many viewed service with the FAU as a substitute for or analogous to the dangers of military service. In China, they were doing a "very masculine job" that demonstrated their manhood and virility.[20] Their commitment to do what they could for the victims of war and their desire to prove that they were not cowards or slackers by putting themselves alongside those who had taken up arms gave these recruits common ground. This first contingent was exclusively male, and none were state-registered nurses. While some had St. John Ambulance training or hospital experience, it was assumed that any additional nursing skills required could be taught after their arrival in China. One distinctive characteristic was their youthfulness: their average age was twenty-three. The Convoy men "shared the anxieties and uncertainties of youth but, more particularly, also its boldness, idealism and hope – and distinctively its question of authority."[21] Non-conformists by nature, these principled young men fiercely defended their right to determine where the Convoy operated and what work it undertook.

By early July 1941, an advance party led by Tennant arrived in Burma and began laying the groundwork for the China section's humanitarian work, although the pattern for its future work did not coalesce until the autumn of 1942. It took time in the field for its administrative structure to settle out as the Convoy boys divided into two camps: Tennant's supporters and McClure's.

McClure was given to making decisions on the spot, and his first challenged the FAU's fiercely democratic spirit. When the ambulances donated by the Americans proved too wide for the Burma Road, McClure sold the ambulances, purchased trucks, and pledged the Convoy to take over all transport for the International Relief Committee for Central China (IRC), the National Health Administration (NHA), and eventually the American Red Cross.[22] The Unit's transport system, delivering supplies to two hundred hospitals, covered over seven thousand kilometres, extending as far north as Suzhou in Gansu Province, southeast to Jiangxi Province, and south into Yunnan Province. This was an ambitious plan. However, the Japanese occupation of Burma in 1942 made its transport work even more important; all medical supplies, fuel, and spare parts had to be flown over the Himalayan Hump between India and Kunming.

For the pragmatic McClure there was no other choice. Duncan Wood, personnel officer of the China Convoy from 1941 to 1944, believed that "McClure was absolutely right, we had to adjust these pre-conceived ideas to the real situation." Transport was a vital service that no one seemed to be providing. Hundreds of hospitals in Free China were operating below capacity because the drugs and supplies were sitting in supply depots in Kunming awaiting transport. Moreover, trench warfare never materialized in China; instead, "there was sporadic fighting, no means of getting an ambulance, let alone a mobile operating unit within 50 miles of where the fighting was."[23] The American FAU physician Henry Louderbough offered a different perspective on why the Unit's original program of ambulance work had to be abandoned: "The simple reason is that the Chinese would not permit it ... The Chinese Red Cross and Chinese Army M[edical] C[orps] do not want outsiders to come in and do something that they won't do themselves."[24] The FAU never operated as a free agent in China in determining where it would work.

Not everyone supported McClure's decision. While some thought that he had been too quick to help out his old outfit, Louderbough believed that the "chief trouble" was that "Bob is not a Quaker and has no background for appreciating their peculiar outlook on the war. At no time has he called everyone together to explain new developments or ask opinions on matters of policy, and the only way to get information about our unit is a stray bit dropped during a casual conversation, or ... when a delegation goes to him and demands definite answers."[25] Many concluded that McClure's style of leadership was better suited to front-line triage than unit command.

Clearly, McClure misread the situation. Dissatisfaction with his ambitious transport plans reached well beyond China. His decision to sell the ambulances, including those donated by the British Ambulance Corps, did not sit well with Philadelphia or Gordon Square. Both cautioned him to operate within approved budgetary parameters to avoid antagonizing either organization's financial backers of the China Convoy. Moreover, his decision had equally disturbing implications for the Unit's future composition. In order to expand the transport work, McClure informed both headquarters that he planned to pair each American or British member with a Chinese counterpart. In McClure's mind, it was "a great scheme" that demonstrated the China Unit's willingness "to co-operate with the government to solve their problems to the best of our ability."[26] Disagreeing, Philadelphia feared that McClure's expansive ideas "would overload the Unit with personnel not selected according to FAU and AFSC standards."[27] From Gordon Square, FAU chairman Tom Tanner's letters to McClure expressed confidence that the "Unit will find its feet ... and perform a valuable service in the spirit of the Friends."[28]

Privately, however, he fretted that the unit would become "just a vast transport company," undermining its original intent to be "a Unit with a definite entity and consisting of a group of men sharing common principles." Others concurred that McClure "may have difficulty holding the Unit together" and questioned whether he would maintain "exactly the right spirit in the Unit."[29]

As rumours spread among the men about promises for work made unilaterally, discontent verged on open revolt. Everywhere, there were "huddles and meetings and righteous indignation."[30] An informal executive committee began meeting during McClure's frequent absences but could not act without his approval. A squad was dispatched to find McClure and bring him back to FAU headquarters at Guiyang to settle the matter. His return in early January 1942 led to heated meetings before the air was cleared and a modus vivendi was reached. The Convoy men acknowledged that it would "have been almost impossible to carry on if he resigned at that stage," and McClure grasped that he could not "ignore the corporate consciousness of the Unit as a body standing for certain testimonies of the Society of Friends."[31] In an attempt to reconcile the need for stable direction of the Unit with McClure's predilection for being constantly on the move attending to practical details, it was agreed that control would be vested in an Executive Council under McClure's direction, with the capacity to make decisions in his absence. The belief that this administrative shakeup marked a "new era in the life and work of the Convoy"[32] would be tested in the months and years to come. McClure's tenure as commandant of the Convoy would remain an uneasy alliance of convenience. Moreover, Gordon Square regarded the new Executive Council in China as a "new and dangerous precedent for local autonomy."[33] But the Unit always maintained that those in China were better positioned to determine the Unit's humanitarian work than either Philadelphia or Gordon Square. The "China Boys" would continue to feel that they were neither understood nor completely trusted. They tottered on the verge of chaos as they threshed out a democratic but realistic way for their scattered members to participate in major decisions while remaining accountable to Philadelphia and Gordon Square.

In a 1943 letter home, AFSC representative John Rich captured the paradoxes inherent in McClure's charismatic leadership style:

He is an amazing man, full of vigour and crackling with ideas ... he comes back bursting with plans for men to work on sanitation, delousing of refugees, engineering and establishing new communities for refugees etc. His ideas are not at all workable and must be checked to verify the connections he wants to establish. But it is invigorating to work with him.[34]

Duncan Wood later recalled the Unit's stormy courtship with McClure: "Most [China] missionaries roared with laughter at the prospect of the most militantly anti-Japanese member of their community being put in charge of a group of pacifists." It took, Wood maintained,

> patience on both sides to work out a happy relationship from this unexpected appointment. The first step would be for the gun-toting McClure to relinquish his weapon.
>
> The convoy benefited from Bob's adventurous spirit and he found among us some of the most unforgettable characters he had ever met.[35]

The stage had been set for a long and bitter civil war in China well before the Convoy started operations, but the Sino-Japanese War changed the fortunes of the Guomindang (Nationalist Party) and the Communist Party of China (CPC). During the 1930s, Chiang Kai-shek had retreated in the face of Japan's aggression, but his preferred strategy of "internal pacification [before] external resistance" that would lead to victory in the civil war was not fruitful. Instead, by 1937 he "wound up fighting all the foes at once, with predictably bad military results."[36] In the meantime, the Sino-Japanese War positioned the Communists to reap the benefits after Chiang and Japan fatally weakened each other.

By July 1937, Japan had launched outright war in China "over an area roughly equivalent to the United States east of the Mississippi River."[37] By the fall of 1938, Japan had taken the five key economic centres: Beijing, Tianjin, Shanghai, Wuhan, and Guangzhou. Contrary to Japanese expectations, however, the Chinese did not capitulate. Instead, "Chiang traded space for time, negating the Japanese strategy for a quick decisive victory."[38] In addition, Japanese forces failed to hold new territories. "Operation victory" went hand-in-hand with strategic stalemate. As soon as Japanese forces left for other battle sites, Chinese forces returned. As the Guomindang suffered defeat in conventional battles, they embraced a new strategy favoured by the weak: Chiang shifted the focus of some troops from positional warfare, which defended cities, to mobile warfare, and from conventional warfare to guerrilla operations. "The combination of guerrilla and conventional forces proved lethal"[39] but not decisive. Neither side anticipated the cost of total warfare.

Japan's military strategy made its economic goals unattainable by causing the collapse of the Chinese economy. Japan failed to anticipate the adverse economic costs – plummeting trade and rising military expenditures – and the nationalism that its strategy fed.[40] By 1941, the Japanese army would become synonymous with the "Three Alls Policy" – kill all, burn all, and loot all – compounding the postwar relief and rehabilitation work that needed to be done.[41] Japan's decision to have its armies live off the land and use poison gas and germ warfare fuelled Chinese nationalism and heightened Japan's diplomatic isolation.

Despite valiant efforts to relocate and rebuild, the Guomindang could re-establish only a fraction of its economic activities, and Guomindang local government income plummeted by nearly one quarter between 1936 and 1940. As Sino-American military historian S.C.M. Paine argues:

> Given all that happened from 1937–1941, it is amazing that the Nationalists survived at all. Within a year of the 1937 escalation, Japan took all or pieces of twenty-one provinces. By 1939 it occupied one-third of China, comprising 40 percent of its agriculture, 92 percent of its modern industry, and 66 percent of its salt fields (the latter a major source of tax revenues). Together this produced a Nationalist loss in tax revenues of more than 80 percent.[42]

Chiang was forced to requisition food to feed the army, and the result was severe deprivation among farmers. The growing shortfall in the revenue stream meant that Chiang turned increasingly to borrowed money to cover military expenses, which meant not future growth but interest payments, thus triggering spiralling inflation when the Guomindang turned to the printing press to cover expenses, and his government became synonymous with corruption and the impoverishment of the Chinese people. This perception coloured the China Convoy's humanitarian relations with the Chinese.

The shift to mobile/guerrilla warfare and inflation wrecked the China Convoy's plans for ambulance-based medical work in a cordon sanitaire recognized by both sides. Moreover, the military medicine system, historian Marvin Williamsen argues, remained insufficiently developed during the first years of the war to provide adequate care for sick and wounded soldiers, despite improvements made.[43] Given the levels of destruction within both the military and civilian populations, Convoy members had little choice. They could either pack up and go home or compromise their ethical concerns over dealing with the military. From its early days in the field in 1941 until it wound up its operations in southwestern China in late 1945 in anticipation of the move to Henan Province, the China Convoy constantly had to negotiate access to those who needed its medical assistance or relief along the shifting battlefront. The unexpected end of the Sino-Japanese War caught the FAU off guard, necessitating reinvention of its mandate and humanitarian imperative. Following the end of the Salween campaign in Yunnan Province, which eventually led to the reopening of the Burma Road in 1944, until its relocation to Henan, the Convoy shifted its focus to civilian medical work and rehabilitation of China's medical facilities as cities were liberated. This shift marks the end of Part 1 of this book.

The China Convoy enabled both Western and Chinese nurses to experience a different way of life and practice in war-ravaged China. The first five chapters of this volume feature the professional and personal vicissitudes that complicated the humanitarian work of the men and women who provided nursing care until the end of the Salween campaign in 1944. Once they were in the field, reality set in, making it clear that, regardless of personal motivation, goals, or pacifist perspectives, the organization for which they volunteered and the unpredictability of war would define what they could do. Chapter 1 recounts the trials of the early medical field teams, including the ordeal of Convoy men during the infamous march out of Burma into India with General Joseph Stilwell in 1942. Burma was a watershed that forced McClure to reconsider how the Unit's medical aid could be delivered most effectively, and contributed to the decision to court Chinese nurses as full members. The next two chapters provide new perspectives on the life and work of the Chinese nurses within a Western pacifist aid organization until the end of the Salween campaign. Chapters 4 and 5 continue the story of FAU nursing from the time the first British nurses arrived in 1944 until shortly after the Unit moved to Henan. Chapter 4 examines their motivation, preparation in England, and initial orientation to medical work at the FAU base hospital in Qujing, Yunnan Province. Chapter 5 appraises the professional, personal, and ethical challenges of their lived experiences as members of a front-line medical team on the Salween front. The stories of

Western and Chinese nurses are dealt with separately because they rarely intersected until late 1944. Cross-cutting themes, probing motivation, coping strategies, individual agency, and acculturation, connect their stories, highlighting simultaneously the similarities and diversity of their experiences. Combined, their narratives weave a vivid historical tapestry of humanitarian nursing as an intensely personal and often stormy journey of self-discovery.

1 Trial by Fire
Early Field Operations, 1941–42

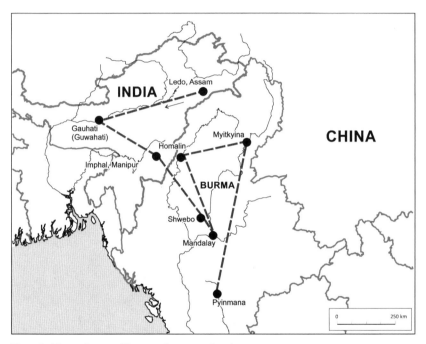

Map 2 The trek out of Burma: Seagrave Section

Burma was a short and gallant adventure, its danger to produce adventurers.

For the Convoy it came at the wrong time, before forces could be marshaled and organized, before the administration could get a grip on what was happening ... In the Unit, each small group had become the master of its own fate, and the sections in China and in Burma had largely fallen apart.

– A. TEGLA DAVIES

Circumstances and character coalesced to make the China Convoy's first year tumultuous. Recruits were still acclimatizing mentally and physically to a nomadic life filled with danger. Typhoid, malaria, and dysentery were so rife that Convoy men were often nicknamed by the disease to which they succumbed most frequently.[1] Within the untried organization, discord simmered about its administration, its survival as a pacifist community, and the direction its humanitarian work should take. The China Convoy reflected individuals' desire to exercise freedom of conscience and to find alternative ways of living that might make war obsolete. For many, ambulance service on the front lines was also their answer to charges of cowardice and their treatment as social outcasts within their home communities gearing up for total war. Those expectations coloured their reaction to China as events unfolded. Often strong personalities butted heads over the Unit's pacifist and humanitarian purposes. The Burma episode simultaneously exposed the deep tensions within the Unit and the courage of individuals to be guided only by their deeply held beliefs. For some, it led to the decision to leave the Convoy.

At the same time, Convoy members had to deal with external events beyond their control. Within five months of the advance party's arrival in China, Japanese forces attacked the United States at Pearl Harbor and the British military forces in Hong Kong, Malaya, and Singapore. Japan declared war on the United States and Britain on 8 December 1941. When Japanese forces overran Burma in 1942, the sole lifeline to China – the Burma Road from Lashio to China – was cut. In the interim, rushing supplies from Rangoon to Lashio before the Japanese closed the port became the Unit's priority, even for the newly arrived American physicians. While Rangoon was under continuous air attack, Convoy drivers frantically scavenged as many trucks and supplies as possible before it was set afire. The last Friends Ambulance Unit (FAU) convoy left Rangoon on 3 March 1942.

With the Unit's medical work on hold, its commandant, Robert McClure, arranged for the newly arrived FAU doctors to work in Ji'an, in central Jiangxi Province, with the 7th New Life Medical Corps (NLMC), composed of "extremely well trained [Chinese] medical personnel," to learn how to work with their Chinese colleagues, how medical practice differed from that of their home country, and what types of war wounds were commonly found in China.[2] Newly arrived British physician Hank Laycock gave the NLMC hospital's medical staff a more mixed review, praising its dedication but noting its shortcomings, especially in the nursing department. Of the seven nurses, only two were trained; the rest compensated for their "amateur" status by their "infectious enthusiasm." At night the patients were "at the mercy of a number of 'non-descript boys' who were as likely to consign to perdition anyone who complained as to fetch help."[3] Cooperation required time in the field and an open mind, for the Unit's priorities changed with the shifting fortunes of the Chinese army and the resources available. McClure had already promised to concentrate the Unit's effort in Yunnan Province when the Indochina-Yunnan border became an active front.

In March 1942, the FAU established two mobile medical surgical teams (MSTs) to visit understaffed hospitals up and down the front lines, intending to stay only long enough to cover the most difficult surgical cases.[4] At full strength, an MST, as McClure described it, would consist of two doctors, to cover for surgery and medicine and the sickness of either one, as well as a surgical and a scrub nurse and a laboratory technician. McClure readily acknowledged that the "usual FAU training of personnel in hospital in England has been good on this score but it takes six months of hard work with a team before a man is qualified for this [nursing] work." He argued that the FAU doctor could train laboratory technicians "with natural ability" on the spot within six months. However, he knew that the FAU teams could not function without either "a man of the country" to act as its quartermaster to secure the team's provisions locally, or the medical mechanic (commonly called "med mechanic") to keep its X-ray and transport vehicles operational and to create hospital equipment from scrap or local materials.[5] The dire circumstances of wartime work quickly blurred strict professional boundaries within MSTs. Often the quartermaster assisted with the dressing and care on the ward, and, in the operating room, doctors relied on lay personnel to give simple anesthesia. As originally envisaged, the local Chinese hospital/

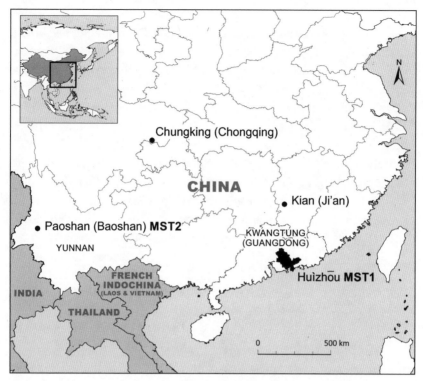

Map 3 Medical Surgical Team 1 (MST1) and Medical Surgical Team 2 (MST2)

army authorities would provide the majority of ongoing postoperative nursing care. Nursing, the Convoy medical corpsmen were to learn, was key to the success of mobile medical services.

Once deployed, the mobile teams had to modify their plans to suit local conditions and mobile warfare. When Henry Louderbough reported that the caseload in Ji'an with the 7th New Life Medical Corps was not enough to keep him and Quentin Boyd, the first doctor to arrive in China, occupied, they were recalled to spearhead MST2 to honour McClure's promise to send help along the Burma border. As the Japanese forces penetrated further along the Burma Road, MST2 was dispatched to the jungle front near the mountain town of Baoshan on the Free China side of the Salween River. In mid-March, the FAU decided to send a mobile team to work with the Chinese 5th Army, which was then fighting in Burma.[6] MST1, the first mobile surgical team, led by Hank Laycock, finally left Guiyang for Burma on 4 April 1942. The timing proved unfortunate.

The Japanese had invaded southern Burma through Thailand in December 1941. The woefully outnumbered, outmanoeuvred, and ill-equipped British and Indian forces defending the British colony retreated steadily. Rangoon, the port through which American Lend-Lease supplies arrived for trans-shipment up the Burma Road to China, fell to the Japanese on 8 March 1942. By 29 April, the Japanese had captured Lashio in Upper Burma. While MST1 was preparing to deploy to Burma in early April, a group of eight FAU transport drivers who were closer to the Burma front went on ahead "without ratification from headquarters"[7] and attached themselves to the field hospital of Burma surgeon Gordon Seagrave, at Pyinmana.[8] When the bridges between Lashio and Mandalay were blown up, a "rogue" advance party of Convoy ambulance drivers and MST1 were stranded. As the withdrawal became a rout, the only escape was over the hills of Assam to India.

MST1 became separated from Convoy ambulance drivers during the trek out of Burma. By 26 April, MST1 had located at Sagaing, close to General Joseph Stilwell's new headquarters at Shwebo but too late to play any useful part in the Burma campaign except during the evacuation.[9] Seven members of MST1 escaped into southern Assam, with the main remnants of the British forces providing the only available medical assistance on the trek westward towards Calcutta. Over jungle roads, through dry and sandy waterways in which vehicles sank and had to be abandoned, they made their way to Kalewa on the Chindwin River, where they found substantial casualties:

> Everything was in a strangely tense and unnatural state ... The only people we saw were Army units and the great tragic hordes of refugees ... They were a pathetic sight, and when one had so packed one's lorry that it was physically impossible to wedge in anyone else, old men and women and mothers with babies literally knelt down on the ground to implore us to help them on their long and weary march.

They continued to Tamu, over the Chin Hills, to Imphal, and finally India. "From here, in consequence of air-raids, the civil population had largely fled; many bodies were lying about in the streets. The Unit turned to grave-digging. And thence they made their way to Calcutta."[10]

For those Convoy drivers who joined Gordon Seagrave, the decision to ignore the order to return to China had been easy. The experience tested their pacifist ideals, forcing some to re-evaluate their positions as conscientious objectors. Despite their orders to stay well back from the action, there were so many casualties, as one British member, Tom Haley, recalled, that "they had to stay and do whatever was necessary, however close the Japs were." Within half an hour of arriving at Kinu during a huge bombing raid, they "operated for nine hours continuously. We worked until the Japanese were within minutes of our position. It was hectic. Those who hadn't survived had to be buried." They packed up moved on, and then started all over again. For Haley, neither the danger nor the hectic pace presented his greatest challenge as a pacifist. Without adequate transport or support staff, how could the team cope with those who were critically injured and likely to die? "We had to use our own discretion because there was no way in which we could leave them for the Japanese to bayonet." There was simply "no way I could reconcile what was necessary to help these men die with dignity with what was in accordance with my belief as a pacifist in the sacredness of human life." It was an ethical dilemma that haunted him long after the war.[11] Burma forced him to confront his pacifist feelings for the troops, many gravely wounded, alongside whom he worked.

Until their arrival, Seagrave had no way to transport the wounded from the front to his advance makeshift hospital.[12] After about a week in Pyinmana, "the town was almost razed to the ground with incendiary bombs, providing us – and Doc and [Burmese] nurses – with much work. The Jap army had advanced to within spitting distance and it was necessary to set off north to take the remaining casualties to a base hospital, then to find a new site."[13] Over the next few weeks, Seagrave relocated four times, setting up casualty stations in a farm, a nice bungalow, and a pagoda deserted by Buddhist priests.

John Grindlay, a young Dartmouth-trained doctor seconded by the American military to Seagrave's medical unit, captured the danger, discomfort, and hectic pace of ambulance work in the final days before the retreat began:

> When the Friends who had driven the 30 Chinese patients to [the base hospital] returned at noon, they reported being "strafed" along the road. Four tires and radiator connector tube hit on one truck and it had to be towed in. Hot and windy-dry. Forest fires and haze. Scorpions and cobras about here. Numerous air alarms – about every half hour a flight of Jap bombers passes down the valley.[14]

Peter Tennant, who had been dispatched "to persuade us (unsuccessfully) to return to China, where he thought we should be," found his return route blocked.[15] Ahead lay one of the most harrowing marches of the Second World War: 225 kilometres of steep jungle mountain trails and impenetrable bamboo thickets, with the Japanese in hot pursuit, before Seagrave's section reached safety in India. Grindlay and others praised FAUers as "indefatigable workers whose valor would be proven time after time in the weeks to come."[16] Despite their own pain, sickness, and exhaustion, they pressed on to provide sorely need first aid and act as stretcher bearers for the sick:

> On the first morning three people cracked up ... Someone made a bamboo raft for all three, and Ken, Eric, Martin and Tom offered to drag it all afternoon. The river was an infuriating one. In some places it didn't reach to your knees; in others it was over your head without warning. The shallow places were the worst because if the raft stuck it was the very devil to dislodge. When it was dark we had to have one, two or three men wading ahead with torches.[17]

Seagrave described the team thus:

> Friends are the funniest Englishmen I ever met. They pick those blood-covered patients up in their arms as if they were sweet and lovely ... The Friends ... are teaching the [Burmese] nurses to call them "Bill" and "Eric" and "Martin." The girls get a great kick out of calling white men by their first names! Well if the girls can get a laugh out of them, it is alright by me.[18]

The two FAU parties that had escaped from Burma remained in India longer than anticipated to care for the recuperating Chinese troops before flying back over the Hump to China. On arrival in India, those with the Seagrave Section cared for Chinese troops and refugees "who had struggled over routes even less congenial than ours,"[19] first at Gauhati in Assam and then at Ramgarh in Bihar. Seagrave later claimed that he had "never seen anything so pitiful as these poor refugees." The FAUers assisted the Burmese nurses in caring for patients who were so "starved and emaciated and suffering so much from lack of vitamin that they can't swallow" and easily succumbed to malaria and dysentery. They witnessed women dying of puerperal fever after having an abortion on the trip out because they had been unable to procure medicines when the railway was washed out. Those who survived lacked even the basic comforts:

The patients slept on mats on the floor, which is what they prefer, and in spite of our nurses being on almost full time duty with flyswatters, in spite of flypaper everywhere, in spite of gallons of Flit, the patients and the floors were black with nasty flies. The dysentery cases are so weak they are incontinent, and that doesn't help matters much.[20]

Amidst all this suffering, the FAU men found quiet satisfaction – they had come to China to help relieve suffering brought on by war. Many wanted to stay with Seagrave, where they felt needed, and returned to China reluctantly. For others, the only answer was to enlist to hasten the end of war.

Once in India, MST1, under Laycock, undertook "the most valuable piece of work ... more by accident than design."[21] He had gone up to Dinjan in Assam with the intent of flying out to China. While there, he was hunted down by the assistant director of medical services for northern Assam and implored to go to Ledo; the vanguard of the 5th Army troops were expected to arrive there shortly and would be in desperate need of medical care. Laycock would "not easily forget" the condition of the Chinese ward in the small Indian hospital when they arrived:

It was a long primitive bamboo hut that contained five beds, one unoccupied because a man had recently died in it and no one wanted to use, and another occupied by a corpse, always a disagreeable sight in the tropics in the summer. The seven living men were crowded at the far end of the hut to get as far away as possible from their dead companion ... In these circumstances, it did not take us long to decide to collect as many F.A.U. members as we could get hold of and get down to work as quickly as possible.[22]

In the middle of August, after the rest of the FAU flew out to China, Laycock remained in Ledo. Travelling sixty kilometres up the trail beyond the railhead, he cared for the stragglers who "had been marching for three and a half months through some of the worst malaria country in the world, and subjected to attacks by hundreds of leeches and the devastating and wasting effect of the local Naga sores."[23] During these days, Laycock saw "many scenes of intense horror. A man dying on the path usually remains there until the rapid assault of ants and other insects reduces him to a skeleton,"[24] but the hundreds of soldiers whom he and his local volunteer Chinese stretcher bearers reached avoided a similar end. As had been typical of the FAU men throughout the whole Burma episode, this work was never part of the program of the FAU China Convoy but was decided on on the spot by men of strong conviction.

After a "good deal of opposing pressure regarding what should be done with them [was] exerted by various authorities, including the Chinese Ministry of Military and Political Affairs and the British and American Armies, the Unit finally recalled its men to Kunming in the middle of September."[25] The China Unit's leaders always contended that "much hard and valuable work was done in extremely primitive surroundings and very friendly relations established."[26] Certainly Stilwell, the Allied chief of staff in the China theatre, was profuse in his praise of them.[27]

After their return from Burma, MST1, reconstituted under the medical direction of Drs. Hank Laycock and Terry Darling, were sent to Huizhou, just behind the lines of the Cantonese Front, where they remained until April 1943. The city was subjected to heavy air attacks and received a steady stream of starving refugees from Hong Kong, creating an urgent demand for civilian work. In addition, several thousand regular troops as well as guerillas were stationed there, but there were no base hospital or skilled surgeons to deal with the wounded. Besides running an outpatient clinic to treat civilian casualties and the destitute refugees, team members made trips into guerrilla country with Chinese troops to retrieve or treat the wounded. Hard work and poor food exacted a toll on the team's health.[28] Lin Sing "Arthur" Yau, a nurse from Hong Kong, was assigned as a probationary member to MST1 in the fall of 1943, but left, claiming that he could not support his family on an FAU salary.

Although the Burma episode had been costly in terms of manpower and equipment, valuable lessons were gained. In some cases, it led individuals to re-evaluate pacifist positions and, ultimately, to decide to leave the China Convoy.[29] The fall of Burma crystallized the Convoy's future direction and highlighted the need for professional nurses. In August, the Unit's headquarters in Guiyang was relocated to Qujing, a convenient hub in which to organize its transport work of hauling 150,000 kilograms of National Health Administration (NHA) supplies from Kunming to government warehouses in Chongqing. By 1942, the cavalier McClure had devised a new definition of an ambulance unit. In China, "instead of carrying the wounded to where the supplies exist, we take the drugs and supplies to where the wounded are."[30] He had a "clear picture of what we are, a team equipped in training and tools to do major surgery in rather advanced positions."[31] Without these FAU teams, McClure claimed, patients often waited for thirty months for surgical attention.[32] Equally important, however, McClure's plan to mobilize several medical teams – purportedly "in order that the work being done was that most desired by the Chinese"[33] – quelled widespread complaints about the lack of real medical work. To give effective medical care on the front lines, McClure argued, required more nurses: "Give us the transport to bring the patients to us, give [us] nurses in the hospital to care for the patients with us and we will do our stuff."[34] Finding and retaining an adequate supply of suitable "girl" nurses, as Convoy men initially referred to Western-trained nurses, would spark continuous controversy until the FSU closed its doors in 1951.

Others echoed the call for fully qualified nurses. The FAU's medical corpsmen who survived the retreat to India after the fall of Burma in 1942 led the campaign. The courage, resilience, and surgical skills of Seagrave's barefoot Burmese nurses, who had helped them survive by collecting edible plants and roots, left an indelible memory.[35] They argued: "There is little sense in doing good surgery then losing the results through careless dressing in the wards. Our own men cannot do this work very well and are not legally qualified to supervise it as would a graduate nurse."[36] It took only a few weeks in the field before other FAU teams witnessed the importance of nursing care to ensure patients' safety and progress: "We have no bedpans, so the patients have either to climb up and down the stairs or excrete in the bedding, in which cases they are likely to be beaten by the orderly. Since there is insufficient boiled water, every patient suffers from thirst."[37] Although the Convoy men had begun training as theatre nurses and dressers, the team physicians argued that it would "be a lot better with a nurse of our own." As teams gained experience in the field, their reports stressed the importance of learning the language, cooperating with Chinese medical teams, and having fully qualified nursing personnel. In fact, all three were directly connected, in their opinion. MST2, stationed near Baoshan, reported:

Things are very much more satisfactory these days, in fact ... the bogy of co-operation has been overcome. I think we are now on very friendly terms. A lot of this has been due to ... one of Wesley May's [New Life Movement] nurses. She is an excellent girl, besides doing all she can to help, she is giving us two hours [of] Chinese a day.[38]

Suei T'ang "Sheila" Iu and "Margaret" Li, rather than British nurses, would be sent to improve nursing care on the team.

In fact, Chinese nurses provided convenient substitutes for "more delicate Western women," whose inclusion "would create innumerable complications." Western nurses, some thought, could not "fit into the Convoy's work unless they have long experience in primitive medical work," and even then would still require a long adjustment period "to the peculiar conditions in China."[39] London and Philadelphia were cautioned that Western nurses would be suited for work only in the better-equipped mission hospitals; their higher standards were not applicable to primitive field conditions, and consequently they tended to become "embittered and frustrated." Moreover, many "quickly marry and quit the job."[40] McClure, however, later claimed that he welcomed fully qualified Western nurses in the China Convoy but opposed bringing out "the girls to get married."[41] John Rich, then in China on a visit for the American Friends Service Committee (AFSC), cabled Philadelphia that it was "not desirable, at present, to consider sending out women." Here, as in the First World War, concern lingered in Philadelphia that sending women would use up limited funds and thereby jeopardize the sending overseas of conscientious objectors assigned to the Civil Public Service camps.[42]

The notion of sending Western women to China initially encountered resistance in both London and the FAU. Gender and racial prejudices most likely shaped attitudes. It remains unclear from the documents whether London and Philadelphia were uneasy about sending nurses into battlefield conditions in an untried organization or about the optics of setting single women adrift in the exotic East. One Convoy member found London's attitude surprising, given that "equality between the sexes is an important point of Friends' principles. The FAU in London ... decided to admit women members, and from what knowledge I have of their behaviour during the London 'Blitzes' I should have said the assumption was justified. If this is the case and we have jobs for them to do overseas, it seems to me unfair to deny them an equal opportunity for serving, with male members."[43] The first British nurses would not reach China before 1944, however.

The convergence of need and opportunity ultimately led to the recruitment of Chinese nurses. Given the continued anxiety over Western nurses' suitability, the expedient solution was to "scour the field for Chinese nurses" essential "to care for women patients and to give prolonged post-operative care."[44] Finding well-qualified Chinese nurses had proven difficult in the past: "Nursing is not, as yet, regarded as a respectable profession, and the few intelligent women who have 'broken over the traces'" were already employed in military or civilian work.[45] When prospects appeared better in June 1942, Convoy leaders made a strong pitch to London to recruit Chinese nurses: "There have been escaping from Hong Kong some of the finest nurses that one could hope to meet in any country." Their escape demonstrated "that they do not lack 'guts'" but were "very patriotic and showed a fearlessness that would make a fine example to their sisters at the front." Heralded as "energetic, capable," and having "a good initiation into war surgery," these nurses, London was told, wanted to work at the front under any conditions for "whatever remuneration will feed them." Since most spoke English, they "would bridge, most usefully the gap that now exists in our work for the wounded."[46] Others agreed that Chinese nurses could furnish badly needed cross-cultural linchpins in the Unit's humanitarian work: "It is certainly impossible for foreigners after a brief residence here and knowing but a few Chinese phrases ... to understand Chinese ways of living" or adapt Western nursing standards "from a perspective of different localities."[47] Fully qualified Chinese nurses were also required in order to bolster the FAU's reputation with local officials for whom paper credentials were paramount.[48] Besides their professional credentials, Chinese nurses provided "'the women's touch' which we have found to be necessary in the work we do."[49] As Robert McClure also candidly admitted, the Convoy would have been unable to meet the British Red Cross relief team's request for assistance without "the new policy of suitable Chinese girl nurses joining the Convoy as full members."[50]

In practice, the Unit quota of twenty "non-pacifists" prevented or delayed Chinese nurses from becoming full members.[51] But the cautious approach towards Chinese nurses reflected deeper anxieties. After a "sticky period in the Spring," Convoy leaders admitted, the experiment of admitting Chinese members to the transport section had been "a limited success," if not its "most shameful failure." Instead of making Chinese members "feel at home," there had been a "tendency to use them as school fags."[52] Never one to mince words, McClure knew what was required "to give a Christian witness in China"; the Unit must "learn something about getting on with our neighbour."[53] He remained adamant that that Convoy members must live close to the Chinese, sharing primitive living conditions and following the Chinese tradition of having only two meals a day to avoid misunderstandings that could negate their work. McClure identified the "greatest barrier" to cooperation with the Chinese: "all the misunderstandings have been due to this – the need for learning the language of the land in which we work – must be put before our chaps always."[54] The Chinese nurses would play a pivotal role in facilitating Unit members' acculturation to living and working in China.

At the same time, American and British Friends were reassured: "[Chinese nurses] living with our surgical teams at the front would not be a problem as Dr. Wesley May, [of the New Life Medical Corps] with whom we are co-operating ... has girl nurses on his staff of the same caliber."[55] The FAU's stringent selection criteria went beyond professional credentials: the ideal FAU nurse would be state-registered, pacifist, and unfettered by family obligations. In the case of Chinese nurses, however, pacifism was equated with being a Christian woman of good character.[56]

As late as 1945, Convoy members would continue to rationalize Chinese nurses' feminine presence in a war zone by casting them in the role of self-sacrificing heroic figures "who had volunteered for the Unit as an expression of their desire to give Christian service to China."[57] Why did Chinese nurses join the FAU in 1942? Once there, how did they construct their identities and relationships within a Western pacifist organization that viewed them as a convenient, albeit essential, source of nursing knowledge and cultural legitimacy?

2 A Marriage of Convenience
Courting the Chinese Nurses, 1942–43

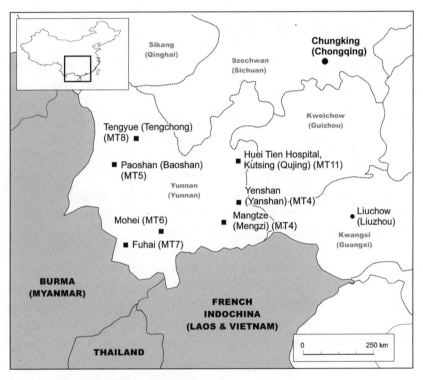

Map 4 FAU Medical Teams, 1944–45

> Here the work is going far better than one would think to hear the reports. First of all it is an amazing demonstration of co-operation but [we] must learn to do more ... Actually things are being sorted out rather well and the vast majority of the surgery is given to our chaps ... The morale of the team is excellent. Everyone gets on perfectly ... The relations with Wesley May [of the New Life Movement] are fine.
>
> – ROBERT McCLURE, MST2 BAOSHAN, 28 JULY 1942

Fostering global fraternity and transferring Western medical knowledge to the local community remained cardinal tenets of the Friends Ambulance Unit humanitarian engagement in China. As a symbolic gesture of cross-cultural blending of lives within the China Convoy, Chinese members were given a Christian name and Westerners were provided with a Chinese version of their surname. However, Robert McClure's glowing account of Medical Surgical Team 2 (MST2) belied the anxieties and tensions that characterized life in the field in pursuit of these sometimes disparate goals. As we shall see, he underestimated the enormous acclimatization required of both Chinese and Western members assigned to the untried FAU front-line teams along the Salween front. In reality, greater flexibility, adaptation, accommodation, and realism than most anticipated would be required of Western members in order to work collaboratively with their Chinese colleagues and local communities. In some cases, their humanitarian exchanges remained clouded with the preconceived beliefs and values of the Western society in which they were reared. FAU teams were appalled by the neglect of patients they witnessed in the course of their humanitarian work. FAUers, as the field staff were known, were morally outraged by the diversion of medical supplies by the Chinese medical staff for personal profit, and stymied by the inadequacies of local healthcare facilities that restricted the Chinese people's access to "modern" medical care or essential medicines. Even with the inclusion of Western-trained Chinese nurses, Western members were ill-prepared to bridge the cultural chasms that divided Western medicine from traditional healers and China's medical system. As the experiences of Chinese FAU nurses told here and in the next chapter indicate, it was not only the team's location and social dynamics with the surrounding community but also the FAU physicians' leadership style that coloured nurses' experience within a male-dominated Western humanitarian agency.

Their stories highlight the fact that physicians could be either "a great help or great hindrance" in determining the team's ability to work in a Quakerly manner that was both efficient and well received by the recipients of medical aid. Acknowledging the magnitude of adjustment required, American MST2 physician Art Barr wrote: "China is a real test of the Christian concept of service. Service here means much more than the work itself. It means sincere harmonious relations with a proud race whose civilization is older than ours and whose heritage is much different." If measuring Chinese by American or English standards, he admitted, "we have full right to become completely exasperated or disgusted." But FAU members "are not living the brotherhood of the American or the brotherhood of the English. We are living the brotherhood of man. It requires great ... understanding, tolerance, patience and humility. Then one may see a people he can respect and enjoy in happy fellowship." He cautioned against drawing comparisons with colonial medicine elsewhere:

> You have probably read about medical pioneers who have so impressed uncivilized peoples with their cures that they are accorded complete and multitudinous appeal. In China the introduction of Western medicine is much different and very difficult. Western medicine must confront a developed civilization with outcomes and practices that have sufficed for tens of thousands of years.[1]

Not all FAU members exhibited the same cultural sensitivity or humility, however. Chinese nurses consequently found themselves cast in new roles beyond traditional nursing at the bedside as they navigated contested personal, professional, and political terrain. Equally important, recovering their lived experiences of nursing with the FAU reveals considerable agency as well as accommodation and assimilation in determining their life choices and work conditions.

Iu Suei T'ang was the first Chinese nurse recruited. The twenty-year-old "Sheila" Iu came from a wealthy Chinese family, spoke English well, and had trained at Hong Kong's Queen Mary Hospital. Despite McClure's intention to welcome Chinese nurses as full members, their admission caused uneasiness within the ranks when the matter was raised in September 1942. When it was suggested that members "should think on it before we say anything ...

the company rather thankfully passed on to the next business."[2] As McClure explained in a letter to his wife, the women "had a positive civilizing effect," but their arrival upset the all-male set-up until the women proved they could live the hard way.[3]

On arrival in Qujing, Iu was hurriedly dispatched to MST2, which was assigned to the 71st Army Hospital at Baoshan, within thirty kilometres of Japanese lines and easy reach of Japanese guerrilla bands.[4] Iu reached MST2 on 20 August 1942.[5] The decision to forgo the traditional orientation period in Qujing reflected the urgency to raise nursing standards and improve cooperation with the Chinese medical teams. By the time she arrived, the team had relocated to Hsiakwan, where it cooperated with teams from the Chinese Red Cross and Wesley May's New Life Medical Corps in anticipation of renewed action along the Burma front. Before Iu's arrival, Michael Harris, who had joined the FAU at seventeen, served as head nurse. A veteran of the ill-fated FAU section to Finland, he had escaped to England in time to work in London during the Blitz.[6] Although Harris depended on and admired the eight young New Life nurses, who seemed to thrive on hard work despite their meagre diet, he welcomed the FAU nurses. However, their arrival unexpectedly complicated the team's cross-cultural relations.

Robert McClure contended that "never in the history of this war with China has a group of foreigners gone so close to the front for work with the wounded and stuck in that position for so long. In Baoshan, I saw the highest technical work done for Chinese soldiers that I have ever seen on any front in five years of war."[7] Years later, he would claim that "for all her youth, Sheila supervised the O.R. in a way that [brought back] my intern's terrors [of head nurses] at the Toronto Western Hospital."[8] In reality, tensions riddled team cross-cultural relationships, making Iu's adjustment to life in the field more difficult than McClure depicted. Similarly, McClure's later observation that "the experiment has proven worthwhile"[9] bears re-examination.

Despite the team's reassuring August report, unrest continued to brew. When MST2 appeared on the scene, the team's original plans were torpedoed, for FAU ambulance work proved redundant; army trucks supplying the front lines transported the wounded coming back. Before MST2 could regroup and salvage beds and equipment to ready the hospital for patients, it had to contain a cholera epidemic raging nearby. There was a far more divisive issue, however. Expecting his to be the only surgical team assigned there, American team leader Hank Louderbough instead found the FAU surgeons competing with the Chinese Red Cross for patients – "a competition in which the F.A.U. has come off distinct second best."[10]

Colleagues, however, laid the blame for the team's strained relations squarely on Louderbough, who purportedly had come "with various misconceptions as to the nature of the Unit." Viewing him as "something of a misfit,"[11] they charged that he "developed a terrible case of Sinophobia, which coloured his relations with Chinese colleagues."[12] He had "been restless for some time as the conditions of work in China did not suit him."[13] Both his unwillingness to "chip in his personal income" to the financial pool that was shared monthly equally among all China Convoy members[14] and disappointment with the lack of surgical opportunities ultimately led to his early resignation.[15] But Art Barr disagreed. In his view, the whole group was "the chief offender," for the FAU group "doesn't mingle much with the non-English speaking Chinese and this leads to misunderstandings."[16]

While the team's strained relations with the other Chinese teams created an uncomfortable working environment, Iu's difficulties settling into Convoy life and her position within the team were more complicated than Barr suggested.[17] According to Louderbough, "there is considerable resentment on the part of other nurses of other groups that she is working with foreigners rather than with a Chinese organization. They taunt her" and "call her the Foreigners' slave."[18] There is some evidence that Iu looked to Louderbough for fatherly protection from her persecutors. On his birthday, she and a New Life nurse presented him with a chocolate cake inscribed with "Happy Birthday Uncle Hank." The expectation that Chinese nurses would naturally be effective humanitarian brokers proved ill-founded, for Iu resisted accepting responsibilities outside her traditional nursing duties. As late as 1943, FAU team doctors complained that "we do not have anyone with us who is a very good interpreter save one girl, Sheila Iu, who refuses to do any interpreting as she says she is only a nurse and dislikes the interpreting job very much."[19] All of these factors explain why the Convoy's leadership in Qujing hoped that the arrival of Iu's best friend, Margaret Li, recruited as a probationary in December 1942, would help alleviate her "trying time."[20] Thereafter, every attempt was made to dispatch two Chinese nurses together, especially in isolated locations.

In June 1943, Margaret Li was assigned to the China Inland Mission hospital in Tali, but Iu, after taking her first leave in Kunming, was sent to the Wei Sheng Chang hospital and then brought back to Qujing to gain additional experience before reassignment. At first glance, this decision is perplexing. At the close of 1942, Iu had been repeatedly praised as "a well-trained English-speaking Chinese nurse who is dandy worker"[21] and as an "unqualified success."[22] Since there was no other physician available to replace Louderbough, MST2 was withdrawn, and most likely the additional training was merely a stopgap measure while the FAU medical teams' new assignments were being negotiated with the Chinese authorities. The departure of Iu's new team, MT4 (the former appellation MST was dropped), was delayed until 30 June 1943 and the team did not arrive at its destination, somewhere near the Indochina border, until 16 July. While waiting, other team members had also received further training.

As 1943 began, life in the field was "one big, blooming, buzzing confusion."[23] In February, the Convoy decided with "considerable trepidation" to try an experiment: "Never before had a foreign organization like ours been under the authority of a Chinese organization for orders."[24] While the FAU publicly portrayed this decision as a reflection of the Unit's desire to perform the work according to Chinese priorities, it had little choice. Its plans to obtain medical supplies through the American Red Cross were thwarted when the US Army placed an embargo on supplies being flown into China to ensure that it had adequate supplies for the Burma campaign. The results devastated the FAU's mobile surgical units. In particular, for MST2 to be mobile for future campaigns, it would have to attach itself to the Army Medical Administration, the Chinese Red Cross, or the New Life Movement to obtain supplies. Necessity dictated that the China Convoy trade autonomy for access to those in need of medical care.

On the positive side, the field report indicated that opportunities for closer cooperation with the Chinese appeared to have improved:

> A certain member of the Unit [McClure] recently had a three hour talk with a high Chinese official during the course of which the latter said ... that despite certain unfortunate incidents, the general view taken of the Unit by the Chinese Government is a favourable one and that if we wished to remain in the country after the war we would be welcome.

It was noted "with a certain amount of amusement that the B.R.C.S. [British Red Cross Society] hospital is at the moment going through the same stage of suspicion and official blocking that we went through this time last year."[25]

In mid-July 1943, Sheila Iu, Wong Kuei Hsien, and (Jane), a Cantonese nursing sister who also trained at Queen Mary Hospital in Hong Kong, joined MT4 in the 2nd Field Hospital of the 52nd Army. The Unit was lodged within the British Red Cross Society Hospital in Changsha, on the railway connecting Kunming with Hanoi and Haiphong in Indochina. MT4 included American physician Ernest Evans, British Red Cross physician John Thompson, and Convoy members Sidney Walker, Christopher Weston, Jackson Progin, Robin Eden, and Bill Rahill. Although a Quaker, Evans proved as controversial as his American colleague Louderbough.

Once again, Iu was assigned to work with an FAU physician widely regarded as "a highly biased person who made no or little attempt to understand the views of the Chinese."[26] Evans's negative evaluation while working with MST1 in Huizhou had resulted in his being placed on probation rather than being sent home, because illness had decimated the FAU medical staff and "we can't spare him now." Described as "argumentative, critical of government, Chinese people," and verging on "developing Sino-phobia," he was "greatly disliked by his co-workers."[27] His lack of tact made him equally objectionable to the Chinese staff. Evans's belief that "conditions should be the same as in New York" and his inability to adapt to local conditions "caused more mental strain on members of [MST1] than, perhaps, a day's dive-bombing!" Depicted as a "go-getter" and a "doer," Evans was condemned for failing to perceive that "the friendships we make in China counts for a lot." It was hoped that he "would turn over a new leaf" on MT4.[28]

FAU physicians did not anticipate that they would have to earn the trust of the local Chinese community, and had difficulties accepting the team's limited capacity to improve patient outcomes or the level of public health services. Viewing the Chinese people through Western eyes as "fettered by the chains of superstitions, tradition and undispelled ignorance," Evans was proud that the local army medical groups had improved the standard of care "under our tutelage."[29] But his dissatisfaction went deeper than his inability to adjust professionally. Evans found the lack of privacy especially disconcerting, as groups of Chinese daily invaded the FAU's private living quarters to "get a look at the foreigners and his [sic] queer ways." The cultural divide made it difficult for him to fathom the Chinese tradition of hospitality. His announcement that he was relieved when invitations to feasts fell off and his hope that "these ordeals will not be inflicted upon us in the near future"[30] indicated his failure to perceive that operating on the cusp of rudeness by Chinese standards compromised his professional relationships as well. Even though Evans realized that his inability to speak Chinese rendered him "pretty helpless," he concluded that the effort required to learn any of the "very difficult jargon"[31] was not warranted for a two-year contract.

For Iu, MT4 brought new professional challenges beyond the operating room, which was well supplied and eventually housed in "a fine set of buildings" in a large compound that had been used as barracks for several thousand Chinese soldiers in a small town near Yanshan. Although the FAU worked in the operating theatre, oversaw the postoperative recovery, did laboratory work, and supervised special diets for soldiers, both community public health and work with civilian patients remained central to MT4's endeavours. Evans wrote home that by mid-August, both soldiers and civilians "flocked to our gates" and over 2,200 patients had attended the clinic.[32] On their heaviest day, the team reported handling 600 cases.[33] A typical day included daily rounds of 60 in-patients, handling 153 outpatients and 110 patients in the eye clinic, and then giving 250 cholera injections in the marketplace.[34]

While some FAU physicians recognized the need for cultural awareness on the front lines, more frequently the Chinese nurses acted as cultural diplomats, fostering unity within the team and facilitating its outreach to the wider community. Despite the heavy workload, Sheila often arranged social evenings with the Chinese orderlies, baking cakes and arranging card games that they especially enjoyed. Often, however, the arrival of the wounded or other emergencies interrupted these social gatherings. An account of their nocturnal excursion to visit an officer's wife in labour conveys the cultural and logistical challenges a small FAU team encountered in rural China despite the presence of Chinese nurses.

Iu and Evans "plodded through the mud that splashed high up the horse's legs and about a half-hour's brisk ride brought [them] to a rather unkempt village and a house equally so." Evans was appalled to find "a young half naked woman there squatting on the floor" in labour. She had endured over forty hours attended by "some filthy little peasant woman, acting as the midwife [who] had attempted to deliver the child forcibly by hand and the dead baby was locked in the mother's abdomen. Flies were everywhere." Unable to deliver the baby but hoping to save the mother's life, they arranged for her to "be carried back to the hospital through the mud on a bamboo litter by a host of men."[35] The deck was stacked against her. The patient was already septic, with a temperature of 104 and weak after her long ordeal, and it was well after midnight before a Caesarean section commenced. The anaesthetist, "who is just one of the 'boys' administered some open ether despite the gasoline lamp we had to have in the room to work by." Fortunately, "there were no explosions and the lady is now recovering ... The fecundity of Chinese women is amazing."[36] Here, as elsewhere, FAU teams struggled to understand why they were called out to deliver babies only after things had gone horribly wrong. Local custom, where childbirth was cloaked in secrecy and overseen by local midwives, limited the team's maternal work. Accustomed to traditional Chinese medicine, in which Chinese physicians usually diagnosed patients only by checking pulse and tongue, women refused to expose their bodies. Moreover, FAU physicians discovered that the traditional Chinese ladylike attitude fostered social reticence outside the home.[37]

Although it appeared to McClure that "we had things nicely fixed for this team," everything went "haywire." He found it hard to fathom why the team had reacted so negatively to the termination of its civilian work: "All they needed to do was to move their civilian opd [outpatient department] to a room on the main street and then get the 'hsien chang' [local officials] to give them a courtyard for their patients. This they seemed to have been unable to do. The result has been a drop-off of work and demoralization."[38] When several members contemplated going home, McClure displayed little empathy. In his opinion, far greater self-discipline was required among this team, and "those who did not like it can lump it."[39] After visiting MT4, McClure claimed that although the inclusion of Chinese nurses raised the level of care and they had proved invaluable translators for the doctors, "they certainly bring a number of problems in their train. They demand, for instance, a far higher standard of living than Unit Members and are pretty faddy about their food, insisting on Chinese food at every meal."[40] And after learning that Sheila Iu wanted to quit after the departure of a team member with whom she was romantically involved, McClure hoped that "Sheila can see the light" and made it clear "that even if she wants to leave she must give us reasonable notice." Otherwise, "we take full liberty to let others know what were the conditions of her leaving us."[41] Sheila remained.

After a few months in Yanshan, the team moved to Mangtze, near the Red River, which flows south through Yunnan to Indochina, and continued similar work with the 1st Army Group. But relocating the team failed to improve relations between FAU doctors and their Chinese counterparts. In early January 1944, MT4 wired Qujing that it was impossible to remain. Evidently, General Ch'iao had "gone behinds their backs" and requested that a Chinese army team replace them. When the Chinese team refused "on grounds of etiquette," the Chinese military officials "just began to freeze us out." They "terminated funds for special diets, stopped delivering firewood and rice ... and finally, said that the Ikwans [Chinese orderlies] were to have nothing more to do with us. Added up, it was quite clear that we were no longer wanted." In an attempt to salvage the team's work, American physician John Perry was sent to replace the recalcitrant Evans.

Bill Rahill, who had worked hard to develop a working command of the Chinese language, described his experience with the Chinese on MT4 very differently from Evans. The American had come to China expecting to help the Chinese, but discovered instead, "on the balance it will be [we] who are helped more than China. A year like this offers opportunities for learning about life and oneself that no College curriculum can boast." In particular, he praised the Hong Kong–trained nurses "who showed us what nursing really meant" and had been integral to making his experience "altogether happy."[42] These nurses' reputation would only grow in the months to come.

When MT4 was finally disbanded in March 1944 "due to a number of difficulties encountered in efforts to maintain it in a useful field of service,"[43] Jane Wong and Sheila Iu were transferred to the FAU's most remote team, MT6, codenamed M. After a two-week trek along a crumbling mule trail built some two hundred years earlier, Sheila and Jane descended on MT6 in mid-September 1944. Here, MT6 worked in anonymity for over a year before its location at Mohei was disclosed to the rank and file.[44]

The local warlord, Mr. Chang, not the FAU, selected the team's precise location. With little action on the Salween front, the team had intended to reinforce the civilian medical work of the Yunnan Provincial Health Administration around Szemao and be available to assist French Legionnaires fleeing Indochina. But when the team stopped overnight at Mohei, it discovered that Chang had established a well-stocked and well-equipped dispensary that had no doctor. When it became apparent that Chang had no intention of allowing them to proceed, physicians Art Barr and Patrick Rawlence secured his promise to build an in-patient clinic if they remained. Despite suspicions that Chang was connected to the opium trade, Rawlence regarded him as "a good man in his own way interested in his people."[45] With the completion of the new in-patient clinic in March 1945, the team was in full swing. Mornings were filled with hospital rounds before doctors saw sixty to seventy patients in the outpatient clinic and made home visits to patients too ill to come for treatment.

Iu and Wong descended on MT6 with a "whirlwind of ideas"[46] and immediately made plans to expand the in-patient work by building a ward on school property, where "relatives of the patients will be allowed to look after them to a large extent, including the providing and cooking of food."[47] Iu was relocated two months after she arrived, but the in-patient work steadily increased as Wong gradually cultivated and gained the local community's trust.[48] Her efforts to recruit and train local nursing personnel encountered resistance, however, because local women were bound by gendered roles of childbearing, household duties, and farming. Although several girls expressed interest in nursing training, in most cases their parents were opposed. Two teenage sisters of the Yang family who defied their parents to train as nurses, wrote Rawlence, did "remarkably well and were of great assistance" in the team's work.[49] Others had a less favourable impression of the younger sister when she was sent for a six-month practical nursing course in Qujing: she was "the best they could obtain locally" but "not very good by our big city standards." The young woman had difficulties settling in far away from home, and after completing only one month of training at the Provincial Health Department clinic she left without notice to work at the local military hospital as a ward maid. She "had to be put back on the rails ... and with considerable difficulty she was finally persuaded to tell us a little more about her difficulties." Ultimately she was relocated to the FAU hospital in Qujing, where she got "as good a training as her brains could possibly absorb."[50] In the meantime, her elder sister, Barbara, had joined MT6 and "seems keen on the work." Wong instructed her in the feminine arts of being a respectable nurse in addition to basic nursing: "Jane is teaching her the elements of nursing and midwifery and teaching her to do hair."[51] Eventually Yang helped with surgeries and did minor operations, such as trichiasis surgery – a simple operation on patients suffering from trachoma to prevent the lashes from growing in to hurt the eyes. But many cases remained beyond her capabilities.

By February 1945, the team medical report noted that Wong remained busy, providing rudimentary nursing education and delivering babies, even when the clinic was not. Once again local birth traditions constrained the team's maternal work despite the presence of Chinese nurses. While MT6 doctors were called for dire situations, such as in the case of a stillborn child, Wong and Yang usually oversaw home deliveries, even when the baby was premature. While Wong was the more experienced nurse, Yang spoke the local dialect. The two often worked all night before starting their regular shifts the following day.[52] In addition to her regular nursing duties in the hospital and outpatient clinic, Wong provided a series of lectures on basic nursing to the girls of the middle school. Whether directly connected or not, Rawlence found it encouraging that, during the team's stay, more girls than ever before went to Kunming University after graduating from middle school.[53] Working long hours in a malaria-infested region eventually took its toll; by mid-July 1945, both nurses contracted malaria.

While Chinese nurses provided vital cultural bridges, here as on other teams their presence could not prevent FAU physicians from viewing China through Western eyes. Patrick Rawlence claimed that through Chang's goodwill and their medical contact with nearly every household, they became part of the community. For him, this social intercourse provided an avenue to determine "the degree to which [the local population's] backwardness is due to inherent racial defects or to lack of communications."[54] Ultimately, Rawlence concluded, "one feels that these people should have been capable of better things than they actually are." Granted that lack of communication with the outside world and the high incidence of malaria "are big handicaps," he still believed "that the air of apathy and hopelessness is largely due to an inherent racial defect." Despite having worked with capable Chinese colleagues and having acknowledged the importance of local support for MT6's success, Rawlence did not believe that "any real advance in hygiene, malaria control, or medicine generally will ever arise spontaneously in southern Yunnan from the Chinese themselves. The area still desperately needs foreign help on these lines."[55] The focus of Western medicine on pathology and disease encouraged a racially biased view of the Chinese community. Conversely, a young Canadian medical student, Edwin Abbott, who joined the team as a lab technician, adopted a public health perspective to identify different underlying determinants of poor health:

> A town such as this needs organization to lift public health, give it water, and electricity, give it access by roads to the outside world, newer types of agriculture with the introduction of better types of fruits and vegetables, better livestock etc., new industries and better leadership.[56]

But again Western development models were seen as the cure for China's ills.

Both Rawlence and Abbott may have overestimated the Chinese people's deference to the assumed superiority of Western medicine and technology.

Despite Jane Wong's Western training, she never entirely abandoned local healing traditions or traditional Chinese remedies. Many FAU teams discovered that the Chinese believed that blood was sacred, and few, if any, would volunteer to give it to save others' lives. Consequently the FAU team often had to donate blood for transfusions themselves. On one of these occasions, Abbott recounted, the transfusion "went a bit haywire" and some remained unused. Jane "could not see anything wasted and so she let it clot and fed it to the beggar lad the next day and he enjoyed it she says. She tried very hard to get me to eat it but I balked ... Of course here blood is sold in the market every day – not a drop is wasted (not human blood of course)."[57]

As honoured guests, MT6 attended lavish feasts of local delicacies: trout, deer tendons, grubs served in a wild bees' nest, crayfish, and snails. On one occasion, Chang dammed the river, caught the fish, and cooked them for a great feast in their honour. But despite their frequent inclusion in local cultural activities and feasts, in many important respects the FAU lived as a Western community within a local community. The Mohei team was lodged in a two-storey house with a courtyard and was provided with a Chinese cook and houseboys to care for them, while Jane fulfilled the traditionally gendered and racial role of managing the team's household routine. She taught the cook how to prepare Chinese food purchased in the local market into "appetizing and satisfying meals" that kept them "remarkably free of alimentary disorders."[58]

Working in isolation from the mainstream of the FAU's work meant that the team created its own family structure and leisure activities. Every effort was made to be inclusive by providing translators for Barbara Yang on these occasions. Daily Quaker worship meetings, evening card games and sing-songs, and occasional hikes in the surrounding countryside provided fellowship and diversion from workday routines. Team members frequently relied on humour to ease their anxiety about working and living in a new culture and to bond with their Chinese colleagues. Ed Abbott's account of Jane's birthday celebration shortly after his arrival illuminates the complex and sometimes contradictory intersection of cultures that cemented the team's familial bonding:

All the fellows dressed in their Chinese clothes [given them by Chang] ... I could not come in ordinary dress so I wore my pjs until Barbara volunteered a dress of hers and then I served as the girl that was needed. I have been a gal all evening. I taught them the 'I went to market game' and half way round Jane changed it from English to Chinese. They really enjoyed it.

While Jane was respected and liked as a colleague, Abbott's private reservations surfaced about the resulting interracial relationship that developed within the team: "I suppose I have given you to understand that David Johnson and Jane Wong are pretty thick. Now I am just being catty but I am glad I am me and not Dave and I don't think they are a very promising match."[59] He never elaborated.

The inability of MT6 to recruit, train, and retain local staff undermined its devolution plans. When the FAU reluctantly withdrew after the end of the Sino-Japanese War, Barbara Yang was left in charge to carry on alone. Only in 1989 would her FAU colleagues learn that she had married and fled to safety in Hong Kong.

Jane Wong remained until the FAU team reluctantly withdrew from Mohei in the fall of 1945. She left armed with a strong letter of recommendation from Robert McClure:

> I have personally known Miss Wong and have had her working with me. I have seen her under the most difficult circumstances and can say that she never lets those circumstances weigh her down ... She is very even tempered and very reliable. She is thoroughly well qualified and an extremely ethical nurse. She has considerable ability in teaching and training others under her. She leaves the F.A.U. only at her own request to visit her parents now that the war ended.[60]

She left intending to sort out her family affairs in Hong Kong and planning to rejoin the Unit, but her return was delayed. Writing back to her FAU family, she shared her shock at what awaited on her return home. "I never expected our family home to be so ruined. From the fourth floor to the bottom, not a single thing is left."[61] Despite McClure's strong endorsement, David Johnson's opinion was solicited when chairman Spencer Coxe invited her to return in 1947. His opinion had been sought because an influential Chinese nurse, Doris Wu, "was dead set against Jane taking her place" in Henan, on the grounds "that Jane is not a good nurse and a difficult person."[62] Johnson's response gives insight into her character and motivation for volunteering, and also speaks to the expectations that Chinese nurses would fit into the

China Convoy's community life and shared purpose. His assessment was qualified on several grounds:

> I would not by any means admit to being an authority on Jane and there is probably a good deal of bias in what I think about her but, in my opinion, she is a very good and capable nurse, hard working and conscientious, who would be excellent in a position where she has sufficient responsibility and hard work.

He was hesitant, however, to "call Jane a good Unit member." She was "not very interested in long discussions about Unit ideals and policy, and section meetings and things like that but she is keen to get on with the job of helping her fellow men and women." He supported Wong's return with a caveat: "I think that she should have reasonable certainty of a pretty solid job to get on with. She didn't have a very good experience with Medical Team 4 and I feel that she might be unsettled by much frustration."[63] A notation in pencil on Johnson's letter simply noted, "Not a pacifist."

Coxe wrote to Jane explaining why he had to take back his earlier invitation to return: "We are caught in a very serious financial crisis and may have to send home a large number of our members."[64] The story did not end there, however. In 1948, Coxe approached Jane as the "ideal person" to take on a very challenging task in the Zhongmou hospital in Henan. He warned her that she would be the only "qualified nurse in the hsein [local or district government] in all probability," and that the Communists were likely to liberate Zhongmou shortly.[65] Wong wisely remained at the Harcourt Infant Welfare Centre in Wanchai, Hong Kong.

In the meantime, in August 1944, Sheila Iu had set out on a seventy-day trek to Fuhai on the Burma border. A notice in the Unit newsletter read, "Team 6 has given birth to a healthy child, MT7, composed of Art Barr, Sheila Yu [*sic*] and John MacMahen that will work with the 93 Division Chinese army medical group that previously had no services."[66] The FAU originally planned to withdraw MT7 at the end of the year, but at the request of the Chinese army authorities it remained until the Chinese liaison group with which the team had worked was suddenly withdrawn from the division. By 15 March 1945, all of MT7 had returned to Kunming.

Fuhai's local conditions, while challenging, offered new horizons for humanitarian medical work beyond McClure's initial hope that the 93rd Division army surgeons "will be better surgeons than when we first took up the work."[67] Typically, McClure praised MT7 for its "perseverance against great odds" and for its "ability to co-operate so well and on such a large scale with every group in the area."[68] Art Barr described the "bad state"[69] of the health services that he and Sheila Iu confronted at the Wei Shen Tuei hospital in a temple several kilometres from Fuhai: "We understand it had a reputation of a morgue ... no temperatures were taken because there are no thermometers but the I-kauns [Chinese army interns] have them to use on their civilian patients." All of the patients "were covered in scabies and lice ridden. There were no mosquito nets and no receptacles for anything. Malaria, dysentery and tuberculosis cases were intermingled."[70]

Predisposed to be more open-minded, Barr found the army officials "very cooperative" because "they realize that disease is their most formidable enemy." Once the team convinced officials "of our sincerity ... all our ideas have received the justice of frank discussion."[71] They helped to choose the site and draw up the plans for the hospital, and secured the cooperation of the military, local people, and magistrate to complete construction in record time. MT7 focused on controlling malaria, dysentery, backwater fever, and other tropical diseases that were decimating the local population. In particular, an ambitious hookworm campaign was also undertaken. Iu's diets for malaria and hookworm patients, "second to none in the Unit," received special praise:

> There is no flour available in the area and the originality, which she has shown in the use of beans and rice flour in making special diets, is most commendable. Over 1600 bowls of rice bean milk are served to the patients each month, 350 bean residue biscuits made into a tasty formula and 530 bowls of blood or liver were produced to treat anaemic patients.[72]

Overworked, Sheila took "a much needed leave" after the team's withdrawal, during which she contracted malaria.[73]

Afterwards, Sheila Iu joined an FAU team sent to the Salachi Leper Home to give treatment and physical examinations to several hundred patients. When Art Barr was needed elsewhere, she helped the Canadian lab technician, Jack Dodds, carry on the work. His diary entries indicate that the two got on well together, and typically she oversaw the household duties at the end of the day, including the preparation of Chinese food the way she liked it.

When she resigned from the China Convoy in August 1945, a simple notice appeared in the weekly newsletter: "Sheila Yu [sic] has resigned from the Convoy with our thanks for her long and valuable work with us."[74] She was, however, one of two Chinese nurses singled out for praise by McClure for his biographer. Documents provide further evidence of her "long and valuable work." After her return from MT7, Iu's opinion was sought, and in some cases it overrode an earlier assessment of a prospective Chinese nurse "as being quite unsuitable."[75] Convoy leaders looked to Iu to help ease Chinese recruits into Convoy life, for at all costs they wanted to avoid negative publicity that might deter other Chinese nurses from joining.[76] Her capacity for hard work, her willingness to live the rugged life, and her nursing skills, combined with her knowledge of local conditions, customs, and language, enabled her over time to become a valuable cross-cultural broker in the Convoy's humanitarian negotiations. Consequently, she too left the Convoy with a strong recommendation for future employment in Country Hospital in Shanghai.[77]

Both Sheila Iu and Jane Wong had a privileged upbringing and education. Daughters of wealthy Hong Kong families, both had learned English while training as nurses in well-equipped Western-style hospitals. Already it meant that the nature of their relationships with the FAU differed from that of other Chinese women who acted as cooks or housekeepers. Their decision to forgo more lucrative employment opportunities suggests that nationalism and the notion of service figured in Iu's and Wong's decisions to nurse with the FAU. Equally important, after the fall of Hong Kong, their desire to find respectable employment in a familiar Western medical setting that allowed greater personal freedom made the FAU a more attractive option than the Chinese military. As Christians and purveyors of Western medical knowledge, both nurses were identified within Convoy ranks as progressive, modern Chinese women who could fit into community life, albeit within accepted racial and gendered boundaries. Although a shared pacifist identify was not officially required of Chinese nurses, its absence remained a criterion for assessing performance and suitability.

Despite their Western training, both nurses found themselves working beyond their normal level of practice and knowledge. The teams' personal dynamics, their diverse geographical settings, and the differing capacities of individual FAU members to understand the importance of supporting and involving local health teams and the community, rather than taking control, coloured Iu's and Wong's experiences in the China Convoy. But despite all the difficulties, they had remained and made valuable contributions to the Unit's work and Convoy life.

Other Chinese nurses assigned to FAU front-line teams during the Salween campaign would prove equally capable humanitarian diplomats and advocates for their own personal and professional destinies.

3 The Salween Campaign
Humanitarian Diplomacy, 1944–45

[MT3] has been a particularly happy piece of work from the Unit point of view. English, American and Chinese have worked well together; many friendships have formed.

– *FRIENDS AMBULANCE UNIT CHRONICLE*

As 1944 dawned, the China Convoy had survived its third year of humanitarian work. The death of two members from typhus and the frequent illness of many others weighed heavily on the Convoy members. Despite the difficulties due to aging trucks, the unpredictability of the military situation, and runaway inflation, the Convoy's medical and transport work endured. However, many of the men still fretted that the very nature of their humanitarian work compromised their pacifist views on the world at war. They experienced first-hand the fact that modern mobile warfare made it impossible to distinguish between civilian and military needs for medical care. The struggle to reconcile individuals' Christian pacifist witness with the practical demands of the job festered, and the Friends Ambulance Unit's purpose of relieving wartime suffering continued to be debated in its weekly newsletter. Many FAU men volunteered in order to transform the image of conscientious objectors as cowards by sharing the dangerous life of the soldier without taking part in the fighting, but instead they found themselves in quiet backwaters doing more civilian work than treating wounded soldiers. But life on the front and within the China Convoy was about to change dramatically.

This year was the turning point for the Allied campaign in southwestern China. In January, Allied forces, including US-trained and US-equipped Chinese divisions in Burma, designated as X-Force, began to attack from India across northern Burma. Meanwhile, in early May, the Chinese 20th Army Group in Yunnan, designated as Y-Force, crossed the Salween River on a broad front about 160 kilometres east of Myitkyina with the objective of connecting the Burma Road with the Stilwell Road being built eastward behind the Allied offensive from Ledo. In late January 1945, X-Force and Y-Force linked up, opening up the Burma Road for truck convoys to Kunming in March.[1] The military plan was straightforward, but the terrain over which it would be executed was one of the most elevated and most rugged battle-grounds in the world.

Since the increased activity on the Yunnan front far outstripped the Unit's capacity to provide additional medical assistance, the debate over admitting European nurses took on greater urgency. McClure's plea for "girl nurses on our teams" emphasized the "great sacrifice" that the current Chinese nurses made in joining the China section, and consequently the difficulty of recruit-ing more. McClure again told London that civilian employment opportunities were more lucrative and promised more rapid professional advancement.[2] For some, British nurses were preferable to recruiting more Chinese women. While McClure unequivocally welcomed well-qualified Chinese nurses as full members of the Convoy, others expressed concerns, especially about the inevitable interracial marriages that would result. Leonard Tomkinson, a former missionary and then the China Convoy's chairman at the time,[3] claimed that he did "not take either of the extreme views." He claimed to differ with both Friends "who tend to greet all such announcements with a romantic enthusiasm" as a step "necessary for promoting internationalism" and those who alleged that interracial marriages inevitably "must have unhappy results." But he believed that these marriages would be unfair to the children involved and had little chance of survival beyond China. "A good deal of loneliness," he argued, rendered the men "unnaturally susceptible to the attractions of anyone who may seem to offer the possibility of mitigating this loneliness." This meant that "marrying in haste and repenting in leisure are greater than usual. That is why we should encourage them to go slow in all cases."[4] Tomkinson ignored the possibility that Chinese women separated from family and friends were equally vulnerable, or that non-interracial marriages forged in wartime could be equally susceptible to failure.

Notwithstanding McClure's gloomy predictions, in the first week of March 1944, Doris Wu (Shih Tsent) and Margaret So (Tsai Hsai), former staff nurses at the Queen Mary Hospital in Hong Kong, joined the Unit. Despite not having completed her training, Margaret So had been accepted on the recommendation of Jane Wong, who described her as "a quiet hard working girl."[5] Their front-line stories, spotlighting how gender, class, race, nation, and place imbricated their cross-cultural personal and professional relationships, capture the diversity of Chinese nurses' experience at a crossroads in the Sino-Japanese War and the FAU's humanitarian work.

Multiple factors figured in the decision of both nurses to volunteer with the FAU. Internally displaced by war, Wu and So looked to humanitarian nursing to re-establish a sense of home and belonging while performing meaningful wartime work that would open future career opportunities. A strong advocate of the New Life Movement's (NLM) approach to modernizing China, Wu was described by colleagues as a spirited and energetic modern Cantonese woman. Chiang Kai-shek's party used the NLM as a tool for national reconstruction and social mobilization through reforms in hygienic and behavioural practices. Elements of anti-communism, Christianity, and state Confucianism coexisted uneasily with the idea of hygienic modernity. NLM was also a key tool for Chiang's forces in preparation for war on two fronts.[6] Like other young Chinese women, Wu embodied the gender contradictions of the archetypical NLM women. She embraced her role in modernizing and revitalizing her nation but did not accept the Confucian view of women's cloistered role of uncomplaining obedience. After graduating from St. Mary's Nursing School in Shanghai, she had joined the New Life Movement and served with the Chinese Expeditionary Force in Burma in 1940. Since Wu and So left better-paying positions with the Chinese Air Force hospital in Kunming to join the Convoy, Unit leaders welcomed them as ideal candidates motivated by the spirit of service.[7] The Convoy offered other benefits over military service. Significantly, the two nurses negotiated their terms of employment: "Unfortunately these two girls insist on working together so we shall have to treat them as a sort of dual personality."[8] So had joined on the understanding that, after six months of service, the FAU would arrange for her to complete her nursing training. In contrast, military service required a longer training period. After completing field service, nurses were required to spend an additional year in the Army Nursing School, followed by several more months in a regular nursing school to cover public health and maternal and child care.[9] In practice, it would be some time before they were assigned to the same team.

Nursing on the Salween front was hard and often shocking. Here as elsewhere, physician/nurse relationships proved crucial in establishing Chinese nurses' difficult and unfamiliar role as cultural interlocutors. FAU physicians' cultural sensitivity and field experience set the tone for the team's relationships with Chinese army colleagues and the local community. All had clear expectations for Chinese nurses' professional and personal behaviour in the field. Their presence signalled better care and patient outcomes. Their commitment to care was expected to override personal interests or comfort. As we have already seen, failure to live up to these expectations might jeopardize their future careers.

Doris Wu accompanied John Perry to help sort out MT4 when a despondent Ernest Evans resigned. MT4 was the first field assignment for both, and was akin to baptism under fire for both as well. During orientation in Qujing, Robert McClure emphasized to Perry: "Our special contribution, as foreign doctors, consists in teaching surgical judgment and technique and the general concept of contamination and asepsis to the 'army surgeons' tactfully and as co-workers, of course."[10] In Perry's view, neither former MT4 physician "had the patience" to act as a model for coaching the poorly trained local talent but "merely banged around on their own, doing all the work themselves and doing too much fault-finding in everyone else's work." As Perry discovered the difficulties of "being a model" FAU team that worked "tactfully and collaboratively," he felt fortunate to have three Hong Kong nurses on his team, all "vivacious girls" and "well trained."[11]

Doris Wu joined Sheila Iu and Jane Wong, but it would be primarily Wu with whom Perry would work initially. On his arrival, Perry received new orders from the local Chinese military commander to set up a small team to handle an outbreak of relapsing fever in a nearby village. Wu accompanied Perry, who was quickly at loggerheads with the Chinese military, local medical staff, and traditional healers before the situation was sorted out. After assessing the situation, he concluded that it was merely a ruse to get MT4 to relocate there permanently. When the Chinese military officials insisted that the team return, more experienced team members, such as Sid Walker, Dr. Terry Darling, and Sheila Iu, also came back to the village to negotiate with local authorities "proper arrangements and agreements as they should be for a decent set-up for work" until the supposed "overwhelming epidemic" ran its course.[12]

Initially frustrated by patients who ignored orders or returned untreated to their quarters to spread the disease, and by his inability to establish orderly hospital routines, Perry was greatly helped by Wu's presence to acknowledge his own humanitarian limitations. He gradually accepted "that you should try to do only what you can, there is a definite limit to this; and that to waste your nerves and break your heart trying for more is only your own damn fault when you feel overcome with frustration and impatience."[13] But his professional relationships with Chinese colleagues continued to be coloured by his Western biomedical perspective of the traditional Chinese medical system as unorthodox and more culture-specific. When the head "Y-kuan [*sic*], ... a kind of cross between Boris Karloff and Thomas à Becket," claimed to have a cure for typhus composed of ten herb powders, Perry belittled the traditional folk remedies passed down in his family for generations: "Poor man: if he only realized this would make him world-famous overnight if it worked." Perry was quick to quash the idea that the local healer had cured his typhus patients with his potion: "I wouldn't let him get away with anything: I explained their fevers were already down."[14] His need to establish his own authority and the superiority of Western medicine was striking.

Given Perry's determination to "have the best dawgone hospital this valley ever saw," and that Doris Wu "has already got started on it, working like a Trojan,"[15] the news that she had been transferred to MT3 came as a devastating blow. The frequent mention of Wu in his letters home attests to both his respect for and dependency on her. Confident in her nursing skills and knowledge, Wu had considerable latitude in prioritizing her nursing activities. Perry observed that she concentrated on bringing order out of the chaos in one ward and launching a program for special diets – despite his preference for making changes in all the wards at once. Doris, he told his wife, had always been at his side in clinic as they attempted "to wrest ... some semblance of a history" from "the befuddled tribesman all foggy with fever and head."[16] Although Wu experienced difficulties with the local dialect, without her the patients' answers had to be pantomimed and dramatized by the Chinese army orderlies.[17] But it would appear that Perry was not the only one who would miss the "buoyant modern northern Chinese [girl]" when she left on 2 February 1944. Her Chinese-American colleague Wes Chin "was in kind of a dither."[18] After succumbing to typhus, Perry was sent back to Kunming in early March to convalesce before being reassigned.

Doris and Margaret were reunited on MT3. Originally set up in an intermediate hospital at Hsiakwan, a former FAU depot on the Burma Road, MT3 worked side by side with the Chinese Red Cross and the New Life Movement teams. Despite their youth and lack of surgical experience, Drs. Arthur Barr, a devout Anglican, and Allen Longshore, raised and educated in the Quaker faith, set a different tone for MT3's professional conduct. As Barr observed, "we could work our fingers to the bone in an individualistic manner and accomplish only immediate good, whereas working in a cooperative manner had a much more far reaching effect. We were to work with the Chinese and not for the Chinese. We were not to order, but to advise."[19]

Although the five-hundred-bed hospital was housed in a school, the wards and diet kitchens were in the nearby village two kilometres away. The already enormous challenge of supervising medical attention over such a scattered hospital complex was further complicated "as the patients often brought their relatives with them."[20] Prior to Wu and So's arrival, MT3 praised the three "New Life Girls" who took care of the special diets and laundry at the hospital.[21] As the team reported, "we have been treating patients in the last throes of chronic illness when all the attention in the world is of little avail," and it was only after the arrival of the New Life Movement nurses "brought about a scientific approach to the problem of diet" that the outcomes of critical patients improved.[22] Welcoming the new arrivals as "quite pleasant" and "good workers,"[23] MT3 physicians thought that "they certainly fill a definite niche in the unit, [but] where we will put them is another problem."[24] As Barr subsequently reported, MT3 was "forging ahead," as Wu and So not only improved wards and theatre routines but also did "other jobs that thrive under a woman's touch."[25] A nurse's worthiness was equated with helpfulness to the doctor within carefully prescribed gendered norms.

MT3 faced a deluge of surgical work under such demanding conditions that five members contracted typhus. Although all eventually recovered, when Art Barr had to be sent back to Kunming to recuperate, British physician John Wilks replaced him. In the interim, the team had negotiated moving to Yung Ping, further down the road near the Mekong Gorge, closer to the front. Dr. Quentin Boyd and Chinese nurse Arthur Yau formed a spearhead team with an advance regiment that had no medical services at all. The rest were not far behind.

Early field reports indicated that Wu and So coped well with monsoon conditions and the steady stream of wounded that poured in day and night. A July 1944 *Unit Letter* extolled their skill and courage and makes it apparent why another FAU team attempted unsuccessfully to raid MT3 nursing staff to improve its own nursing standards and relationships with the wider Chinese community: "There is a rumour that the two girls may have to be withdrawn as the area is said to be unsafe for women; as they are both doing a wonderful job and putting up with the discomforts with complete cheerfulness, it most likely that the order will be forgotten."[26] The prediction proved correct.

Wu and So rejected the American military commander's caution "that they may not be able to stand all the hardships" and "not to take the risks ... You see, not even our foreign girls have yet crossed the Salween River."

Both nurses found his arguments "simply ridiculous." Viewing themselves as "modern Chinese women," with "more courage and endurance than other nations' women," they were determined "[to rebuild] our nation with our men together whatever the risk." It is noteworthy that the article carefully pointed out that neither "clamoured for equality with men and yet, in every respect, they are not inferior."[27] The implicit message was that women could be patriotic within prescribed gendered norms of women's role in war. They were playing the traditionally accepted role of nursing the wounded in wartime.

Despite the danger, Robert McClure never considered withdrawing nurses from forward positions. As he explained, "if the girls are properly chosen," they worked well, even though the "life is rugged and considerable physical endurance is required not only in spirit but for sustained effort under difficult conditions." "The girls," he warned, must be "sensible and willing to put their hormones on ice during the duration of their stay at the front."[28] As events would indicate, that seldom happened. The men, however, never appeared to be given the same advice. On many occasions when "some trouble with hormones" erupted, the Canadian medical missionary would be cast in the role of "father confessor."[29] Given her military experience in Burma, Doris Wu had a more realistic understanding of the gruelling journey ahead, but even she could not have predicted that an enduring love could be forged amid such human carnage. Doris would marry John Wilks.[30]

When Y-Force crossed the Salween front near Myitkyina, MT3 moved to Yung Ping to handle major military casualties. But the Japanese counterattacked the Chinese river crossings, making effective use of the mountainous terrain and monsoon season, and halted Chinese advances in June. MT3 witnessed first-hand the dogged determination of the Japanese troops in what culminated in a bloody but decisive land campaign for the Chinese forces. The team took to the rugged hills with the armies in May 1944 and reached Tengyue in August only hours after the Japanese had evacuated.

After crossing the Salween River, Doris Wu and Margaret So climbed hundreds of *li* (half a kilometre) over the Kolikun Shan and finally arrived at a forward dressing station ten *li* from Tengyue. By then they had "laboriously dressed over two thousand wounded soldiers under heavy gunfire."[31] A teammate's vivid, poignant, and often shocking account of the daunting trek to Tengchong explains why Wu and So earned "a reputation for the Unit over the whole of this front":

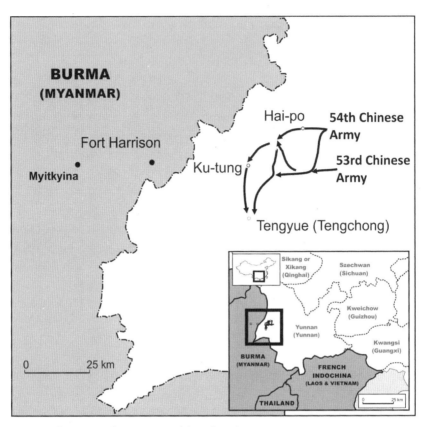

Map 5   The MT3 trek to Tengyue (Tengchong)

The road was ... so steep and muddy it was almost impossible to keep one's [footing]. As we came over the mountain ridges we heard the rattle of machine-guns, the explosion of shells and the "plump" of mortar fire ... Stretcher-bearers with camouflaged hats were waiting by the hundreds; gun crews half naked were reaming off round after round ... and I found the girls and John [Wilks] surrounded by stretchers of wounded men. They were the only qualified group ready to deal with the situation. The girls worked wonders. They fixed each case calmly and systematically as it was brought up. Every man was given hot water to drink and had his blankets tucked in around him, fractures cleaned up and splinted and loose flesh cleaned away. All seemed to be done in such a matter of fact way, it was like London all over again. There was no initial muffing that one finds under conditions such as these.[32]

Other unforeseen dangers and lurid images of battle lay ahead. On 22 May, MT3 relocated to a small mountain village recently evacuated by the Japanese and began a gruelling trek:

> The path up the mountain was a torrent of water; grass up to our waist brushed against our clothing making it sopping wet. As we climbed it became cooler. Towards afternoon, we were shivering, covered with mud and soaked with rain. The girls could still laugh and joke – they were more far more cheerful than the rest of us ... [The city had] only two houses standing ... our room had two holes in either wall that a steam roller could pass through. Judging from the smell of the floor this place must have been a morgue ... spent the evening trying to dry ourselves and bedding around the fire.
>
> Girls were plagued by fleas – hardly slept all. Ordered to move at 7:30. Breakfast of salt and rice and we started off in the pouring rain ... We could not see more than ten yards in any direction and everything took on an eerie appearance.[33]

On 23 May, Pip Rivett's journal captured the emotional fortitude required to cope with the unremitting violence and cruelty:

> Sometimes we could smell a corpse ... [We] saw a Japanese corpse hanging from the tree where he had strapped himself ... We climbed for about two hours when we came to a horse station left by the Japanese a few hours before. The stench of rotting flesh hung everywhere ... Horses had been slaughtered ... almost three hundred had been slashed by the Japanese and left to bleed to death. Here and there, a hand showed from a fox-hole; shoulders and heads stuck out from the mounds of earth.[34]

At times the harsh conditions en route to Tengyue turned unexpectedly life-threatening:

> The rain increased: we scrambled on, up and up. Towards mid-afternoon we reached our new location – a place without buildings exposed on a mountain range. A bitter wind was blowing and the rain stung. We were all wearing light clothing – it was all we could carry, and so we waited around shivering. We pushed our way into a fox-hole ... we crammed around the fire and no one spoke ... We waited in this small cave for about an hour when, without any warning, the hillside collapsed almost burying Doris and Margaret.[35]

The same teammate acknowledged that "generally speaking the girls have worked harder ... [and] can stand heavy marches, poor diet, long hours and difficult working conditions better than the average convoy member." Yet he continued to believe that "nurses in forward positions are a good improvement provided that they are not too attractive and relatively unemotional."[36] Despite Wu's and So's demonstration of skilled nursing, courage, and resilience, the gendered stereotype of women as a distraction in combat zones persisted.

The pressure intensified and conditions showed little improvement by early June. Wilks, Wu, and So "experienced even worse conditions on the top most peak of the range; they were busier than we, though their diet was almost as bad."[37] When Tengyue finally fell at the end of August 1944, with hardly a Japanese left alive, MT3 was among the first to enter the scene of utter devastation. In November, John Wilks described Wu's and So's contribution to the "unending struggle" to establish in-patient treatment for sick soldiers in a disused temple: "By unremitting pushing and cursing, we had at the end of eight days a few bamboo frames made for beds, some straw and an apology for a latrine." Wilks complained that "the [Chinese army] nurses knew nothing and had to be taught by Doris and Margaret how to do dressings and take temperatures and at first all of their work had to be supervised." After Margaret resigned, "all the work fell on Doris and she made a very good job of it. We spent a lot of money on special diets, which was greatly appreciated by the patients and did them a lot of good; this again was Doris's work."[38]

The simple announcement in the *Unit Letter* that Margaret So had been released from the Unit in December 1944 to complete her nursing studies at the Canadian Mission Hospital in Chongqing did not tell the entire sordid story. McClure's belligerent handling of her request to leave left her feeling bitter. She "never expected her relationship with Unit would end with a rupture." So had agreed to serve for six months on the explicit understanding that she would then be released to complete her nursing studies. When pressed, she agreed to extend her contract until a replacement could be found. Once the team "went into the wild country beyond the Salween," no one was willing to make the long trek through the jungle to join the team. When So broached the subject of leaving, McClure at once "adopted a high handed manner. He said that in view of the existing personnel situation, he is not prepared to consider giving leave for anyone and that the only way for anyone to leave is resignation. He added, however, that resignation in the midst of the campaign would spell ruin to my future." So stood her ground.

As she explained to Chairman Duncan Wood, she was "always willing to serve [the] general interest, even if necessary at my own expense, it is my opinion that nothing could be more humiliating than my submission to such a threat. Consequently, I decided to resign." Wood most likely agreed with So's assessment "that the situation would have been entirely different if it had been handled by another person."[39] In closing his letter of apology, Wood hoped that anything McClure said at Tengyue did not create the impression "that we do not appreciate the excellent job that you have been doing with the Unit."[40] He ensured that Margaret So left with a strong letter of recommendation[41] and had secured a place in a mission nursing school. She later married fellow MT3 nurse Arthur Yau.

The remainder of MT3 was left to deal with the outbreak of plague south of Tengyue. With the withdrawal of most of the team for leave or permanently, the FAU anticipated winding up MT3 but was forced to change its plans. Given the insistence of the Chinese divisional commander, "short of an open rupture of relations," a small team had to be left in place.[42] In March 1945, MT3 ceased operations after the military division with which it was working was suddenly reassigned, and the team "was notified that its services with the division would no longer be required."[43]

After her leave, Doris Wu was eventually reunited with John Wilks in MT5 at Baoshan in the spring of 1945. Housed in tents that became ovenlike when the sun came up, the team got a "bit restless" after four months of expecting to move any day.[44] After Doris took over the ward from a departing British Red Cross nurse seconded to the team, her dedication and skill again drew praise for improving nursing standards and patient care: "Doris presides over the FAU ward and it is spotless. It is amazing what can be done with bamboo walls and a mud floor."[45] With "her customary drive," she began "[to train] the orderlies to [do] more of the actual work."[46] Chinese nurses were appraised against Western medical standards stressing cleanliness and serenity in the wards.

Sometimes as staff assignments were juggled and two pieces looked as though they should fit, they didn't. Robert McClure claimed that Doris Wu and Sheila Iu could not be assigned to the same team because they "will not work at all happily together."[47] Without specifying any specific reason, Wu had made it clear that while she wanted to continue working with the Convoy, "she would prefer not to be on the same team as Sheila Iu."[48] Towards the end of June, Wu was sent with the advance team to launch the new Nantan hospital in cooperation with the United Nations Relief and Rehabilitation

Administration (UNRRA), the newly minted but untried relief organization. MT12 was composed of two physicians, John Perry and Philip Hsiung, laboratory technician Jack Dodds, and two nurses, Doris Wu and, later, Juliet Chiu (Ting-hsin), one of six university students who had recently joined the FAU "as an alternative to getting into all sorts of peculiar army jobs for national service."[49]

Excited by the prospect of launching the "first medical UNRRA project actually to set up in China,"[50] Perry and MT12 met unexpected setbacks in their plans to quickly construct and devolve a community hospital. New players with different agendas had arrived on the scene. The team arrived in Nantan to discover that it had to share accommodations with an UNRRA medical team "in one of the town's few intact buildings, a dingy hole of a place, with mud floors." Perry found the living arrangements unacceptable on other grounds: "They were quite cordial in their invitation for us to take the remaining upstairs room; their doctors and nurses were living in alternative beds in the next room, and they seemed to have forgotten that there were other ways of going about these things." Instead of "letting the bars down and lifting our heels against those protective conventions of ours," Perry gave Doris the room and the two men took "the mud hole"[51] below.

Other aspects of the team's relationship with UNRRA were far more unsettling. Dodds wrote a scathing review of UNRRA's reconstruction efforts throughout this reoccupied area of China: "The same thing is happening here as has happened in so many countries that UNRRA has moved into. This whole policy is so tied up with investigation, red tape and presenting budgets that by the time they are ready to start, the greatest need is past and inflation has thrown the budget all to hell."[52] MT12 quickly discovered that the town already had four Chinese doctors sent to it and that all buildings suitable for a hospital were occupied by the Americans or the Chinese army. Through skillful negotiations, along with a modicum of luck, the Americans relinquished the building that used to be the county hospital.[53] Undaunted by the repair and improvements required before opening, Perry forged ahead and engaged the local community with his ambitious plans for hospital construction:

Then we got after the railway people, to make a bargain with them about coming in on the plan with us, and making a third of the project their own ... And Bob [McClure] came in just then, and with his barrage of speech sold them on the idea with no trouble at all. So we upped the budget again to make use of these extra funds.

Ironically, the Chinese National Relief and Rehabilitation Administration (CNRRA, the Nationalist Chinese distribution wing of UNRRA) increased the budget: "they'd put the budget very high for the Chinese run hospital and didn't want to create the impression that foreigners can get by on a smaller budgets because they don't expect squeeze [pay-offs]."[54] Diplomacy, bluff, and preserving face converged to swell the hospital's construction budget. Its devolution would be no different, except this time Wu and Chinese physician Philip Hsiung would be tasked with handling the prickly situation when Perry washed his hands of the situation to deal with another crisis.

The end of the war in August 1945 changed FAU priorities in Nantan. McClure was eager to reallocate the team to other projects that offered more exciting and urgent opportunities for medical work. But just as MT12 prepared to devolve, "the bottom seemed to fall out of everything at once." The Chinese National Health Administration (NHA) team that was to take over the hospital "was suddenly ordered out, leaving us stranded holding the baby." The NHA team was sent to where the FAU planned to set up next, perhaps out of rivalry or "the need to show up at the front and all."[55] UNRRA, CNRRA, and the NHA could not agree on the Nantan hospital's future, "so that the FAU has really got itself saddled with the thing until they can make up their minds, and that involves much political diddling."[56] In an even more bizarre turn of events, a local health team arrived and announced it was to take over. When Perry discovered that there were no nurses among them and that the young Chinese doctor had graduated but never practised, he was prepared to "[throw] the meat to the dogs again, and decided to get out." When the rest of the team moved on to Liuzhou to battle the cholera epidemic, Doris Wu and Philip Hsiung were left "to battle it out for a few weeks. "It takes a Chinese to find his way around the complications of a mix-up like this, and to unravel it without offending people."[57] Eventually a provincial health team appeared without warning and simply took over. "The problem of devolution was solved but the mystery of the hidden wheels was beyond the [team's understanding]."[58] Wu remained on duty until the team withdrew during the first week of September, and arrived back in Chongqing "all set for [her] next expedition to Honan."[59]

Jack Dodds's and John Perry's descriptions of the team's handling of cholera, smallpox, relapsing fever, and accident cases prior to the Nantan hospital's official opening suggest that they viewed and treated Doris Wu as they would any member of the team, as part of the "we," not the "other."[60] Recounting the flurry surrounding the "first bit of surgery," an accident victim "with a badly mashed lower leg, already half a day old, needing amputation pretty quickly," Perry wrote: "We pulled the stuff out of the boxes, and set up on boards on trestles for a table and packed up my bed out of the room ... and pretty soon Doris had the place set up quite like the most orthodox of ORs."[61] Dodds had wakened Wu to prepare the morphine shots and stabilize the patient before transporting him, and her postoperative nursing care was credited with ensuring that there were no complications.

While the records corroborate the competence, courage, composure, and diplomatic acumen of the Chinese nurses, Doris Wu was particularly remembered as "a powerful advocate" in negotiations with Chinese army officials in Baoshan and on the march to Tengyue.[62] Her reputation most likely accounted for her inclusion in the advance team to get the Nantan hospital project rolling. Nor was this the only example of Nurse Wu's agency. In January 1945, the Unit leaders acknowledged her fundraising efforts on what was supposed to be her leave: "The biggest news of the week is the result of Doris Wu's time in Chungking [Chongqing]: a grant from the Friends of the Wounded Soldiers to the Unit teams of NG140,000 per month for special diets, over a period of a year."[63]

According to Bob McClure, the Convoy developed the "highest respect" for Doris Wu and John Wilks. The 25 June *Newsletter* announcing the couple's engagement heralded it "as an entirely new category of GOOD THINGS ... HURRAY!"[64] Wu and Wilks married in Henan on 30 November 1946 in a ceremony that, as was common in the FAU, was immortalized in song, skit, and poetry, even if not everyone in the organization was equally enthusiastic about other interracial unions.

Wu continued to be a key player when the Unit shifted to Henan. Their arrival in December 1945 coincided with what McClure characterized as a period of gross "bureaucratic incompetency," with the result that the FAU base hospital had no power plant, no sewing machine, no blankets, and no winter clothing for his staff. According to his biographer, with the couple's arrival, McClure "began to relax."[65] Once again, she deftly negotiated additional supplies from the military for the FAU during a cholera outbreak. An active recruiting agent was dispatched to Chinese universities, and Wu was also credited with easing both Western and Chinese members' transition to Convoy life. The negative side was that many of the best Chinese nurses were reluctant to remain once the couple moved on to other FAU projects as mission hospitals were devolved. Doris and John Wilks returned to England in January 1948; Doris was simply not comfortable working at the FAU's only remaining Henan hospital at Zhongmou once it was "liberated" by the Communists.

While McClure respected and valued the skills, service, and sacrifice of the Chinese nurses in the FAU, he could be a tough taskmaster. He knew the kind of Chinese nurses that he wanted as colleagues on the front lines. One of a series of articles about the heroic Chinese published for the United Church, "Tales from China," is a telling example of the idealized standards he expected Chinese nurses to meet during war. McClure, a master of weaving compelling stories to draw the public's financial support, recounted how he had mistakenly stereotyped Miss Li, a Chinese nurse, "sitting back in a safe city" at a "cushy job" looking after a drug warehouse. When he commented to a Chinese colleague, "That girl illustrated why the Chinese were going to lose the war," he was quickly reprimanded and informed that the nurse had been gravely wounded. Skeptical, he challenged the young nurse to tell him her story. She simply turned around and showed him "a hole in her left chest large enough for me to put a fist in. It was still discharging."[66] Three months later, she tracked McClure to a hospital where he lay recuperating from an accident and demanded, "Sign this slip because I am going on your truck to the front tomorrow." She waved off his protests that she was not fit to go to the front, saying, "Fit or not fit, Doc, they are having a hot time at the front and they expect an awful lot of us Christians." McClure told his audience that they would never have this girl as a colleague: "Two weeks later they got her by a direct hit." However, there were "thousands like her in China who have come through the heat of a modern war, who have been tempered by having passed through the fire and are available to work with us as colleagues in building a new world."[67] Nurse Li epitomized the good nurse, an angel of mercy who sacrificed personal interests to care. His intimidation of Sheila Iu and Margaret So, threatening to effectively blacklist them from future employment, indicate that McClure had little patience for "bad" nurses who did not live up to the sense of Christian service and professional ethics demonstrated by Nurse Li.

Convoy life produced new boundaries and expanded frontiers for these Chinese nurses. Serving with the FAU gave them greater autonomy to acquire skills and implement them far beyond regular hospital nursing practice. Patient outcomes, it was widely acknowledged, improved with the presence of trained, knowledgeable Chinese nurses. Their skilled nursing care and preparation of specialized diets reflected their Western training and scientific knowledge but adapted to local conditions, customs, and resources. Chinese nurses proved to be dedicated, courageous, and capable soldiers of peace in dire circumstances on the battlefield and beyond. After work in Henan, they joined the teams removing landmines near the hospital compound. Chinese FAU nurses' front-line experiences suggest that gender operated in such a way that women's wartime experiences continued to be simultaneously liberating and constraining. On the front lines, they embodied normalcy, using their "feminine touch" not only to provide solace to the patients but also to arrange the team's recreational activities. But for nurses such as Wu and So, wartime service challenged proscriptions around femininity. Chinese nurses' presence on front-line mobile medical teams or as single women assigned to remote locations contravened stereotypes about women's suitability for dangerous assignments or their capacity to function without a strong support network. It had become clear that without their presence the physicians' medical outcomes would have been compromised.

Reflecting on the FAU wartime experience, McClure admitted that the China Convoy "had a long process of 'bedding in,'"[68] but its members "learned how to live more or less 'off the country' and, most importantly, to work *with the Chinese* not merely *for* the Chinese."[69] All ranks conceded that Chinese members played a pivotal role in their acclimatization, recalling fondly "our nurse-maids who helped us through all the trying, pettifogging problems that you encounter when you are working with a people whose history and background are so different from ours. They taught us the 'Chinese art of making do'; helped us accept that the Western standards could not be achieved and the limitations of our personal humanitarian capacity."[70] Others acknowledged that "without them our work would have had little significance, for the success of the convoy is not only judged by the material help by which we gave ... but [also] by the way in which we have succeeded in co-operating with the Chinese people and Chinese organizations."[71] In retrospect, other Convoy members were reluctant "to say that we have solved all the problems inherent in admitting Chinese into membership of the Convoy ... We have given them the hard end of the bargain and have not always been sensitive to their needs and views. But at least it can be said that they have taught us that international brotherhood is a two-way business, and that we have made some good friends among them."[72] As we have seen, the FAU record of cooperation with the Chinese was mixed. While their ability to act as cross-cultural bridges matured with experience and confidence gained in the field, a few Chinese nurses could never mitigate the prejudice of some FAU physicians or override the priorities of Chinese military authorities.

Skilled nurses such as Doris Wu, Margaret So, Sheila Iu, and Jane Wong, who understood and were respected by both cultures, exercised considerable agency within the gendered, racial, and political limits of a society being radically transformed, caught in the grip of global war. As skilled cross-cultural brokers, each balanced "bridging social capital," which is outward-looking, with "bonding social capital," which fosters a "shared organizational and professional identity." Both are crucial for humanitarian agencies seeking to foster enduring and effective cross-cultural ties.[73] Being graduates of recognized Western-based nursing schools who could speak both English and Chinese enabled them to develop and nurture such ties despite the limitations of China's diverse dialects. Their careful selection as respectable, young, highly trained professional Christian women who shared a commitment to relieve China's wartime suffering enhanced their acceptance within the Convoy.

For Chinese nurses, the Convoy presented expanded opportunities and at the same time significant cross-cultural challenges. For some, such as Sheila Iu, working within a Western medical relief agency entailed the unexpected personal costs of being ridiculed and belittled by their own compatriots. The teams' diverse geographical settings and the varying abilities of FAU physicians to understand the importance of supporting and involving local health teams and the community rather than taking control coloured Chinese nurses' experiences in the Convoy and with their compatriots. While FAU community life and relationships were based on the Quaker principles of equality that celebrated difference, as well as congruence in one's outer and inner spiritual lives, as we saw earlier, neither Henry Louderbough nor Ernest Evans practised these ideals in his intercultural relationships. The Unit's treatment of Sheila Iu and Margaret So and the leadership's assessment of Jane Wong were not always aligned with its foundational values. Others who developed cordial working relationships sometimes failed to consider other hardships, level of education, understanding of Western medicine, or different attitudes towards pacifism that coloured Chinese views of the Unit's humanitarian endeavours. Still others, such as Bill Rahill, who understood the need for cooperation rather than domination in working with their Chinese nursing counterparts, left China profoundly changed. They developed a new appreciation for the resilience of the Chinese people. Chinese nurses had proven to be valuable cultural bridges who fostered morale within their teams and cooperation with the surrounding community; they could mitigate the cultural and racial divides but could not eliminate them.

Capturing the Chinese FAU nurses' stories complicates the historical narrative of the FAU's cross-cultural humanitarian exchanges prior to August 1945. Unpacking their stories reaffirms that postcolonial frames do not always fit the study of Western-based humanitarian initiatives that implicitly regard the beneficiaries as passive entities. In fact, working with the FAU enabled the Chinese nurses to advance personally and professionally. They exercised considerable agency as they charted new beginnings, personally and professionally, in Free China. They negotiated the terms and duration of employment and the risks they were willing to assume, even though they were sometimes constrained by the gendered realities of war or their need to find respectable work that might lead to better prospects. By depicting China's nurses as victims or ignoring their agency in nation building or their contribution to Western humanitarian work, Western scholars run the risk of recolonizing them.

Unfortunately the details of the Chinese members' contribution and the challenges they encountered remained blurred by time and the lack of Chinese voices in the official records. There were, for example, no laudatory articles in the Convoy newsletters covering Arthur Yau's gruelling work on MT3. The few letters that do survive speak to the contribution and the determination of women like Margaret So to use employment with the FAU as a bridge to a better future.

For Chinese women who served with the FAU in other capacities, volunteering opened the door to other educational opportunities. Nellie Wee, the daughter of a self-made wealthy banker in Penang, was forced to abandon her studies at the University of Hong Kong in 1941. She escaped to China on a truck, selling most of her possessions to fund completion of her undergraduate degree at a Chinese refugee university, Tahsis, in Guiyang. Wee joined the FAU in July 1944 as Brandon Cadbury's secretary somewhat by accident. As she recalled, the FAU hosted teas on Saturdays for anyone who could speak English. Being hungry and speaking English, she turned up regularly until she was hired.[74] In February 1945, she left with a strong character reference and financial backing to study in England. As Colin Bell explained in his recommendation, "community living especially in the abnormal conditions of wartime China tends to reveal the strength and weakness of its component parts in no uncertain fashion. Nellie is one of our assets here. She is adaptable, hard working, good tempered – altogether a well balanced person."[75] Even when funding had been arranged through the Colonial Office on the understanding that she would return as an educator to her homeland of Malaya, a persistent cough threatened to derail her plans. Despite Robert McClure's caution against going to England on health grounds, a determined Nellie arranged her exit permit and completed her university applications. However, she never returned home after completing her studies in English literature at Bedford College; instead, she worked at the BBC in London and embarked on a very happy marriage with fellow Convoy member Len Bonsall.

Other Chinese Convoy members encountered more difficulty in making their case for financial support to study in England. Teresa Hsu Chih served with the Convoy as a bookkeeper for four years. According to her celebratory autobiography, she came from an impoverished background but, by combining domestic work and night school, she acquired basic secretarial and bookkeeping skills that opened the door to employment with the FAU.[76] After her FAU fiancé, Brian Sorensen, died in a plane crash en route back to England, Teresa wrote Colin Bell requesting assistance to study nursing in England. Before making any commitment, Bell had "a long talk" with her "to test the sincerity of purpose in connection with her nursing career." He stressed that it would "be an extremely hard thing to start as a Probationer at the age of 33," and that for "a person of her temperament" both "the rigid systems and somewhat archaic traditions associated with 'Nursing Standards' would prove irksome." He also warned that she might feel "victimized on a racial basis" by some of the "hard boiled nursing sisters." His efforts to dissuade her or to have her consider hospital administration as an alternative proved futile. She "stuck to her point that she wanted to do nursing for humanitarian reasons ... and because she did not want to remain an amateur office worker." Bell commented, "She is determined and independent in outlook," and he had "no doubt at all that as far as the technical side [of nursing] ... is concerned she would make circles [around] a great many of the girls at home."[77] His evaluation proved correct. With the backing of the FAU and Brian's parents, Lord and Lady Sorensen, Teresa entered the Royal Free Hospital nursing school on 22 March 1947. She became a state-registered nurse in 1950 and later qualified as a midwife. Her nursing credentials became an internationally recognized passport to a life of humanitarian service. Affectionately known as "Singapore's Mother Teresa," she would receive numerous awards, including Singapore's Special Recognition Award in 2005, in recognition of her lifelong dedication to helping the sick, aged, and destitute.

Unlike British nurses, whose stories follow, Chinese nurses had lived, been educated, and worked in a cross-cultural environment before joining the China Convoy. The inclusion of Western nurses would further complicate the contested power relations in negotiating and providing patient care on the front lines and within the newly liberated areas. They too would find that Convoy life would follow a winding road filled with unexpected detours.

4 "China Needs Good Men, and Still Better Women"
British Nurses, 1943–44

> The principle of women in China was originally accepted with much reluctance and misgiving. Among some older members that feeling has crystallized into the feeling that on the whole the decision was a mistake ... on the whole, they prefer the life of the Convoy before the arrival of women.
>
> – COLIN BELL

By 1944, the China Convoy "was going full blast. Military work is way up and civilian work is increasing and entering on long-term policy work." According to Robert McClure, "things were never better."[1] The Unit's long-term plans proved unpredictable, dictated by the circumstances of war and the adroitness of its humanitarian diplomacy. As the Chinese mounted a major offensive across the Salween River, more FAU nurses were needed. This chapter examines the controversies over selection of the first three British nurses directly recruited for the China Convoy, their motivation for joining, orientation before leaving, and initial acclimatization to Convoy life. Their experience on a front-line team, as purveyors of Western nursing services and as respectable Christian young women far from home and family, round out their stories in the subsequent chapter.

As early as June 1943, Unit leaders had concluded that there was "a definite job to be done," and they renewed the request to London to recruit women for China. Their attempt to "cash in" on the flow of refugee nurses from Hong Kong had been unsuccessful; only one Chinese nurse remained, "and even she was a bit doubtful about continuing with the Unit." As the personnel officer, Duncan Wood, candidly admitted, "the peculiarities of the Cantonese temperament that make it rather difficult for these Hongkong [sic] girls to work with us" had not been considered. While the need to admit Western nurses became more urgent, the request to London and Philadelphia to recruit nurses provoked lively debate on all sides. Duncan Wood remained adamant that only suitable women qualified for a definite job would be accepted; in no circumstances should they be sent to provide "companionship."[2] Disagreement erupted over the relative importance of pacifist values as opposed to nursing credentials. London's decision to send Connie Bull, who was not a state-registered nurse (SRN), triggered a heated exchange of letters and cables. In August 1943, Robert McClure and acting medical director Art Barr had already "made it quite clear that the requirement is for fully trained nurses and we should only have any who are not fully trained if they are supplementing the former."[3] Philadelphia, however, demanded to vet prospective nurses' pacifist views, especially those who were not state-registered nurses before they were approved for China. Accordingly London was asked to search for two SRNs outside the FAU, but, given the wartime shortage of nurses in Great Britain, their recruitment proved more difficult than Gordon Square expected. During the war, the FAU was not permitted to recruit fully qualified nurses until a designated overseas posting had been identified, and since FAU members received only a very modest monthly allowance, there was little financial incentive to volunteer.

Tempers flared when McClure recommended seconding British Red Cross nurses or mission personnel to fill the immediate need. McClure chafed at the reluctance of London and Philadelphia to use seconded personnel who did not subscribe to the Convoy's pacifist ideals. Again, Philadelphia consented to accept mission personnel, provided that "they are interviewed by our Home Committee, to ensure that preference is given to people who share our views" and would "fit into our community." Philadelphia recognized that "the FAU differs in important respects from Missionary Society" but maintained that seconded personnel "should, nevertheless, be prepared to give their first loyalty to it [FAU] during their initial period."[4] While McClure did not want to be "accused of diluting the pure flame of idealism that glows in this Unit," he thought that "the purity of the flame is not always very accurately gauged during the interval between staff meetings or when we are further away from the section fireside." Pointing out that "we are in such a serious way for nurses and doctors," he implored, "if we co-operate with the military of all types and the mission staff ... I do not see why, in order to get the work done, we cannot co-operate with these people."[5]

Nonetheless, as late as 1945, London prioritized women's character over professional qualifications:

We would certainly welcome a few if they were free to enter and if they were reasonably young, deeply dedicated, strong in health, even in temperament, and with their emotions well under control. A person of real calibre can be of enormous value to our work and to the community life out here. A person who is not completely dedicated and balanced can be a real danger to herself and all others. China needs good men, and still better women.[6]

As we shall see, neither Philadelphia nor London ever deviated from this position.

By June 1944, four British women had arrived in China to join the Convoy: Margaret Briggs, Connie Bull, Elaine Conyers, and Rita Dangerfield. Conyers, the only non-nurse, was recruited as the Unit's secretary. Unlike the Chinese nurses, who had been educated and worked in a cross-cultural environment, the British recruits were innocents abroad. While London and Philadelphia believed they held pacifist ideals, in practice a number of factors, as individualistic as the women themselves, motivated each to join. Their sense of adventure and their personal and professional goals added to the humanitarian enticement to venture abroad.

Elaine Conyers, then secretary to FAU chairman Tom Tanner in London, was at the vortex of the debate over sending women to China. Always "keen" on China since her student days, she was fascinated by the heroic stories of the Unit's trials in Burma and its medical transport work. The China Convoy was "an adventure" she wanted to experience. Coincidentally, she was well positioned to help change headquarters' attitudes towards sending "delicate women" to China. Once she was in China, transforming the views of the "Cockloft," as the Convoy men referred to themselves, would take more time. The introduction of women, the men complained, would disrupt the "old boys" manly style of Convoy life. Curtains would be required for showers, and nudity and rough language would become a thing of the past.[7]

Margaret Briggs, a birthright Quaker and a fully qualified SRN and midwife, was the poster FAU nurse. From her account, the decision to volunteer appeared straightforward. Simplicity, equality, empathy, personal responsibility, and forthrightness were all part of the Quaker philosophy that underpinned her family life and Quaker education. Raised by a devout family in Birmingham, she entered Sidcot, a Quaker boarding school, at eleven, and for the next six years returned home only for the holidays. Adopting a progressive approach to education for the time, Sidcot encouraged students to think critically rather than simply absorb lectures. Like her brother, who had registered as a conscientious objector, Margaret never questioned Quaker values that saw God in everyone or her pacifist convictions that killing was wrong. As she later admitted, she was not a "very thinking person ... that was how I was brought up and how I felt."[8]

By the time war broke out, Margaret had completed her preliminary nursing qualifications and was about to start midwifery training in Oxford. Wanting to be involved more directly in wartime relief work on the home front, she accepted a job running a home for evacuated children for two years. Then, deciding it was time to go back to nursing, she returned to Birmingham as a night sister at the Queen Elizabeth Hospital. While she was there, Michael Cadbury, a childhood friend who was a member of the FAU executive, wrote asking her to go to China. After considerable soul searching, she turned down a coveted promotion at the hospital to fulfill her quest for a more meaningful wartime contribution. She knew nothing about China. Cadbury simply told her that the "untrained boys" were doing a super job but needed the assistance of trained nurses to run the hospitals.[9]

For Connie Bull and Rita Dangerfield, the road to China bore some similarities, but in other ways their paths differed remarkably. Neither was a Quaker or pacifist while growing up. Their austere backgrounds forged self-reliant women who viewed nursing as a marker of personal success, self-worth, and social respectability. Despite the dangers, both young women had thrived in wartime London because they believed their nursing work made a difference. Nursing offered them the prospect of economic independence and social respectability denied in their youth.

Later in life, Rita publically cited her strong memories of the "horrific stories" told by her father of his time as a gunner in the First World War – tales of human fodder sacrificed to the stupidity of military leaders as the source of her pacifist convictions. Growing up, however, Rita had witnessed first-hand the long-term psychological and emotional damage that war could cause. Her father's spotty employment record and strained family relationships bore the scars of war. Her family's impoverished circumstances meant that despite her abilities she could not continue her education. After working in a factory for two years, she became the youngest probationary accepted at Mile End Hospital Nursing School in London.

According to her later recollections, the twenty-year-old nurse's views on pacifism crystallized only during her training in London during the Blitz, where she met FAU orderlies at Midland Hospital. Rita was fascinated by their stories of becoming pacifists and admired their moral courage. When she decided to volunteer, the matron demanded to know why she was join-ing a pacifist organization when she had three brothers serving in the armed forces. She recalled, "I am a practical person. When there is a job to be done, I will go ahead and do it." Fundamentally, she "loved helping people." While she was "delightfully surprised" when the request came to go to China, she admitted that she had initially hoped to be posted to the Middle East, where her brother was stationed.[10] Service for this deeply religious young woman was certainly a motivating factor in her decision to volunteer with the FAU. But the China offer was attractive for a more personal reason. Rita, still grieving the unexpected loss of her mother the previous year, probably regarded China as a new beginning.[11]

Reticent by nature, Connie Bull had neither the benefit of a happy family life nor the opportunity to complete her nursing studies before leaving for China. Orphaned at sixteen, she was left destitute with nowhere to live or anyone to care for or support her. Nursing school offered free accommoda-tion and a respectable profession. Entering nursing and midwifery school in Scarborough, however, meant severing her few remaining ties in her home-town in Gloucestershire. Whether motivated by loneliness or the search for adventure, Connie left nursing school in 1940 without finishing. Instead, she eagerly reunited with a favourite cousin, Vivienne, who had been forced by the outbreak of war to return from Europe to find employment in London. Both eventually found work with the FAU during the Blitz. Connie joined the 4th FAU Women's Training Camp on 8 July 1942, then, after completion of her training, she was transferred to the London Relief Section, where she worked until her appointment to the China Convoy. Although she received additional nursing training at the Hackney Hospital, she spent most of her time caring for the children who had been evacuated from Gibraltar.

By joining the FAU voluntarily, Connie became eligible for military ser-vice and had to appear before a local tribunal to justify her demand to be treated as a conscientious objector.[12] Her application to be registered as such in August 1942 suggests that her view of war – as an inherently unjust polit-ical construction that destroyed basic human rights of the common people – rather than a desire to bear Christian witness determined her pacifist stance:

> I believe that no human being has the right to kill another. I think that the slaughter of thousands of human beings is unnecessary and irrelevant, when presumably the aim is to destroy Nazism.

Nazism, like all other social evils, is the result of the private greed and lust for power of individuals, and the ignorance and apathy of the majority. It therefore seems to me that the remedy can only be a universal change of outlook and realization of international responsibilities. War can achieve no good; it can only destroy. It destroys the common people, not their rulers. Rather, by uniting the people in racial hatreds, it strengthens their rulers.

With practically the whole world at war, with each nation deluding itself that it is fighting for freedom, the human race is intent on self-destruction.

The FAU offered adventure with the secret promise of a better future in keeping with her pacifist views and genuine desire "that her life should be of service to others."[13]

Elaine Conyers believed that an important part of their training at the women's centre at the Rowntree home involved talking about what "Go anywhere, do anything" actually meant for women. They wanted be certain that "we had our feet on the ground" – indeed, make sure that "[we] did not have family obligations that would encumber [us]." British female recruits left their briefing at Gordon Square with a clear message: they were being sent to China to do a job, not to find a husband. Elaine recalled being told that it "cost a lot to send them" and that they were on their "honour" not to succumb to sexual temptations. "They could not say: you can't fall in love but they tried." As the only non-nurse selected for China service, she remained acutely intent on using her "humble little skills" of dictation and typing and not disappointing London. But as she said, some kept that promise better than others.[14]

During her time in London, Connie Bull became romantically involved with one of the FAU men, Ron Condick, who joined the China Convoy. From Calcutta, he sent her a hurried note proposing that she join him in China. "This calls for faith to believe. I want to re-meet you – and I judge the same for you. We both want foreign work." In going through the files that were being sent to China, he discovered, "China cheeses feel women would help men (FAU) in China. Proposed that only after two years should men ask for womenfolk to join them." There were conditions, however:

Seems we must have a sort of official engagement which could be done entirely from this end as soon as you write and accept this my proposal of betrothal. That I will work and wish for you to come out is something I want more than any other thing. You have qualifications nursing – relief work –

garage – driving – farming. It's best not to be too modest – bluff will carry us thro.

Once in China, Ron made a powerful plea to include Connie in the first group of nurses sent:

> I was invited to give all the helpful information I could and – perhaps apology is needed for what may seem a little presumptuous – that you had had at least 18 months hospital training (the minimum) that you wanted to work in China because this gave opportunities for types of work that were not always open to women in England ... The work will probably [be] surgical work at some advance post or other and should give you all the new interest you are ever likely to want.[15]

Ironically, Rita Dangerfield had assured London that she was neither engaged nor emotionally attached, only to become engaged to a young missionary posted to Iraq whom she met aboard the *City of Exeter* en route to China. Connie Bull and Rita Dangerfield would leave the Convoy to marry, Margaret Briggs would wed on the eve of her departure from China, and on her return from China, Elaine Conyers would marry Colin Bell, the former chairman of the China Convoy.

Travelling to China first class seemed at first like a lavish holiday after the wartime rationing that ended when the real adventure began. After surviving attacks in the Mediterranean, Rita's convoy was one of the first through the reopened Suez Canal. The uneasy juxtaposition of a travelogue with the near-death experience portended the contrasts of human courage and cruelty ahead. The physical beauty of the Chinese landscape, all four women would discover, masked the devastating realities in war-torn China.

Most FAUers were fascinated by China but, as cultural outsiders, they were largely unprepared for the constant readjustments required by Convoy life. Even while attracted by its novelty, raw beauty, and strangeness, each struggled to find the key to get in. For some, frustration, disillusionment, and a longing for the familiar would follow the honeymoon period filled with enthusiasm and enchantment. But for all, the gritty, gruelling but at times inspiring experience of humanitarian nursing was life changing.

All three British nurses agreed that much of their orientation proved irrelevant for navigating the new professional and personal terrain in a war-torn country where "poverty was rife" beyond anything imaginable.[16] The mountain-climbing equipment, recommended as essential gear, lay unused. Although nurses were assumed to be professionally competent, limited specialized training, such as in identifying different types of malaria slides, was provided. Most British recruits took Mandarin lessons at the School of Oriental and African Studies and in London, but still required months of further practice in China before they could handle patient care without a translator. Years later, Rita Dangerfield recalled that great emphasis was placed on Chinese customs and hospital etiquette, especially the importance of knowing how to save "face."[17] Warned not to adopt a direct or aggressive approach, she was encouraged to respect Chinese history and civilization.[18] In reality, as they were about to learn, cultural adaptation could not be taught but evolved differently for each individual within the intimate contact zone of providing patient care and joining in team life.

Despite their China briefings or previous wartime experience, none of the nurses were ready for the profound cultural and professional shock they experienced. All three received their introduction to the Chinese medical world in the FAU's Huei Tien Hospital in Qujing. Described as being "somewhere between a hospital on Western standards (like the Canadian Mission Hospital in Chungking [Chongqing]) and the crudities of the usual Chinese Army hospital,"[19] this was the Unit's first attempt to run a Western-style hospital in China. They were briefed on Chinese hospital procedures and familiarized with the spectrum of tropical diseases and wounds they would regularly encounter in the field. In reality, recruits often took on new responsibilities that they may have preferred to defer until "they found their way around in such strange conditions."[20] Equally important, the hospital's origins epitomized the ethical dilemmas all three nurses confronted in China. The Qujing Sick Bay scheme, providing free medical care, received approval in November 1942 largely because FAU members had found it difficult to leave wounded or ill Chinese soldiers on the roadside, but they knew that "if you pick them up and give them a lift, trace their unit, and take them back to it that what happens is that you leave them to die in another place."[21] To most new FAU arrivals, the Chinese people's apparent disregard for their countrymen's suffering appeared cold and callous,[22] but to the impoverished Chinese refugee trying to save his family, there was no alternative. Chinese custom dictated that caring for their compatriots made them responsible for their burial or lifelong care.

Although Rita Dangerfield had nursed through Blitz, the twenty-one-year-old felt totally unprepared for the squalid hospital conditions or for improvising in a chaotic situation without supplies or backup. She had "never seen such a filthy mess in all my life."[23] It was "so completely different from what [she had] experienced in London."[24] She found it difficult to focus on the unfamiliar tasks at hand rather than on the horrific nature of the wounds. For the first time in her career, she "scrubbed and assisted at the amputation of a hand. Very nervous, hope I didn't show it."[25] Chinese hospital etiquette was equally unfamiliar professional terrain. She was prohibited, for example, from asking a patient's age directly when working up patient histories. Despite her reservations, others noted that Rita "had made the best of the unsuitable conditions" in the outpatient clinic and "had done useful work in the operating room and wards." The full story of her awkward initiation into ward work was related in the *Unit Letter:* Rita was giving back rubs, in themselves something of a sensation, when she came to an old man, "'Bing hao jowle,' she said in her best Florence Nightingale manner; must be something wrong with my tones; 'Bing hao jow-ow-ow-le'; still no response. The other patients seemed highly amused, so she looked more closely at the old man; he was dead."[26] Whether or not the account is fictional, Rita later vividly recalled her struggle to learn enough Mandarin so that she would be able to make "simple diagnoses" on her own, aided only by her independent clinical observations. A simple diary entry captures the emotional toll that first month: "Walked solidly for 5 hours, am very unhappy and lonely here."[27]

All three British nurses quickly found themselves in situations beyond their level of practice or knowledge. During their six weeks there, many recalled the one emergency that "would always be vivid" in their minds.[28] Just seven days after her arrival, Rita Dangerfield was rudely awakened before dawn to respond to a rail disaster sixty kilometres away. A troop train had derailed while negotiating a viaduct; the locomotive and most of the cars had plummeted fifteen metres into the stream below. Fifty-nine soldiers were killed and sixty-six were seriously injured. Once there, surrounded by the "injured and dead scattered everywhere," the young American physician Allen Longshore and Rita quickly began triage before beginning to cope with survivors' injuries. A simple "M" or "T" written on the victim's head indicated who had already received morphine or tetanus shots.[29] Working all day in the pouring rain, Rita struggled to keep her patients comfortable; painful memories of that night endured, such as of a severely burned boy with nothing to keep him warm but his soaking wet coat.[30] Some images seemed surreal. Just as she had sprinkled sulphonamide powder into the compound fracture of a soldier's leg, a little black pig came rushing out of the nearby sty and jumped over the leg. Startled, she "sat back and roared with laughter." Then, and in the months ahead, humour provided a much-needed "moment of relief." It wasn't until after dark that the wounded had been evacuated to the Chinese army hospital in Qujing. During the five-hour ordeal of loading patients into the evacuation train, she later acknowledged, "we had to break all the St. John's rules to drag them inside." While triage had taken its physical and emotional toll, what made the whole experience even more "macabre" was that the Chinese Red Cross left the scene to prevent the FAU from "losing face." They attended the living while the Red Cross carpenters built coffins across the road for the dead.[31]

But the "terrible day" was not yet over. With the walking wounded gingerly loaded into the FAU truck, the team began the drive back over roads that had become "a skating rink." Unable to rest when she returned to Qujing, Rita looked in on the patients temporarily housed at the FAU hostel and then went to check on the progress of the accident victims taken to the Chinese military hospital. She was appalled by the horrific conditions and lack of nursing care provided there.[32] On this and many other occasions, she found it difficult to transition from the Chinese patients' world to the relative comfort of the FAU hostel. On another such occasion, she recalled, after returning from treating a destitute burn victim in the village, she was unable to eat the birthday feast that had been prepared in her honour.

Arriving in Qujing on 1 April, Connie Bull was horrified at the sight of human skeletons scattered between coffins waiting for burial. Later that week, when returning from an FAU picnic, she witnessed a local man being tortured by being hung by his thumbs outside his home. Connie's first walk around Kunming provided a glimpse of the healthcare challenges ahead: the rows of white hand imprints on either side of the door to ward off evil spirits that brought cholera, and a beggar lying prone by a brook, the local toilet, with an open sore the size of a saucer on the back of his thigh. In the days that followed, the source of the high patient mortality became clearer after her tour of the Qujing hospitals:

> They have uneven mud floors and the beds are of wood on which the bedding is a straw mat and a pookai [quilt] ... but apparently the bedding is never changed. In the maternity ward, the baby shares the mother's bed, and a rat

ran along the floor as I looked in. The one in the town has one larger ward but there seems to be practically no nursing.

At the Army Medical Service base hospital, "the soldiers just lie on straw on the floor, all of course fully dressed including caps ... a few were squatting in the corner killing lice with charcoal."[33] What appears as a perfunctory or even callous diary entry of her second visit to the army hospital that week noted: "There was a man lying under the table in the big room with no clothes on to whom no-one paid any attention. I can now machine in a straight line." Many Westerners had difficulty processing the sights, sounds, and smells, but more particularly their Chinese colleagues' apparent indifference to their compatriots' suffering. Focusing on familiar activities became a way of injecting some normality into the chaos.

Connie returned to Kunming the first week in May to await transport to Tali, on the Burma Road 150 kilometres east of Baoshan, where an FAU team was assisting at a mission hospital. She would receive further training here while awaiting a team assignment. Separated from Ron and uncertain of what the future would bring, Connie succumbed to a bout of melancholy: "Have done nothing but finished a letter to Ron, and read all day. When living in the unexciting reality of this small attic room ... with a gray day of drizzle and dim shapes outside; then it is I know the error of my yearnings." Lacking close family to write to or be encouraged by, Connie found that her diary remained an important vehicle to filter and internalize the wild wash of emotions that swept over her.

Margaret Briggs's memories of the Qujing hospital and her work there differed from those of her compatriots. Downplaying the squalor, she characterized her work as "interesting but nothing very dramatic."[34] In all likelihood, Briggs, a more experienced nurse, was designated to remain at Qujing to raise the nursing standards. The Chinese matron and two staff nurses, in the FAU's opinion, were not "up to the standards" of the nurses the FAU had hoped to secure in Hong Kong.[35] Longing for more challenging work after six months, Margaret pushed to be transferred to the front line.

Qujing provided a brief introduction to the personal, professional, and ethical choices inherent in humanitarian nursing, albeit within the controlled environment of working in an FAU hospital and living in the relatively comfortable FAU hostel. The real test still lay ahead. All three British FAU nurses would eventually be reunited on MT5 near Baoshan, on the Salween front.

5 Baoshan
Professionalism, Pacifism, and Proposals, 1944–45

Why should I like this hour of the day?
At this hour something comes over me
Resistance, courage, is that it?
Failures and hopeless aspirations
Then crowd in to mock.

– CONNIE BULL, OCTOBER 1944

In April 1944, when the Salween campaign was being fought in the jungle-covered Qinghai Mountains, a new medical team, MT5, initially composed entirely of Friends Ambulance Unit staff, was established at Baoshan. Chiang Kai-shek had finally yielded to pressure from the US government and issued the order to cross the Salween River on 14 April 1944. By mid-June, the Chinese had encountered stubborn Japanese resistance and suffered heavy casualties. None of the British nurses joined MT5's forward team that crossed the Salween, but worked instead in MT5's Intermediate Hospital – something between a field dressing station and a casualty clearing station – in huts seven kilometres from the town.

Rita Dangerfield and Connie Bull arrived at MT5 in the first week of June 1944. Connie's poem, quoted above, reverberated with her feelings of being emotionally overextended and exhausted by team life. Neither nurse was prepared for life on the front line. Japanese bombers frequently strafed the hospital compound, dropping bombs on nearby towns. They risked becoming casualties on their daily trips to market to obtain food for the team. Patients who had survived the ordeal over mountainous terrain arrived in terrible condition, displaying symptoms of life-threatening gas gangrene, tetanus, and malnutrition.[1] Their chances of survival were further compromised by the diseases of the region: malaria, relapsing fever, tuberculosis, tetanus, and dysentery. The team was constantly stretched beyond its limits. Team dynamics and the extreme conditions, aggravated by cultural and professional clashes, made front-line nursing simultaneously exhilarating yet frustrating. For all, it involved an unforgettable experience in faith, pioneering, and cooperation that was life changing.

The *Unit Letter* announcing Connie and Rita's departure, replete with bawdy overtones and emphasizing the quantity of their baggage, appeared to trivialize the importance of the event. It also reflected the perceived contradiction between placing women close to danger and the maternal image of nursing as a caring and comforting occupation. Such gendered discourse negates the independent choices women made and the risk they were willing to take. All three British nurses arrived with clearly delineated professional expectations, views of citizenship, and obligations of service; life in the field would test their choices. The daily realities of attempting to provide adequate nursing care in extremely difficult conditions brought unprecedented personal, professional, and ethical challenges for all the British nurses. As we shall see, other factors contributed to the women's heightened stress levels. FAU nurses were expected to make all aspects of team life run more smoothly. Their stories, complementing those of the Chinese nurses told earlier, probe how war affected all aspects of the women's life and enhance our understanding of the China Convoy's tangled humanitarian endeavours.

On the way down to Baoshan with a General Loo (Lu Kyo Chuan), Connie recalled, they passed a swollen black corpse. The general paid a man in the next village to bury it, but the incident was a disturbing prelude to the human drama about to unfold. Once the nurses arrived, their reception was not quite what they had anticipated. Returning from town to MT5 after their "splurge, feeling reborn," Dr. John Perry and Ron Chapman were greeted by what they took as a practical joke, "one of those games inventing a story about some nurses having come." Everyone "had a good chuckle," but they kept it up "very obstinately" the following morning, just convincingly enough "to make us quite sure it was a fable." So Perry and Chapman played along and "actually started calling out in falsettos for 'Rita!' and 'Connie!'" Just as Perry hung his bare body out the window to brush his teeth to show he did not believe it, "well damme if they weren't there walking up the patch big as life."[2]

Despite his flippant greeting, Perry proved a stable and supportive team leader. During earlier field experience, he had come to accept the limits of his own humanitarian capacity and the fact that there would be tensions and misunderstandings in the team's dealings with the Chinese. He developed several maxims to stave off burnout:

Try for one thing at a time and keep trying doggedly day in and day out for that and it will finally happen; bringing order out of chaos is a very slow and gradual process, depending entirely on patience and in order to maintain your sanity; you have just to adjust yourself to the facts, and adjust your medical conscience to the knowledge of what you can and cannot obtain.[3]

But gradually he became "acclimatized to it" and "found I don't mind it so much." Success in China, he confided, "involves first admitting how perfectly disgusted you are and then making adjustments accordingly."[4]

Perry was elated by the arrival of Bull and Dangerfield. Without adequate nursing staff, he had been experiencing "all the unusual difficulties getting things running properly." Daily, he and his fellow physician, Eric Waddington, spent hours admitting and classifying cases to be operated on the following day, only to find "that they had been whisked away" on trucks down the road by the Chinese orderlies, "who make their own lists according to their own lights and vague impressions of what's going on ... that gives them a feeling of security, that it's sure enough their show no matter what impression we may be trying to make."[5] His daily "polite little visitations," however, had recently led to a compromise: the FAU team would control the forty-bed ward nearest the operating theatre as their "own little shooting match."[6] "But o what a difference," he found,

to have these girls, one running the ward, the other the theatre so as to make the place really hum with efficiency, keeping two tables going hard at all times; and the stretcher bearers will bear with us once more; and temperatures will be taken regularly, and the wounds dressed and backs rubbed and orders will be carried out and operative schedules will go off by the clock, and we'll have supper at seven and get to bed when a guy should. And besides it is quite a change having some feminine touch around.[7]

Those were tall orders to fill. The 150-bed hospital eventually accommodated three hundred to four hundred patients; makeshift straw beds cluttered the aisles wherever space could be found inside or outside in extra tents. Over the summer months, the "top really blew off" without moving the team closer to the front. "All types of cases that had died in the older system and routes were now just pulling through to [them], definitely more interesting and acute."[8] Bull's diary provides glimpses of the team's "interesting life" of working far into the night to assess and treat hundreds of cases daily. In addition, the team was always on call to deal with civilian casualties when planes dropped bombs on Baoshan. Under these circumstances, adaptation, both personal and professional, was the core coping mechanism for survival. Would the British nurses step up to the challenges of making constant readjustments required by team life on the front lines?

Dangerfield took charge of a surgical ward of fifty-six beds in a bamboo hut, with a mud floor and thatched roof. Bull assisted in the operating theatre. Quickly finding themselves outside their normal level of practice and knowledge, the two nurses had to be more creative when working with minimal resources and to accept that the level of care would be different. Both knew every day that patients had to be passed along untreated. Patients who arrived "with wounds with large green maggots in seething clusters etc." gave Bull "a real shock." Like the team's Western physicians, both struggled to come to grips with inattentive Chinese orderlies who passed by grievously ill patients. If the soldiers were "too weak to ask for food no-one bothers to feed them."[9] Nursing routines had to be adapted to makeshift equipment. Startled soldiers awoke to discover their fractured leg hung up by parachute cord and adhesive tape to a big wooden post, and traction was provided by bricks tied together at the end of ropes. In the operating room, a "big three-legged gadget" was jury-rigged to suspend fracture patients in the air to allow the theatre staff to wind the hip spica plaster that covers both legs from the ankles to the belly button.[10]

The scarcity of antibiotics and dried blood plasma or hospital equipment was not the only obstacle to the effective practice of Western medicine. Language barriers and cultural differences added to the difficulties encountered daily. Neither nurse anticipated that Western medical knowledge would be challenged or that they would have to gain their patients' trust. Chinese patients did not meekly submit to Western medical authority. Rita Dangerfield grew "weary" of delousing soldiers only to have them put their contaminated clothes back on top of their clean pajamas for fear their clothes would be stolen.[11] Wounded Chinese soldiers regularly pulled off casts because they believed that if they died they would have no leg in heaven because it was bound in plaster.[12] It was here that Rita struggled to reconcile traditional Chinese medicine with Western practice. Patients preferred local herbal remedies to those offered by Western physicians. She recalled her astonishment on seeing a "witch doctor" placing metal discs on a patient's chest, but the team's FAU physician, John Perry, wisely instructed her not to interfere, as the surgical dressings were not touched.[13] However, Rita found it difficult to remain complacent when traditional Chinese remedies were harmful. One such case was a child whose hand had been badly damaged while playing with a grenade. The injured hand had been encased in chicken feathers bound by banana leaves in the hope that the spirit of the live chicken would save the hand. It did not. Surrounded by suffering, foul smells, and unruly patients, Rita became "sick to death of maggoty wounds" and "longed only for breath of fresh air and to discover the hills around here."[14]

It seemed, however, that every time staff felt overwhelmed, new members appeared, allowing the team to keep pace with the heavy caseload. As MT5 expanded, it had to accommodate outsiders' perspectives and demands. In early August, the team grew to twelve members when Bob McClure arrived with two British Red Cross nurses forced by the war to abandon Changsha: Edna Kenneth and Judy Grieve. He immediately changed team nursing assignments. Arguing that Connie "is not up to theatre standards," he placed Edna in charge of the OR and Connie "under Rita on the wards," "which is a big job, and smelly job, and rather thankless job but very important." Arguing that "we must have more wide-awake and thoroughly trained people" to run the theatre efficiently, he believed that "Connie is now in her right place and the spirit of both the girls is fine."[15] But he misread the situation. Bull had found theatre work rewarding and did not like ward nursing "half so much."[16] Nor does McClure's assessment accord with earlier reports that "the addition of the two girls to the section was most welcome and they have been working very well indeed the last few days. What an amazing difference it makes to a section to have the Female Touch."[17] Moreover, Rita Dangerfield and Ron Chapman were not the only ones learning their theatre job on the spot; the young FAU physicians John Perry and Eric Waddington "were learning their surgery so fast they can hardly keep up with themselves."[18]

The new arrivals adversely affected team morale, in Perry's opinion:

> We had been having a good team atmosphere until these British Red Cross Society girls came along, a couple of the fussiest old hens you ever saw. The second day they were here they blew up and asked to return immediately to Kunming because our "standards" were so low, meaning that we have no sheets and pillow cases, a floor that you could not scrub in the O.R., and too few rooms to work in and too few Chinese coolies around to lift things for you.

The trouble, in Perry's view, was that they "come from the BRCS Changsha background, which is a pukka little hospital, such as you would find in any western town, with their spiritual Maginot line protecting them from any encroachment of the Orient upon Occidental ways. We'll learn them! I hope."[19]

But the reverse appeared to be the case. With the secondment of two more British Red Cross nurses, Barbara Tawn and Peggy Toop, in September, the team reached nineteen. Fortunately, the latest additions appeared "a bit more youthful and a bit more gifted with the spiritual pezazz [*sic*] that makes this kind of life a good thing rather than a burden."[20] Now, at least, the team was able to assign a nurse to assist with the dressing and lighter cases on the Chinese wards. Just as important, it meant that drugs could be released to these patients without the fear of their being sold on the black market.

Having more specialized teams in the hospital to handle the increasingly complex caseload appeared to be a mixed blessing. Perry began to "sense the feeling of a 'tree when it grows rigid and strong, and is about to die.' The hard and the strong are companions of death, the supple and the weak are companions of life." MT5, in his view, "lost a certain spark of initiative and willingness to go out of its way to meet pressures and urgencies, and in order not to lose our BRC contingent, we bowed to a rule of thumb and superficial regularities, the patients have paid for it more than once."[21] But other FAU visitors believed that ward sister Peggy Toop and "ward brother" Bill Emslie did an excellent job of "ministering to the sick under the strangest nursing conditions of all of their experience."[22]

In October 1944, Margaret Briggs joined MT5 as the Salween campaign wound down and the well-organized medical team turned its attention to mop-up surgery. Edna Kenneth and Barbara Tawn covered the operating theatre, and Margaret worked with Peggy Toop, Rita, and Connie on the wards and oversaw the special diets program. Reports that Peggy and Margaret were "doing good work" also noted that they did not have an "easy task with the ward orderlies who with few exceptions are the average lazy uninterested crowd, but they are getting the best possible out of them." But it was Peggy who was singled out for praise: "The patience Peggy has shown in building up good relations over a long period is bearing fruit."[23]

Perhaps Margaret's arrival, coinciding with a larger nursing staff, makes more understandable why years later her memories of the primitive living conditions, arduous practice setting, or difficult cases differed from those of others. Her professional adjustments were minimized in her later recollections, but not in the Unit's weekly newsletter. Years later, in recounting a particularly "difficult" maternity case involving a Japanese prisoner, Margaret censored the tragic outcome that had been widely reported at the time. In spite of the nurses' "pep talks and psychological treatment to awaken her maternal instincts," the Japanese mother strangled the child.[24] In her later recollections, however, Margaret spotlighted the professional autonomy that she was given while working on the front lines: "You would never do anything like that if you were in England at that age and at that stage. It was an extraordinary experience." She knew only enough Chinese to get things done or to say a few comforting words on the wards; equally, her lack of fluency in Chinese limited her exchanges with her Chinese colleagues. Although she wished that she "had done lots more finding out about things," her experience, as she said, was in "a hospital and that was it."[25]

Although the Convoy men, such as Ron Chapman, provided essential front-line nursing services throughout the war, few recollections survive in the official records, and only scant references to their work, such as that cited above, appear in the weekly newsletters. The account of American Clement White's training in Qujing and subsequent time with MT5 in 1944 is an exception. White's medical education consisted of learning by doing under supervision, and studying on the side between language lessons. He did surgical dressings, assisted in the wards and operating theatre, and gave a few anesthetics. White was then sent to MT5 to get additional training in preparation for his appointment as section leader in Qujing when the Unit shifted its headquarters to Chongqing.

With only limited training, White was given extraordinary nursing responsibilities at Baoshan. Describing MT5's field hospital, he wrote: "We live and work all the time in surroundings much like the hospital scene in 'Gone with the Wind' or like the paintings of Florence Nightingale in the Crimea. Only the pictures do not do justice to the sound or to the wonderful fortitude of most men." He modestly described his main responsibility in "a little ward of seventeen filled with critical cases." There his nursing duties included administering sulpha drugs five times a day; dressing wounds and amputation stubs; and monitoring and recording the patients' vital signs, especially watching "for the dreaded bleeding or gas gangrene that may be fatal in a few minutes or hours." In addition, White helped out in another ward that had over two hundred patients and, at other times, assisted with "the sulpha schedule" on a third ward or in the operating room.[26]

He had "many vivid mental pictures" of administering drugs on night rounds:

> The room has an air of quiet, but the illusion of the monoliths [patients shrouded in mosquito nets] is broken by the sounds from invisible patients. Some men moan all the time. The steady rasping comes from a man breathing through a tube in his neck, or from a whistler – one who gets his air through torn flesh in his chest or back ... And some are so still I have often startled moments of fear lest I may have overlooked some deadly sign on the last round.
>
> The attendants usually are asleep under their canopies beside the door. I may leave them there, though sometimes I waken the more willing one. When I do he holds the flickering lamp and passes bowls of water while I struggle with the netting and get the patients in a position so that they can swallow ... But the well-meaning attendant tries to rush the patients and shouts at them so much I usually let him sleep.
>
> It is hard for some men to understand how a few white pills can help a shattered jaw or leg that isn't there. There is a great game of wit and will every few hours. Their sleight of hand is so skillful, I have to pop the pills into their unwilling mouths lest they be found later on the floor or in a crack in the mud wall. Even that does not always work.[27]

White found satisfaction in his work and developed a genuine affection for the Chinese people, some whom he hoped to have as lifelong friends. This was not to be. Clement White died in 1945 after a fall from a Convoy truck.

One of the few other references that went beyond identifying the geographic location where FAU men acted as theatre or ward nurses confirmed that male nurses' work often extended well beyond their medical knowledge or skill: "In a temple, a mile down the road [from the MT5 main hospital], Derek Cox and Frank Willsher continue to supervise a medical ward containing up to 60 patients. Their main job is laboratory test followed by the requisite treatment. Relapsing fever, typhus, typhoid and dysentery are all found here."[28] What the account did not mention was that often laboratory stains had to be improvised or were not available at all.

The relative silence about men's nursing work in the weekly newsletters raises important questions. Did the prevailing gendered view of nursing – as an extension of the women's sphere – inhibit men from valuing their contribution or considering it as heroic as that of the Convoy drivers whose tales and poetry filled the newsletters' pages? Male nurses, "or ward brothers," did not fit the normative gendered narrative; their exclusion makes it difficult to assess men's contribution or gendered experiences in war.

Housed in a series of rat-ridden and lice-infested rooms, Connie Bull and Rita Dangerfield had little privacy or comforts of home to provide much-needed respite at the end of a long workday. The nurses were expected to "sleep rough"[29] and subsist on two meals a day, as was the Chinese custom. Although the bamboo walls were covered with paper, there were a lot of holes. Rita recalled that she often had an audience at bedtime as she dusted herself with DDT and slipped quickly under the mosquito net that covered her bed, which consisted of boards with a straw mattress and a sleeping bag, and then "listening to the sounds of bullfrogs calling each other and Yunnanese rat eating our precious English soap."[30] Despite John Perry's continued efforts, for a long time the nurses "had no mofung [outhouse] ... At least, one has been erected, but resembles a transparent meat safe, so it's still unusable." This means that when the nurses "have squitters [diarrhea], as we do very frequently owing to cook trouble, they have to go dashing out to the highways and byways." But Connie took their rough living conditions in stride; their room was "not at all bad, the beds of course are just planks but we have fixed up bamboo on which we hang our clothes and have a chair and table. Lice and fleas are rampant – all the soldiers have lice and we get them on us when we lift them etc." More problematic was the lack of leisure time: "We have so far had very little time free for writing letters ... or washing. And, when it comes, we are tired."[31]

John Perry's subsequent letters, written in the fall of 1944, corroborate Margaret Briggs's later recollections, painting a more sedate portrait of team life. "You ought to see this team now; how the old baby has changed," Perry told his wife:

> You remember how it was when we started with six, and were reinforced after a time by a couple of girls, and meals were irregular and we got sick all the time; and the place here looked like a pig-pen because we had so little time for fooling around and making things look like home ... Well, last night our team of eighteen sat down to dinner prepared by our housekeeper, one

of the nurses on fulltime, with a couple of brass hats guests at a table with a white spread; the table cloth being composed of a number of squares of operating cloth ... it really looked pretty pukka with a colourful touch added by the "bat boy" who likes to wear white BRC pyjamas for uniforms ... But what I am proudest of all is the change in room decorations. I went through all the copies of *Life* and others I could get my hands on, and finally ran across some reprints in color of Giotte's [Giotto's] Fra Angelica and Bellimis [Bellini's] and another of Raphael's of Madonna of the Ronda; so it really begins to look civilized at last.[32]

Life within this larger team was being constructed as a civilized Western en-clave sheltered from the more chaotic Chinese society that reigned within the hospital.

In addition to the professional and physical challenges, Convoy life pre-sented new gendered frontiers. Even before they left Qujing, the arrivals of three English nurses and one "office gal" in Qujing, Allen Longshore had observed, "are boosting the morale no end and the U.S. Army is also taking notice of their arrival!!!"[33] When some consideration was given to what the women FAU members should be called, "i.e., 'Unit-ettes' or some other tricky handle," Longshore suggested that they should be "fondly known as the 'FAU-cets.'" But his humour went largely unappreciated, as his British col-leagues most commonly said "tap" or "spigot." As he said, the women "were here to stay regardless of what we call them." According to the editor of the weekly newsletter, the arrival of Rita, Connie, and Margaret in China heralded the end of bachelorhood: "So that for which we have been waiting has come to pass. A new era has dawned; stirring times are upon us; and the unfit must go. Misogynists!"[34] The new recruits would have to adjust to more than the ribald poems and songs that characterized life in the Cockloft, however.

Convoy life involved complicated choices about sexual conduct and male friendships. Defining appropriate social relationships was often emancipat-ing and exhilarating but, at other times, equally disturbing. As Margaret later recalled, being thrown into the FAU hostel in Qujing "just full of men" long-ing for female attention was "quite frightening." She quickly determined to avoid any permanent entanglements that might cause strife within the tightly knit Cockloft. In any case, she too remained wary that "this strange situation" made it impossible to discern whether the attraction was genuine.[35] Keeping that promise was quite another matter!

Connie had come to China with the understanding that she and Ron Condick would marry the following November. While Connie's pre-existing relationship with Ron perhaps protected her from unwanted advances within the Convoy's ranks, there were no official policies or channels to protect non-combatant nurses from sexual harassment on the road. During one stopover en route to the mission hospital in Tali, an uninvited American soldier, believing she was asleep, "put his hand under the bed clothes – Luckily he went meekly when [she] turned round and told him to go." Like other victims of sexual assault in wartime, she was reluctant to report the incident for fear that it would reflect badly on her conduct or the Unit. Instead, she chose to sublimate the incident in her diary by focusing on the next day's diversion of driving a military Jeep.[36]

Connie, like other women on her team, enjoyed the attention she received from a host of admirers.[37] But life away from the hostel involved negotiating more challenging social relationships with the American military community. John Perry's letters attest to the "sudden new popularity [MT5] acquired since the girls arrived."[38] While Perry may have enjoyed "the quick jerk back to the good old ways and days" visiting and dining with American military, for the women, it was a mixed blessing.

Connie's diary records the conflicted emotions that she as an engaged woman experienced trying to provide social companionship for the men in the field and still be fit for duty in the morning:

> Rita and I go out about five out of seven nights a week. At least that's what it feels like. It's sometimes very difficult to know what to do about this woman shortage. I refused an invitation to have dinner with two American lieutenants and so the weapons carrier they used to send up to take us to the flicks no longer comes ... Rita and I have had dinner three times with Ravenholt and Col. Nanse, the first two were mostly spent discussing pacifism and the wine didn't affect me much, but last night it really went to my head; and A.R. did not behave.[39]

Unaccustomed to all the attention, Connie's initial exhilaration was quickly replaced by guilt:

> I am getting doubts about R[on]; so try not to think about it, but of course that is not the most honest thing to do. I am not sure how serious they are but feel I must write soon to him, and ask him not to speak to Duncan [Wood]

re November. The truth is I'm just not worthy anyway, I'm much too shallow, fickle, and seem to lack any deep feeling. Am capable only of superficial attractions to all sorts of people.[40]

November was approaching and team assignments were also changing; she would soon have to make a decision.

Life after MT5 took each British FAU nurse in a different direction. As the Convoy began a new phase in the fall of 1944, with the rehabilitation of medical facilities in recently liberated cities, a new MT8 was formed and located in Tengyue, where efforts to build and devolve the hospital to the local guild were being planned. Rita Dangerfield and Margaret Briggs would eventually be sent there. Other adventures awaited Connie Bull.

Whatever doubts lingered, Connie decided to start a new life with the man she had followed to China. With great fanfare, the *Newsletter* announced "the first all Unit marriage" of Ron and Connie and later recounted events of the wedding in detail. In contrast, Connie's diary entry on her wedding day simply noted: "19th Oct: Were married by Bishop Hall."[41] By the end of November, Ron had an exciting new assignment to oversee the building of a garage and hostel in Lushien, while Connie was relegated to the role of a supportive wife and stripped of nursing duties. Despite her happiness in being with Ron, the Lushien interval was a dark period for the young bride cut off from family and FAU friends and faced with little prospect of finding work as meaningful as nursing on MT5:

Have become at times since being here very tired of this pretence of liking China and the Chinese specially when the weather is extra foul; the diet, smells, food; and *ding hous* [I am fine] every time one walks down the street become wearing. This is chiefly due to not having a hostel, or many foreigners about ... and we see very little of any Americans. But to talk of universal brotherhood is a good deal easier to do from inside England: but at least I know that now and wouldn't have known (or believed) it without coming.

For some reason I am not receiving any letters from England, not that there is anyone who cares a damn, but hell it's something just to get a letter. Whatever happens now, I feel I have made an absolute failure of working in China. First in giving up medical work. Second, here I am sure I am not doing anything like half a job. As soon as Ron gets at all busy it's very obvious that I am in the way. All the same, there is nothing else to do, so I suppose I shall have to go on pretending to work here, after all, I am lucky in only having that mental degradation; to be in China (or rather to be outside Europe) and to be with Ron, though I'm a very inferior sort of "assistant."[42]

As time passed, she felt increasingly guilty at her growing despondency: "I feel vaguely that it is traitorous to write down that although being married brings a kind of peace and warmth, it also is in these circumstances stultifying."[43]

For a long time, Connie remained surprisingly unaware that another factor contributed to the emotional roller coaster that she had experienced in the last few months. After seeing Dr. Karfuncle on 19 March, she wrote: "He said it's pretty certain I shall have a baby, but I still can't believe it."[44] The couple's request to be repatriated was granted, but lack of transportation made it impossible for them to get home before the twins were born. In the interim, work was found for Ron in Calcutta. "It was with joy and sadness"[45] that the *Newsletter* announced on 3 November 1945 the birth of twin boys to Ron and Connie, and the death of one son three days later. Since both parents were too ill to leave the hospital, the twins were being cared for in the FAU hostel in Calcutta. She finally arrived there only to learn her son had died earlier that day.

As the *Newsletter* notice said, "it was not easy to face such extremes in so short of a period of time."[46] It was an equally fitting epitaph for Connie's difficult and troubled life from her early childhood to her time in China. Her ingrained lack of self-worth and brooding personality made her acclimatization to Convoy life and marriage beyond the honeymoon stage more difficult. Unable to share her real feelings about China, even with Ron, Connie found that in many respects the China years were best forgotten.[47]

In the meantime, new adventures awaited her teammates. The trip to join MT8 in Tengyue stood out in Rita's memory. Departing on 31 October 1944, travelling as far as possible by truck and then weapons carrier, the group drove through a "battery of shell fire" en route and saw US dive bombers attacking Japanese positions at Dehong after crossing the Salween. As she trekked the final hundred kilometres towards their destination, Rita remembered passing the time with Robert McClure and Doug Crawford by singing "Guide me O thou Great Jehovah ... What our Chinese companions thought, I do not know." It was, as Dangerfield remembered, more "of a climb than a walk and we crossed a mountain range, the coolies all the while telling me it was a short cut!"[48] No special concessions were made for Rita: "Our coolies shared the same roof with us, at very little remove I must say ... After supper, footsore and weary we laid our sleeping bags on the rough floor and slept like proverbial logs."[49] The trek was a prelude to the city. Tengyue "presented an appalling sight." Most of the city "had been razed to the ground. Ditches and wells were filled in and bodies of men and mules were lying in shallow graves." The public health tasks had to come first. To meet the immediate needs of the refugees swarming back towards their homes, they opened a clinic in a shop, "under the floorboards of which they found a live grenade."[50]

John Perry described the conditions in the Confucius temple being renovated as a hospital, where Rita Dangerfield and Margaret Briggs attempted to introduce basic nursing services while acting as the team's housekeepers: "The accommodations have been crude of course and we look forward to the blessed time when we no longer have to scrub up in the court outside and do the sterilizing over the kitchen fire and operate in a room with very unluminous windows, amid, we regret to observe, great buzzing of flies."[51] Despite the primitive conditions, Briggs remembered the early days of building a hospital in Tengyue as exhilarating. Their first patients were for the most part victims of the mines and ammunition that lay scattered in the town, and then the local people suffering from the maladies common in Yunnan started coming back. It was "really super." Put in charge of the theatre, she increasingly functioned as a surgeon's assistant to McClure. It was an extraordinary experience – one that earned her his praise as the finest surgical nurse with whom he had worked.[52] Again, Margaret Briggs depicted team life there as "very much involved in our own group," with few contacts beyond the hospital compound.[53] At times, she functioned as a troubleshooter, dispatched to deal with a plague outbreak south of the city, where she gained a greater appreciation of the importance of community cooperation for FAU's future success. Both Margaret and Rita left MT8 before runaway inflation and local politics soured relationships.

Rita Dangerfield married Reverend David White in June 1944 in Basra, Iraq, but only after Duncan Wood in Gordon Square had written her sister for approval.[54] Rita's public accounts speak of leaving in response to David's pleas for her support in his missionary work, but her diaries reveal a more conflicted choice. In mid-July, American "photographer-lieutenant-geologist" Charles Schwepp began courting Rita. By early August, expecting to marry Charles, she had broken off her engagement to David. But David continued to press her to join him in Iraq. Throughout the fall, she remained emotionally torn about what she termed "the mess." "When [Charles] is around I love him dearly, but just as soon as he goes I'm back to where I started from with the same old fears and worries." Doubts lingered that he would have proposed under "normal" circumstances or prove a reliable husband. Although she had shared more experiences in wartime China with Charles, by December Rita chose "safety in the arms of David and his spiritual life" as a "good" cleric wife. Like Connie, Rita also questioned her worthiness. "I've given up the hope of becoming a good Christian, afraid I joined the ranks of the strayed a long time ago. Oh, how I'd love to be a Really Good, and unselfish person." Marriage to David promised social respectability, a purposeful life of Christian service, and a happy family life for which the deeply religious young woman had always longed.[55]

Despite her unhappiness at times, Rita carried passionate memories of her China years. Looking back, she believed that she had acquired a "breadth of vision," a great love and admiration for the Chinese people, and a different perspective on her privileged Western lifestyle.[56] In Dangerfield's later years, she regularly attended the meetings of the China Society in London and with its support published her redemptive memoir, *South of the Cloud*, describing her China odyssey. In recognition of her work in China, the British government awarded her both the Burma Star and the Badge of Honour.[57]

Margaret Briggs's selection as MT8 representative at the Yearly Meeting of the China Convoy in Qujing in the last week of September 1945 attested to her growing stature. For Briggs and the Convoy, the four-day meeting was a watershed. Despite her determination not to become personally attached, Margaret celebrated her engagement to Al Matheson at a special banquet that coincided with the final night of the meeting. No one suspected what the feast was really for. Once the news broke, the "revelry department began with a series of speeches barely heard over the cheers and huzzahs ... Song took up where words left off ... It was all part of a monster effort which had to be absolutely the biggest and best ever ... chorus followed chorus until the streets grew quiet and we knew it was late." Everyone "felt a share" of their new life.[58]

Expected to be a "pillar" of the FAU's future hospital work, Margaret left four days later with Robert McClure to kick-start the Henan-area project. She recalled their surreal meeting with a Japanese general who still occupied the mission compound selected as the FAU's future headquarters. As Margaret remembered it, McClure said "out and we got it." She remembered thinking, "Is this real? Is this me?"[59] However, the *Newsletter* suggested that the negotiations were somewhat more protracted: "The Japanese are still in occupancy at the Baptist Hospital, and negotiations for the team to take over are full of snags, not least because it is suggested that the Japanese still have plenty of face locally and since everyone is being so nice about the whole thing it seems a bit much to turf the boys out."[60] Shortly afterwards, Briggs was dispatched to survey the damage to other Henan mission hospitals. Interestingly, Doris Wu was the head nurse in Zhengzhou charged with organizing a nursing school. Margaret acted as warden and ran the operating theatre. Along with Philip Hsiung, she became part of McClure's refurbished mobile surgical team that travelled between mission hospitals to handle major surgical cases.[61] Although she could have left when the war ended, she remained until the end of her two years in March 1946. With Doris Wu as her attendant, she married Al the day before leaving – as she said, travelling home together unmarried was simply not an option.

Margaret found her China years rewarding and professionally exhilarating: "I would never have believed that I could have got so completely absorbed, in a group so quickly as I feel I have done out here. I certainly am awfully glad I was given the opportunity of coming, and that most of the fears that I had before coming proved groundless."[62] Her almost breezy characterization of her pacifist motivation and experience once in China consciously distanced her from the Victorian notion of a benevolent lady providing charity to deserving individuals. The epitome of a respectable Quaker woman, she drew personal strength from the pacifist convictions that took her to China. As a Quaker nurse, she took a sensible, practical attitude towards war, poverty, and distress. Although McClure described her as "good-natured,"[63] developed a great affection for her, and admired her take-charge attitude, not everyone did. One of her New Zealand colleagues in Henan summed up his feelings:

> Margaret is 29 and rather overbearing – likes to have her own way. Everything for her is first priority and must be done immediately ... I bristle often underneath and I am getting to the stage where I stall in principle to her demands and object sometimes rather pointedly because of the demanding attitude. Her voice seems terribly hard to me now, maybe the warden's job has done that. I may add that although I would not call her fat, she sure does fill out her slacks she has been wearing.[64]

Strong-minded women in positions of authority still had to negotiate the male-dominated organization where gender expectations dictated that women exhibit a sense of decorum and deference.

While cognizant that the Convoy's contribution was at best "a drop in the bucket," Margaret Briggs believed that the presence of Western nurses raised the standard of care as they worked alongside their Chinese counterparts and ensured that the best possible care had been provided under extraordinary circumstances. Like other Convoy members, she left China with indelible memories of the resilience of the Chinese people and a lifelong comradeship forged with a like-minded group of globally recruited pacifist humanitarians who epitomized youthful hope for peace. Other Western FAU nurses who followed, however, found that their China years would either be more personally traumatic or less professionally transformative.

The war opened up new frontiers for the British FAU nurses, enabling an exciting journey of self-discovery and maturation. Connie Bull, Rita Dangerfield, and Margaret Briggs did things that they had never dreamed of, but growing up also carried different costs for each: physically, emotionally, personally, and professionally.

Combined, the historical vignettes of the Chinese and Western FAU nurses paint a richly textured picture of the diversity of their lives and humanitarian work in wartime China. Executed in the midst of social, cultural, and political cleavages, the FAU's contested humanitarian exchanges were a highly negotiated process in which the Unit's integrity and operational autonomy were balanced against the need to gain access to those in need of medical care or relief. As Sheila Iu's treatment as a social outcast by her compatriots demonstrates, race played itself out in ways that do not easily fit into the binary stereotype of Westerners versus Chinese. Nurses' experiences and their relations with FAU physicians suggest that some Westerners could become "authentic knowers" who share the struggles of those among whom they work, but not always.[65]

What factors shaped Westerners' acclimatization and acculturation? Were team size and geographic locations the primary determinants? Chinese nurses served primarily on smaller teams, composed of three to five Western and two Chinese members. These teams tended to be placed in more advanced front-line positions or remote locations. Conversely, the seven British nurses on MT5 gradually functioned within a larger team of eighteen members that was more "self-contained." Doris Wu joined the team late in its history, and her Western education, proven record, and engagement to John Wilks buffered her cross-cultural relationships. At one point, however, McClure considered sending Margaret Briggs back to Baoshan because the British Red Cross nurses wanted her as matron instead of Wu. As the Convoy discussed its future work in light of its past experience, its members debated whether the team's size influenced the "expression of those ideals of service under which the convoy works": to work *with* rather than *for* the Chinese people. Arguing that it was necessary to look at not only "the great differences in the manner of their work but also the great differences in the manner of their living," British physician Terry Darling argued that the dichotomy between small and large teams mirrored the two camps within the Convoy ranks. He distinguished "between the man with a special 'concern' for China and the growing idea of long-term service in China and the man with the short-term ideas who has come to China because it provides opportunities for expressing his pacifist ideals – an opportunity which might equally be found in any other needy country."[66] While his overall assessment has historical merit, as noted earlier, MT6's life as a small team differed dramatically from that in the two spearhead teams that operated within MT3 during the Salween campaign on the long trek to Tengyue.

In Darling's opinion, small teams offered the best option for working with the Chinese because they were required to live as completely as possible with and on the same level as Chinese medical staff, with members "to whom they become personal friends and co-workers." This, he noted, "involves eating as nearly as possible on the 2 meal a day system and sacrificing much that makes up the familiar Western way of life, but it makes possible integration with the Chinese community." In contrast, he believed that large-team life resembled "a foreign community, insulated for all practical purposes from the Chinese community," that recreated as far as possible "something of a Western way of life," and its members chose to socialize with the US Army or other Western relief workers. Several factors predisposed FAU personnel to cocoon themselves: "inadequate language; the size of the group which centres the social interest of the members in group life and created a distinctly foreign atmosphere; and, lastly, the self-sufficiency of this team as a specialized unit." Darling's complaint that FAUers "[take] for granted that Chinese staff are incapable of serious surgical work" and consequently turn their attention to "making up the lack by independent effort" rings true for MT5.[67] Here and elsewhere, impatient FAU physicians often tried to carve out an FAU ward to control practice patient flow and maintain higher standards than within the larger Chinese hospitals. Certainly Darling's evaluation of team life is similar to both John Perry's and Margaret Briggs's description of MT5. Western FAU nurses on MT5 tended to navigate the cultural and professional divide within the parameters set by the FAU physicians. None, however, had to contend with the likes of Ernest Evans or Henry Louderbough.

As we shall see, the debate over the FAU's postwar direction and the continued relevance of its pacifist purpose exacerbated tensions within its ranks. As membership broadened, it remained to be seen whether the new nurses recruited from Canada, Britain, New Zealand, and the United States would find the experience of humanitarian nursing even more conflicted and complex than the first wave of Convoy nurses had. Later it would also become clear whether, in peacetime, they would challenge the views of physicians and Convoy leaders with which they disagreed. As with their predecessors, the diversity of practice settings, team size, geographic location, and combination of politics and personalities imbricated their experience of humanitarian nursing until the Convoy closed its doors. Again, the question arose as to why some would become "authentic knowers" while others simply left.

PART 2

Navigating New Humanitarian Frontiers, 1945–51

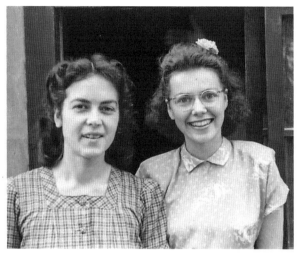

Elizabeth Hughes and Margaret Stanley, Zhengzhou, 1946.
Source: Douglas Clifford Collection

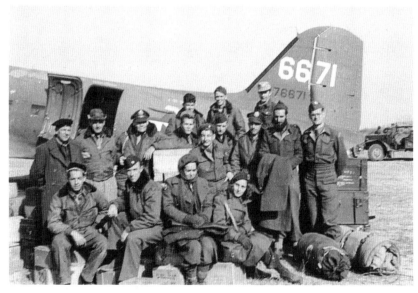

MT19 arrives at Yan'an airfield on 2 December 1946. *Left to right – front row:* Joan Kennedy Woodrow, Elizabeth Hughes. *Middle row:* Douglas Clifford, US Airman, Eric Hughes, Peter Early. *Source:* Douglas Clifford Collection

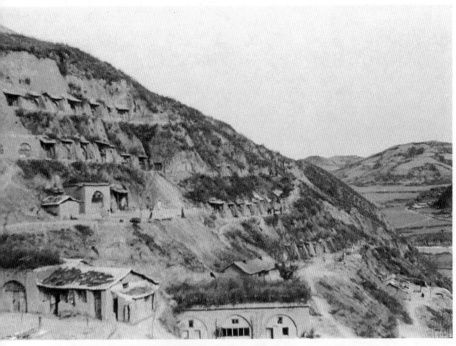

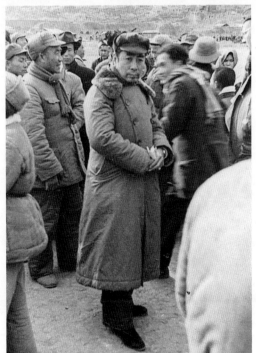

Looking towards the Gates to the International Peace Hospital, where MT19 expected to be stationed. Wards were in the caves scattered across the hillside. *Source:* Douglas Clifford Collection

Zhou Enlai on the airfield in Yan'an, February 1947. *Source:* Douglas Clifford Collection

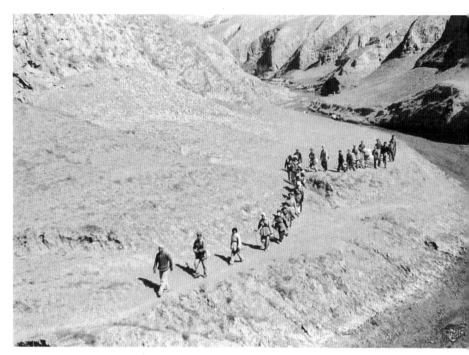

The "girl nurses" leave Si Huai Jia village. *Source:* Douglas Clifford Collection

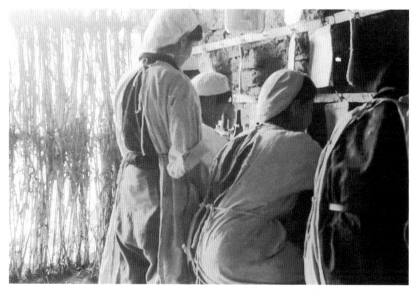

Looking into the nurses' office at Tu Jia Chu. At each village, caves were cleaned out and a new mobile hospital set up. *Source:* Douglas Clifford Collection

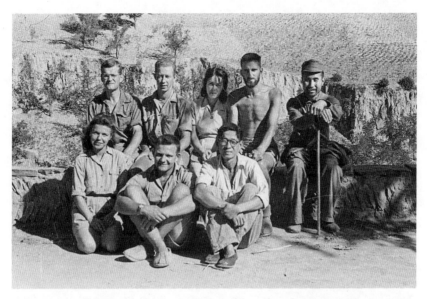

The section at Li Chia Ke J'ai, 12 July 1947. *Left to right – front row:* Margaret Stanley, Frank Miles, Lee Shing P'ei. *Back row:* Unknown, Eric Hughes, Elizabeth Hughes, Jack Dodds, Peter Early. *Source:* Douglas Clifford Collection

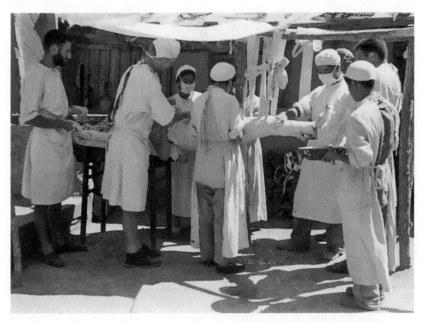

Putting on a plaster hip spica – at Li Chia Ke J'ai, 18 July 1947. *Source:* Douglas Clifford Collection

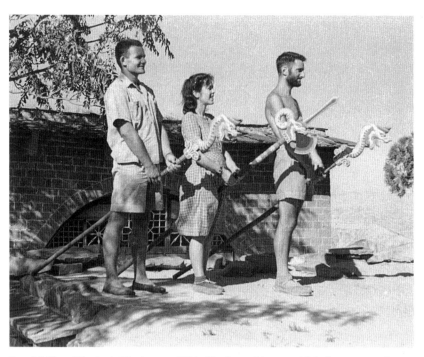

Frank Miles, Elizabeth Hughes, and Eric Hughes with some idols from a temple, 18 July 1947. *Source:* Douglas Clifford Collection

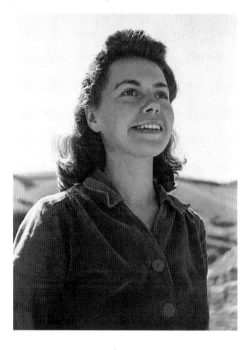

Margaret Stanley at Hsia Pai T'ai, 16 September 1947. *Source:* Douglas Clifford Collection

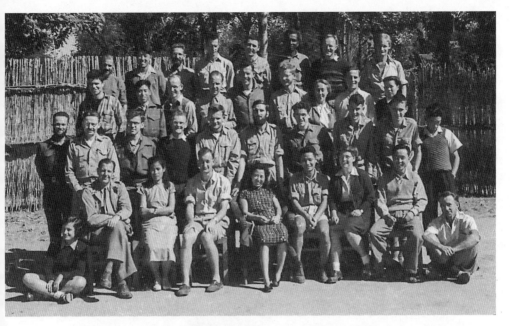

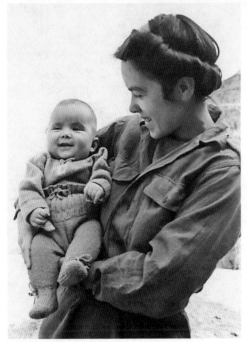

Elizabeth Hughes with son David, age 3½ months, 9 March 1948. *Source:* Douglas Clifford Collection

FAU staff at Zengzhou, 1946. *Left to right – front row:* Doug Turner, George Yang, John Brown, Henry Stokes, Dick Ruddell, John Peters, Delf Fransen, Lindsey Crozier, Johnie Johnson. *Second row:* Mark Shaw, Wang An Min, Dennis Frone, Charlie McDonald, Tim Haworth, John Rue, Cathy Green, Roy Lucas, Julie Chan. *Second front row:* Melvin Rigg, Alf Sidwell, David Jarman, George Theuer, Frank Miles, David Spillet, Charles Cadbury, Peter Mason, Chinese teacher. *Front row:* Kathleen Stokes, Griff Levering, Doris Wu, Neil Johnson, Emma Yang, Choe Sh Yeu, Margaret Renner, Michael Yih, Doug Clifford. *Source:* Margaret Stanley Tesdell Collection

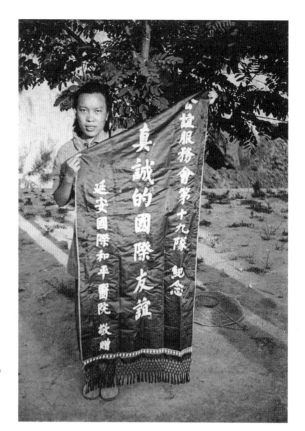

Banner of Friendship made by International Peace Hospital nurses and presented to MT19 on its departure in 1948. *Source:* Douglas Clifford Collection

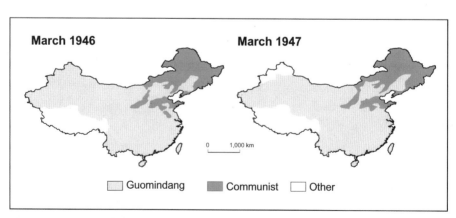

Map 6 Communist-held areas, 1946–47

Military campaign maps cannot fully capture the human tragedy in China between July 1937 and September 1945. The fighting demolished political and administrative institutions, devastated the civilian economy, displaced hundreds of millions of Chinese, and wreaked profound collateral damage. By the spring of 1945, as the Chinese began recapturing Japanese-occupied cities in the interior, and refugees began swarming back to the devastated cities, neither the Chinese government nor the international community could ignore their plight. Rival factions within the new giant international aid agency, the United Nations Relief and Rehabilitation Administration (UNRRA), and within the Chinese government vied for involvement in postwar relief and rehabilitation. Keenly aware that their political, economic, and strategic interests were at stake, all were determined to put their stamp on humanitarianism. In the fall of 1945, the China Convoy shifted its headquarters to Chongqing to lead an ambitious area relief and rehabilitation project, centred primarily in Henan Province. Rehabilitating and running the mission hospitals until their staffs could resume control along with epidemic control would be the first priority.

Between 1945 and 1947, impartiality, neutrality, and organizational integrity continued to be the hallmarks of the Friends Ambulance Unit's pacifist witness. To meet the changing needs of the Chinese people, it strove to carve out new frontiers of humanitarianism, both geographically and intellectually. Convoy leaders reiterated:

> We wish our work to be not merely useful and efficient but rather at all times to be an expression of our Christian Pacifist way of life ... [We] always endeavoured ... to work as far as possible alongside the Chinese peoples working with the Chinese ... The very familiar cliché expressing this intent is working *with* the Chinese people and *not merely for* them. As part of this philosophy, we wish our work to be ... a lasting contribution to China in her effort to rebuild and secure a promising future. Whether it is in the institutions we create, or whatever technical or professional skills we may pass on to our associates, we always hoped to use our small numbers to give the maximum of lasting use to this future. Hence our desire to fill the needs that are not met by others.[1]

The China Convoy, equally determined to create its unique postwar humanitarian niche, now became increasingly planning-minded as it turned its attention to longer-term postwar humanitarian development. The Unit's transition from direct relief to helping people help themselves mirrored the trend within the changing global humanitarian architecture originally anchored in European relief. International direct relief agencies working in Europe ultimately exported their experience to the Middle East and Southeast Asia. These voluntary agencies that had become development agencies had also adopted the philosophy of self-help and were predicated on the twin pillars of humanity and impartiality, purportedly determined by need. As the FAU redirected its humanitarian endeavours, it risked being viewed as politically aligned, not only because of who its financial backers were but because it was moving from direct emergency relief to development work, from emergency work to self-help development projects. Building local capacity and competencies had profound political implications in a country no longer fighting a common enemy but increasingly divided by civil war. Aid became viewed as a political weapon.

Although many agencies "increasingly committed themselves to the principles of impartiality and non-discrimination, in practice they had to decide who had first claim on their resources and identity remained a powerful criterion."[2] As a small faith-based aid agency, the Friends Ambulance Unit and its successor after 1947, the Friends Service Unit, were never immune to those considerations. As international relief agencies, missionary societies, and other private relief organizations crowded China's postwar humanitarian landscape, where to use its scarce resources and distinguishing its unique pacifist identity remained a powerful criteria for determining the future directions of the FAU and FSU. Anxiety among FAUers to avoid entanglements that compromised the Units' institutional integrity and autonomy triggered lively debates of where and with whom to work, especially given the continued need for partnerships to fund their operations. Nowhere was this more apparent than in the Units' relations with UNRRA. The Units' leadership had no intention of allowing the Convoy to be viewed as an appendage of UNRRA.

The creation of the UNRRA by forty-four nations on 9 November 1943 was a defining moment for postwar global humanitarian governance. It heralded the expansion of tasks beneath the humanitarian umbrella: peace and nation building. UNRRA, whose mandate was to coordinate Allied relief, was viewed as a test case for future patterns of international organizations.[3] Designed to prime the liberal economic order and foster democratic governments to preserve a peaceful world order, it was conceived as a vital program not only to save lives but also to safeguard American and British strategic interests. For many of its creators, UNRRA "reflected their faith in the ability to bind compassion and technocracy, to create a muscular, modernized, spirit of progress."[4]

As humanitarianism achieved a global reach during the Second World War, what was happening in China could not be ignored. No UNRRA mission presented a greater challenge than China. The desperate effort to salvage something of the ally that had been propped up in the UN Security Council as a "great power" was ill-timed; China was already imploding economically and politically. It was soon apparent that international aid agencies would confront insurmountable odds in helping the Chinese restore the country's public health programs and medical facilities, even to their prewar levels. The magnitude of its relief task in China, apparent only after the end of the Japanese occupation in August 1945, outstripped UNRRA's capacity, given its other commitments. By the end of the war, half of China's hospitals and field health stations had been destroyed and there was only one physician for every 40,000 patients and one nurse for every 75,000 patients.[5] UNRRA's medical tasks were further complicated by the need to prevent or control epidemics among the millions of Chinese driven from their homes whose immunity had been compromised by malnutrition and who were now swarming homeward without adequate sanitation facilities or food supplies en route. The emergence of cholera, smallpox, and the plague for the first time in over eighty years highlighted the collapse of the quarantine service and public health service in the wake of war. Moreover, before UNRRA could begin to deliver supplies, the "transportation and communication system would have to be rebuilt throughout vast territories roughly equivalent to the entire area overrun by the Axis powers in Europe."[6] The war-induced shortage of supplies, the uncontrolled inflation of the Chinese economy, which fuelled a dramatic increase in black market activities in medical equipment and supplies, and the lack of adequate medical personnel hindered UNRRA's medical initiatives from November 1944 until its wind-up in November 1947. The quality of Chinese medical education had declined dramatically during the war and was symptomatic of the pervasive wartime corrosion of the public health system nationwide. In China, as elsewhere, UNRRA "underwent severe growing pains; a greater degree of organizational stability was achieved only after many administrative shake-ups, including major changes of policy by the Administration and by the Chinese government, along with a series of operational crises accompanied by a rapid turnover of personnel."[7]

Not surprisingly, UNRRA's trials tainted its relationship with the FAU and constrained the Unit's ability to deliver humanitarian relief. Whatever its reservations about UNRRA's checkered performance, "being a small organization with very limited resources," the FAU depended on UNRRA for assistance.[8] With the establishment of UNRRA, however, charitable organizations in the Middle East and Europe, which were required to work under its umbrella, had become "subservient to Allied occupying armies and international agencies."[9] That was especially distasteful to the independent-minded FAUers. The heated debate over its relationship with UNRRA peppered several editions of the FAU's newsletter. For some Unit members, it was tempting to become part of the UNRRA machinery – "a dozen of the most experienced of us could get fat jobs tomorrow, and in those jobs we would be doing a far bigger service for China." There were equally strong reasons for resisting the temptation to work under UNRRA. If the Unit remained determined "to make a witness based on its beliefs," then it "must preserve its identity in a clear-cut fashion, and also its right to choose the sort of work which can give expression to that witness."[10] While the early days of UNRRA/FAU cooperation were fraught with difficulty on both sides, by May 1946 the Unit had established a permanent agent in Kaifeng to coordinate its efforts with the both UNRRA and the Chinese National Relief and Rehabilitation Administration (CNRRA). Over time, the FAU would develop a symbiotic relationship with UNRRA, seconding personnel to staff UNRRA/CNRRA programs and drawing on it to fund purchases of medical and relief supplies vital for its rehabilitation and development programs.[11] At the same time, it took every opportunity to ensure that Communist areas under the jurisdiction of the China Liberated Areas Relief Association (CLARA) received UNRRA supplies denied by the CNRRA.

Other changes were also brewing that further complicated its humanitarian exchanges. "A garden of dragon's teeth was sprouting" as McClure headed for Henan in the fall of 1945.[12] Maintaining a semblance of neutrality, impartiality, and autonomy of action as civil war spread throughout the country presented a new set of challenges to the FAU. General George Marshall, representing President Harry Truman, was given the unenviable task of building a coalition government comprising all contending political/military parties in China. By the time he arrived to negotiate a ceasefire, the country had been embroiled in a civil war for two decades, and the power bases of the two sides had shifted after the Japanese invasion. Recently, revisionist historians have emphasized the damage that the Sino-Japanese and Pacific

Wars did to Chiang Kai-shek's prospects, thereby setting the stage for the rise of the Communist Party.[13] Despite the uneasy anti-Japanese alliance between the Guomindang and the Communist Party of China (CPC), neither lost sight of the Asian war's implications for the civil war. Neither was prepared to relinquish control over the territories it had seized in the wake of the Japanese surrender. In fact, the Communists, who controlled wide areas in north and central China, quickly extended their control of Manchuria when the Russians withdrew. The Americans, endorsing Chiang's regime as the government of all China, began airlifting Nationalist troops into cities that had been under Communist control. Despite repeated efforts by General Marshall to broker an agreement for a coalition government, by 1946 the two sides were engaged in a full-scale civil war. The termination of the Marshall mission particularly affected the fate of the FAU team that had been dispatched to the Communist wartime capital, Yan'an.

Moreover, the old guard was changing within the Convoy. The repatriation of the original "holy forty" founding members, the majority of them British, during 1945–46 marked a watershed in the China Convoy's history. Their departure heralded the transition of its administrative control from London to Philadelphia. As important, by June 1946, Robert McClure's time with the Convoy came to a close. Acknowledging that his departure left a "very large gap on the Council," Griffith Levering, then chairman of the Convoy, speculated that it would be "difficult to find elsewhere the energy of planning and the China wiseness, coming from more than thirty years of residence in this country which have been available to us from Bob."[14] But would the departure of the old guard be accompanied by change in the Convoy's ethos predicated on its non-evangelistic pacifist witness? The postwar organization would certainly be more international. The influx of New Zealanders, Canadians, and more Americans brought new energy, skills, and enthusiasm. The newcomers were, however, as strong-minded and colourful as the original "holy forty." While they owed their allegiance to the Unit and were purportedly sympathetic to its pacifist principles, few abandoned their nationalistic characteristics or pacifist perspectives forged in very different circumstances. Clashes in personality and divergent perspectives on its mandate threatened the pacifist fabric that had tenuously bound the fiercely democratically minded group together. Disputes between the "faith" and the "work" factions peppered the debate on where and how the Unit should work.

The prospect of longer postwar service terms rekindled heated discussions over other long-standing controversies. The Unit's cardinal philosophy of working *with,* not *for,* the Chinese people would continue to be questioned as a pattern for its postwar work. As one member admitted:

> I am on touchy ground now, but I think that there has been too much wooly thinking about "getting close to the Chinese." I think we should frankly realize our limitations in this area and avoid unnecessary frustration. It is one thing to "understand" the Chinese, and another to "become" one. Become is perhaps too strong a word for the position ... Attempts to undo the cultural fabric that is woven into us and then adopt Chinese culture and all it implies seems to me to be wasting our energies.[15]

Other Convoy members voiced renewed concern over the questions of couples, especially interracial marriages, and women's safety and health during pregnancies. As Bronson Clark put it, "children being raised in Shanghai are one thing; in the field is quite another. The dangers to health are so great that many problems arise. Missionaries have not constructed walls for nothing. Yet we in the [Unit] oppose these walls, and rightly so. But let us clearly understand the price."[16] One nurse's decision to have a child while campaigning in the field highlighted this dilemma.

After the decision was reached at the September 1945 Yearly Meeting to concentrate FAU efforts in the Henan region, McClure led a spearhead team to survey prospects for an area project that encompassed eight separate schemes. In addition to rehabilitating mission hospitals, the Henan project prioritized an ambitious epidemic control program for kala-azar (also known as visceral leishmaniasis), a disease spread by sandflies. Plans were also considered for the care and control of refugees all over Henan Province through establishment of ten transit camps with medical services and five industrial holding camps for longer-term care and rehabilitation of refugees – this at a time when the damage caused by the breaking of the Yellow River dikes prevented refugees from returning to their homes.[17]

The Convoy, however, left a diverse legacy that included programs outside the Henan area. Gripping stories of its work in medical transport continue to command scholars' attention.[18] Innovative programs to train medical mechanics, laboratory technicians, and physical therapists seconded to the Union Hospital at Hankou were also an important part of its medical legacy.[19] Not all can be included here.

The vignettes of nurses' humanitarian work featured in this section were chosen as representative of the ethical and logistical challenges that FAU- and

FSU-run projects encountered in attempting to deliver humanitarian aid across political, cultural, and institutional lines from the summer of 1945 until the FSU assumed control in 1947. Clashes in perspectives pivoting on the treatment of Chinese colleagues marred the humanitarian exchanges of Western Convoy nurses wherever they worked. Most of the new recruits lacked cross-cultural experience. With time in the field, some gained greater appreciation of why Chinese nursing practice differed; others simply got on with the job at hand or left.

The shift from emergency medical work to relief and rehabilitation began well before the move to Henan; in fact, FAU leaders viewed the experience in building and devolving hospitals in southwestern China as models for their future work. Chapter 6 therefore examines the contested experiences of Chinese and Western nurses during the transition from wartime to the establishment of the Unit in Henan. It offers new insights on how these devolution experiences shaped the decision to relocate to that province. Chapter 7 appraises nurses' conflicted roles in the Unit's efforts to rehabilitate mission hospitals in Henan and its repeated attempt to negotiate access to work within both Communist-held and Nationalist territories. After early rebuffs in Henan, it was the only Western humanitarian organization to deliver tons of medical supplies and to send a medical team to Yan'an, the Communists' wartime capital. Chapter 8 follows the story of MT19's unanticipated work as a mobile army surgical hospital (MASH) unit with Mao Zedong's 8th Route Army across northern China. It examines the personal and professional challenges faced by humanitarian providers working across cultural boundaries and, deliberately or not, venturing into the world of politics.

6 The Road to Henan
Plagues, Cholera, and Devilish Devolutions, 1944–45

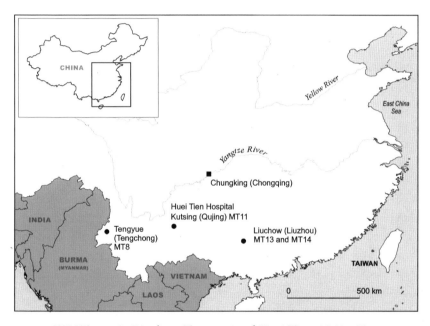

Map 7 FAU Teams in Liuzhou, Tengyue, and Huei Tien, 1944–45

For the first time it was becoming apparent that Chinese troops
could be expected to push the Japanese out of their strongholds.
The Unit was thus faced with an opportunity for work much after
its own heart, that of relief and rehabilitation where the hand of
war had recently been ravaging. A very comprehensive policy
emerged, largely, it is fair to say, out of Bob's [McClure's] inspiration
and knowledge, but in quite a natural way appealing to the Unit
universally. It was that our teams should act as forward units for
rehabilitation, to follow close on the heels of advancing armies on
any front, and step into the re-occupied cities to set up medical
facilities. We should establish hospitals in a way that local authorities
would consider them their responsibility, and that local staff and
support would be found during the FAU period upon which it could
"devolve" at the end of half a year or year. We would bring with us
an accumulation of experience in the special requirements for
setting up hospitals ... and most of all, bring a foreign type of "push,"
which is often not native. What could be a more fitting expression
of our wish to serve? It is work that is lasting in effect, an expression
of good will in practical terms and of the desire to serve where
there is suffering from the effects of war and it is work to which
we are especially suited perhaps more than other organizations.

– JOHN PERRY

John Perry presumed that China's health services could be rehabilitated
and modernized without being contaminated by politics. Several factors not
mentioned in his account contributed to the Friends Ambulance Unit's shift
to civilian medical work. As the Chinese military assumed greater administrative control over medical work, opportunities for military work dried up.
The FAU could not meet the Chinese military's new criteria that called for
mobile hospital units of over thirty personnel.[1] In July 1944, the Unit was
informed that "no further teams were required and with the end of the war
shortly afterwards finally closed this chapter of the FAU's medical work."[2]
When civilian work in southwestern China subsequently encountered unexpected roadblocks, the Unit reconsidered where and how it would work.

Typically, Robert McClure had taken it on himself to create the blueprint
for future United Nations Relief and Rehabilitation Administration (UNRRA)
hospitals by building one. According to his biographer, the turning point in

his career came in 1944, with the building of the Tengchong hospital in Yunnan Province. "He was finally feeling the exhilaration of dreams come true. The Westerners were finally working not for the Chinese but with the Chinese." McClure wrote: "This is our idea of what an UNRRA hospital should be, and the fact that it is not yet adopted by its rightful parents doesn't bother us in the least." Tengyue, Nantan, and Liuzhou were viewed as testing the UNRRA scheme as an opening for the FAU's future work. Arguing that "no other organization in China has tried to do this type of work," McClure felt totally justified in using Canadian Red Cross money to equip the hospital. "The Canadian Red Cross, like U.N.R.R.A., was still blissfully unaware that it had gone pioneering with McClure."[3]

The experiences of Harriet Brown and Doris Woodward on FAU spearhead teams in recently reoccupied cities take centre stage to illuminate the opportunities and perils of humanitarian work that ultimately led the Unit to relocate to Henan. As the only two Western FAU nurses involved, their stories are unique; nonetheless, there are issues that resonate across Western nurses' earlier work elsewhere in the field. The stories of Brown and Woodward intersect with those of the Chinese nursing students recruited by Doris Wu from Lian Ta University (United College of Yunnan) to meet the China Convoy's dire need for nurses. The six "Kunming girls," as they were affectionately called, regarded the FAU as a stepping stone to medical careers or a better life. More immediately, they elected to work for the FAU for one to two years as an alternative to serving with the Chinese Army Women's Corps. Liu Lung-chien (Jean), Hsu Kwang-hsin (Elizabeth), Shen Ming-chen (Constance), Chiu T'ing-hsien (Juliet), and Hoh Kwang-ch'u (Ruth Ho) were all well-educated Christian women. Three of the Kunming university students who received rudimentary nursing training with Brown and Woodward provide a critical lens with which to explore Chinese nurses' cross-cultural relationships and contribution to the life and work of the Convoy. Collectively, their stories from the field demonstrate how gender, race, and politics shaped nursing as it was imagined and practised at a hinge point in the history of China and the Convoy.

In the spring of 1944, while recuperating in Canada from a bout of relapsing fever, Robert McClure fired up efforts that had been under way for over a year to recruit Canadians for the China Convoy. McClure masterfully spun stories of a unit that offered opportunities for "adventure, danger and service that was in line with the most demanding conscience."[4] Recruiting conscientious objectors eager to serve overseas was just the first step, however. His assistance was required to overcome the reluctance of the Canadian government to issue permits for the conscientious objectors to serve abroad and, more significantly, to allow nurses to leave Canada during wartime. Audaciously, McClure told Canadian officials that sending two nurses to China now would do more to redress Canada's tarnished image in China – for having sold Japan strategic war materiel – than ten nurses sent out later "under some government appointment." Even after Ottawa granted approval, "the Government carefully demanded secrecy to avoid public attention and possible discussion of this pacifist endeavour."[5] More than a year would pass before those who answered McClure's call to service arrived in China.

For the first Canadian nurse to volunteer for work with the China Convoy, the road from nursing school in Toronto to Henan would set the course for her future. When war broke out, Harriet Brown was a nursing student at Toronto's Hospital for Sick Children. Having absorbed her pacifist views from an elder brother, accepting his argument that "it was wrong to kill, no one wins in a war," she supported his decision to take a stand against war as a conscientious objector. Canada's entry into the war forced Harriet to confront the strength of her own Christian pacifism. Although a devout member of the United Church, attending services when preachers were blessing the departing soldiers in flag-draped buildings "turned me off and I stopped going to the established Church." Years later, recalling her defiance when summoned to the nursing director's office to explain her reluctance to volunteer for military service, she remained adamant about her feelings: "I was sure about what I felt, and was glad to tell her why." In 1944, while doing public health nursing in Toronto, she began looking for avenues "to serve mankind" without violating her pacifist convictions. A former classmate, whose fiancé had served with the China Convoy from 1941 to 1943, directed her to the Canadian Society of Friends. Understandably, she was amenable to the idea of service to heal the wounds of war, "so I simply signed up to go to China."[6]

The delay associated with getting a visa for a nurse to China in wartime Canada meant that she joined the second Canadian party in April 1945 at Pendle Hill, the Quaker Study Center near Philadelphia. Her time there was followed by additional briefings at UNRRA's Maryland training centre. Like other Canadians, she believed that the Pendle Hill backgrounders were superior to those offered by UNRRA staff. "Old China Hands" with extensive and recent experience in doing medical work in China, such as Ken Bennett, gave detailed instruction in Chinese language and culture, and FAU work in China. But for Harriet Brown, "the loveliest and most important thing that happened" at Pendle Hill "was the development of group life ... sharing work, study, recreation and worship with the common desire of expressing the spiritual life." They were "determined to find a way of living which did away with the causes of war [within] a brotherly community."[7]

At Pendle Hill, Harriet came into contact with Canadian conscientious objectors whose idealistic brand of pacifism had been "expanded to include not only the traditional religious witness to non-resistance but a growing social activism as well."[8] By the time of her departure, she had become engaged to fellow Canadian recruit Walter Alexander, a conscientious objector with leftist political leanings. After graduating from college, Walter had a job for several years helping people in rural areas to work together, and his experience dispelled the idea that the "world could be changed by any kind of social order 'without spirituality.'"[9] Marriage during wartime, they were told, was out of the question, so Harriet enthusiastically agreed "to be dispatched, encumbered only by the knapsack on her back, wherever necessary."[10] Her personnel file from Pendle Hill indicated that she had made a good impression as a "deeply concerned and responsible person." The twenty-seven-year-old Canadian nurse was described as "quiet, unobtrusive rather 'English' but more 'efficient than surface appearances' suggested."[11] And, as predicted, "inexperienced in travel," Harriet would find China "a very big adventure."[12]

It took her some time to find her feet after her arrival in March 1945 at the FAU hospital in Qujing (MT11), where all FAU recruits were routinely oriented to Chinese medical conditions. Having enthusiastically imagined "what this new life and work [would] demand of us,"[13] Harriet later admitted, "hospital life here was a great shock to me – coming from the orderly Sick Children's."[14] A simple wooden structure, it had bare floors and no windows except in the operating rooms, and its beds were only planks on trestles. Hospital nursing routines bore little resemblance to those of Toronto. Patients' families stayed to cook their food at a small fire near the bed. In this hospital, where instruments were sterilized in boiling water over a charcoal fire, she "learned to do without all the things [she had] thought were essential back home."[15] For the first time, she faced the grim reality of medical work in China: "We have to leave much undone and yet try not to lose our ideals of caring for the sick." And gradually she came to accept that, with training on the job, "a United Church minister can make a fine anaesthetist and a farmer can learn to do a dressing as tenderly and skillfully as a trained nurse."[16] Her difficulties in adjusting and constant need for assurance left some colleagues initially questioning whether she was cut out for Convoy life.[17] She would prove that she was.

For Harriet, Christian pacifism provided a moral compass to navigate her overwhelming feeling of "being suddenly reborn into an ancient civilization." There was a significant caveat, however. She cautioned others against trying "to compare or use our standards here," for it "only serves to confuse and cause misunderstanding," especially when conveying the Christian message. In her view, rather than imposing Western theology, Christianity must be demonstrated in a practical way that held meaning for the Chinese people. Her personal cultural shock was mitigated by "a deep feeling of unity and fellowship" within the Unit that "stems from our common will to show the love of God to others by our way of life."[18] Her time in China began as a personal spiritual odyssey to bear witness and share China's suffering, not to proselytize.

As Harriet Brown wrote home from Qujing, her arrival in China coincided with a watershed in the Convoy's history: "Unit plans are changing – old members going home – thirty new ones arrived and others en route – type of work and demands and needs greatly changing ... We never know when or where we are going."[19] As the Japanese retreated from towns, the FAU teams entered and negotiated with local officials, UNRRA, and the missionary societies to provide emergency medical relief, epidemic control, and public health education. Eagerly anticipating "the happy plans ... afoot to push eastward and help re-establish refugees in towns,"[20] she was instead dispatched to Liuzhou, a devastated city teeming with cholera. The third-largest city to be recaptured from the Japanese, over three-quarters of it had been destroyed.

Along with UNRRA personnel, MT13 and MT14 (as the Liuzhou teams were designated) organized delousing teams, set up temporary refugee hostels, and gradually instituted more orderly routines within the makeshift hospitals. Before Harriet and the bulk of the team arrived, Robert McClure flew down to set up two temporary cholera hospitals, one on either side of the river, and unilaterally made arrangements for their funding from the Chinese National Relief and Rehabilitation Administration (CNRRA).[21] According to John Perry, assigned to oversee Unit operations, "Bob had left things rather a mess as far as personal relations went, with almost every other body in the city feeling offended and resentful." Consequently, Perry set aside medical work in the cholera hospitals until he had rebuilt the frayed relationships.

Harriet Brown was on the spearhead team dispatched to the cholera hospitals. On the north bank, American physician Art Barr set up in a burned-out Roman Catholic monastery. On the other side of the river, in an open compound with bamboo beds and bamboo poles holding "infusion bottles," Harriet did triage with a New Zealand physician, Graham Milne, who had been seconded to the FAU pending the return of South China Mission staff. Two Unit members "trained in some basic first aid procedures" salvaged buckets and other items, and kept a drum filled with water from the river full and a fire going to boil instruments and provide safe water. The two took turns caring for the patients at night.

Each day, the nurse and the doctor went back across the river to sleep, returning the next day with more supplies. Their daily journey offered harsh reminders of the difficult decisions and exhausting day that lay ahead. Almost every morning, "a yellow bloated body was carried past them ... It was easier for the refugees making their slow return home to use the waterway to carry their dead."[22]

Harriet Brown and Graham Milne made a strong team. Each respected the other's professional skill, but there was affection also, for they had learned "to care for each other's welfare on the road, in coping with the disease and wounds of those they had been sent to help." Both were altruistic but humble; both perceived their humanitarian mission as "sharing their talents with folks in need."[23]

Her circular letters, written to share with family and Canadian Friends, admitted: "Those were grim days ... Cholera patients are a horrible spectacle when you see them for the first time."[24] Careful to avoid any disappointment in her performance, she emphasized that "seeing life return to a corpse-like figure was encouragement enough." In reality, all too often families simply abandoned their kin to die in the hospital courtyard.

How the young nurse coped with unremitting human suffering was captured in Milne's tender memoir written after his return home, "Two Women." Milne recalled that a mud-covered skeletal body left to die inside the gate did not repulse Harriet; rather, she saw only the hopelessness and terror on another young woman's face. She explained, "I know I can't do much, but I would like her to feel some love from another human being before she dies." She gently removed the rags "from her emaciated body, washed, wrung dry and covered her again. The hair, encrusted thick with black mud, was washed clean ... and softly combed. Harriet sat crossed legged beside her, holding her hand, moistening her mouth, one hand touching the brow and sunken cheeks. She sat otherwise motionless, looking only into the gazing eyes in a pool of stillness that separated the two women from the heat and turmoil around them." Then, as he watched, Harriet slowly raised her head, acknowledging the woman's death "by gently closing the eyelids ... and kiss[ing] the cold lips." Her colleague moved a few yards to meet and comfort her. "With tears brimming in her dark eyes," she squeezed his hand and said, "Thanks, I'm OK. Let's get on."[25] While this was an intensely personal encounter, Harriet Brown's ability to provide compassionate care at the end of life's journey sustained her through the tough days ahead. Word of the young nurse's compassion and composure during the cholera epidemic spread throughout the Unit.[26] It resonated because others also understood the human cost of caring.

The team extended its stay beyond the height of the cholera epidemic to support the CNRRA's medical services to returning refugees. Harriet Brown joined John Perry to start a small cottage hospital in Liuzhou to deal with malaria, dysentery, and malnutrition among the refugees. Here, she gradually felt a closer connection with the Chinese community and was exhilarated by the work. Publicly, she described the early days of the hospital as "a game – setting it up from nothing, working together as a team (and a quite happy one at that), the thrill of receiving our first patients ... Our patients were firstly refugees in terrible states of starvation and disease, and then the permanent citizens of the city began to come."[27] But to her fellow FAUers she painted a starker picture of coping with the heavy caseload of critically ill patients: "The mortality can be called definitely high ... since the conditions in which the patients arrive is low to extreme and we get only the sickest of the most destitute refugee population. Many cases are sent in, quite frankly, at death's door to die here ... the medical stores are hopelessly inadequate to handle this situation."[28] Significantly, in her public account back home, she failed to reveal that she had contracted malaria from overwork.

Similarly, her description of their "adventure" in devolving the hospital, written for the Quaker Friends and Unit members' families in Canada, was more upbeat than John Perry's account. While she also admitted that "difficulties no end beset you – political, financial, and technical, and every day the situation was critical and different," she emphasized that "things have smoothed out now though and there is an almost complete Chinese staff of varying abilities. It was encouraging to us to see this new kind of China, progressive, enlightened, educated, after the backwardness of Yunnan."[29] In contrast, the more skeptical Perry described the doctor designated to take over the hospital's administration as "not only a know-nothing, but a crook as well; besides he hasn't got the funds to pay his staff, and stands a chance of losing them all." Perry was trying to "wriggle out of our commitments to him" and devolve the hospital to the county medical staff "headed by a German-trained man, with a lot of pep and go." The process, he admitted, was akin "to cross[ing] a pot full of eggs by walking over them without breaking any."[30] In the end, the team pulled up stakes to begin work at another mission hospital without assurance that the hospital they were leaving would survive.

Jack Dodds, one of the last FAUers to leave Liuzhou, provided perhaps the most judicious appraisal of the Convoy's experience there. Reflecting on the team's contribution and the challenges they faced, he wrote: "UNRRA/CNRRA has not worked out so well. If it had not been for the [FAU] staff sent down ... and the co-operation of the American army, there would have been no treatment for cholera patients from the coast."[31] Dodds, like Perry, was proud that FAU teams responded more quickly than the CNRRA, which they charged was entangled in red tape and politics.[32]

Harriet Brown's orders were different from those of her teammates, however. She and Walter Alexander received separate instructions to proceed to Qujing, where they were married on 27 January 1946. As Harriet said: "When the [FAU] Council says get married there is nothing to do but obey!"[33] She remained in Qujing for several weeks, helping at the hospital in preparation for its devolution as the Unit made ready to move to Henan. Following their honeymoon, the couple joined the Unit in Zhengzhou, Henan Province.

En route to Zhengzhou, Harriet and Walter spent two weeks at Keinshui to discuss plans for the rehabilitation of the hospital's physical plant and the opening of a nursing school. Both considered their time there well spent. During their stay, Harriet typically discussed nursing procedures and began training a dresser while covering the outpatient department.[34] The Alexanders' time as a married couple in Henan would be short-lived, however, for they left China on 27 September 1946. The Unit was informed simply that Harriet's poor health forced their early repatriation. Actually, her pregnancy complicated the treatments available for her repeated bouts of malaria.[35] When treated with Atabrine (mepacrine), she exhibited "signs of severe drug intoxication," and the alternative, quinine, was contraindicated during pregnancy.

The memory of an FAU physician's suicide due to Atabrine poisoning clearly informed the decision. There was no choice but to repatriate the couple so that Harriet could "obtain more effective anti-malaria treatment."[36]

Personality, individual faith, and training shaped Western nurses' individual adaptation to Convoy life. Gendered and professional expectations coloured others' evaluation of their private and work lives. From the perspective of Convoy leaders, Harriet Brown was the epitome of a respectable Christian woman of "great ability and the deepest motivation."[37] While British nurses had also commented on the sexual tension caused by their presence, Harriet always believed that as an engaged woman she was regarded as "off limits" from unwanted sexual attention, and the "brotherly" protection she experienced within the FAU family provided a safety net that mitigated her loneliness far from home and from Walter.[38] Unlike the British nurses who attended separate women's training camps, Harriet also had the benefit of being part of the Canadian group that had bonded during their stay at Pendle Hill.

In responding to human suffering, she found her ideas about nursing practice altered. Western perceptions based on hygiene, notions of efficiency, strict hospital routines, and careful patient observation collided with the realities of "bare bones" nursing in China. The Qujing hospital's devolution in particular was disappointing, in Harriet's view. Believing that it would "completely fold up," she found it difficult "not to come out of it bitter, cynical and defeated." In her opinion, "with a great effort and, in a short time, we could build up and run ourselves a Western hospital but we did not even approach the real problem of training Chinese to take over themselves and to even want to have to make the necessary sacrifices for it." The experience triggered considerable introspection. There was, as she realized, "much more in living and working here, most of which we haven't yet discovered."[39] Relying on nursing's core value of caring, she found it easier to accommodate Western nursing standards to primitive China's hospital settings than to reconcile her spiritual quest for peace and social justice with the legacy of the Convoy endeavours.

Harriet left China grateful "for the lovely experiences with the Chinese and with our fellow-foreigners," but more for this "period [that brought] us face to face with the bitterest human problems and urging us to a growth in faith which must result." She was changed by her humanitarian exchanges within Chinese communities. Her idealized version of humanitarianism, "to show the love of God to others by our way of life," did not fit the real situation in China, and she became disappointed by the corruption and seeming indifference to human life that she witnessed in Nationalist China.[40] In all likelihood, the young wife increasingly identified with her husband's growing desire for a stronger exposition of the Christian message in conjunction with the Unit's relief work – a position that was decidedly unwelcome among the majority of Convoy members.[41] The Alexanders were linked to other dissident Convoy members who were considering the possibility of forming a small Christian-based community to undertake long-term work in China.[42] After they returned to Canada, they "could not go back to living just for ourselves and our families ... we had to find a bigger purpose." In joining the Bruderhof, an international Christian communal movement, in 1954, they made a commitment "to living in service to others and finding relationships of trust and sharing with those around us."[43]

For one British nurse, Doris Woodward, the challenge of maintaining an acceptable lifestyle proved more difficult than the professional transition to humanitarian work. While she and Harriet Brown had parallel experiences with unsatisfactory hospital devolutions, their professional and personal journeys were remarkably different. Doris's experience reaffirms that Convoy life simultaneously recast and constrained women's gendered roles.

Originally intent on doing missionary work, Doris Woodward was a fully qualified state-registered nurse with additional training in ophthalmology. The records offer little insight into the strength or origins of her pacifist position. She had considered missionary work. In all likelihood, volunteering with the FAU offered more immediate prospect for overseas service than mission work during the Japanese occupation.

Doris arrived at the FAU's Huei Tien Hospital in Qujing on 23 September 1944. Acting as matron and theatre sister, she shouldered considerable responsibility. In addition, she was expected to cover the hospital's maternity work, which had increased dramatically. Her efforts to westernize the hospital received praise in the January 1945 *Newsletter,* which noted that

> as matron she has effected some remarkable improvements in the nursing side of the hospital, the discipline of the staff has been improved; the wards are clean and tidy and the patients are regularly washed, blanketed, and bathed. All the hospital laundry is boiled after laundering and the other bedding is deloused. The nurses now distribute the food, instead of the servants, and the nurses are encouraged to give more attention to the patients.[44]

While Doris Woodward's initiative and the arrival of trained Chinese "refugee nurses" were credited with the improvement in patient care and number of patients treated, a new hospital delousing station and the greater availability of bedding and drugs certainly contributed to the improvement in nursing services.[45] The hospital had also received a windfall of supplies from the US Army as it prepared to withdraw from the city.

As it turned out, plans to transfer Doris Woodward from Huei Tien were complicated by several considerations. She had been scheduled to go to MT5 at Baoshan, but only if Doris Wu did not "jib too severely at going to MT8 at Tengchong [Tengyue]."[46] While the preference was to find a Chinese nurse to lead the nursing school there, Woodward was viewed as "most likely to make a much better job than any of our other foreign nurses in the Tengchung [Tengchong] situation." She had "an excellent record in management of the Chinese staff at Huei Tien and in the training of people like Miss (Mohei) Yang, and it is that sort of quality which Tengchong [Tengyue] seems to need just now."[47] But her transfer to Tengyue had to be postponed when the Chinese nurse, Miss Pun, proved incapable in the Unit's estimation of taking over the matron's job in Qujing. "Were Doris [Woodward] to leave now, the nursing standards would slump rapidly."[48] The difficulties in devolving Huei Tien reaffirmed Robert McClure's view that the Unit should adopt a more practical approach to training medical practitioners that anticipated China's future barefoot doctor approach to primary health. "Our medical staff can train junior staff, our nurses can train sub-standard workers for smaller clinics."[49] As we saw, Tengyue became the FAU's trial balloon for the Unit's postwar community work.

It was June 1945 before Doris Woodward replaced the British missionary seconded nurse Nancy Harris at Tengyue. At the time of her arrival, the hospital's facilities had been upgraded, and there was much talk of opening a rural clinic, expanding maternal health programs within the hospital, and training local midwives, as well as sharing the hospital laboratories with local practitioners. The training program included four Chinese university students on a short course, as well as the regular program leading to accreditation. There were high hopes for the nursing school: "The teaching is impressive blackboard and all. [Chinese physician] Jim Chai taught first aid and physiology, [New Zealand physician] Douglas Clifford taught bandaging, [British Red Cross nurse] Peggy Toop general nursing, [American Chinese physician] George Yang anatomy, and Dave Stafford English, with set hours for lectures and assignments."[50] While Doris was not directly involved in the formal teaching, she oversaw instruction in the wards. Equally important, she solicited McClure's aid to secure financial support for local Chinese girls who wanted to study nursing.

Unfortunately, Woodward arrived after the end of what staff referred to as a "happy-go-lucky period" and remained through the acrimonious devolution, characterized by continued financial shortfalls and growing staff shortages.[51] As the optimistic vision for the hospital as the centre of a wider community-based program gradually dissipated, morale plummeted. Earlier arrangements to cooperate with local organizations, "again under Bob's steering hand,"[52] began to unravel. The FAU had negotiated with the Yunnan Burma Highway Engineers working nearby on road construction to dedicate one third of the hospital facilities to care for their employees if they guaranteed one third of the equipment and operating cost of the hospital. The FAU would also train their clinical staff. But when the Highway Engineers pulled out, the hospital lost both key financial backing and staff.

The high levels of staff turnover took their toll. When British Red Cross nurses Fern King and Peggy Toop were repatriated, two trained Chinese nurses replaced them, "proving valuable additions to the team especially in the training program."[53] However, the Chinese sister tutor who had come from Qujing remained for only a short period:

The departure of her husband [who had been working with the Yunnan Burma Highway Engineers] probably influenced her, but in addition she did not like the place much, there wasn't a proper lecture room, there were no proper nurses quarters, there were no teaching accessories, there were no textbooks, or charts or any of the paraphernalia required for the job.

By July 1945, the local girls were reluctant to enrol in a nursing program "unless it will eventually make them qualified nurses." The prospects of finding a replacement sister tutor were not good without "a good school to come to, with enough pupils to justify her existence there."[54] On 6 October 1945, the *Newsletter* reported that all the trained Chinese nurses had left, and it was proving impossible to replace them. "It is too isolated a place for nurses to work and live contentedly, unless they are really concerned people with a desire to serve in a very deserving place."[55] Their exodus again speaks to

Chinese nurses' ability to assess and seek future options that were more advantageous.

The FAU staff struggled to provide rudimentary nursing training to students who remained. The team's hope that the Border Mission of the Church of Christ in China would run the hospital were dashed in late December. The mission wanted to avoid possible tensions with the CNRRA, which planned to do work here, "chiefly as usual, because they have vast stocks in Yunnan and it is either inconvenient or too expensive to send them to the newly liberated area."[56] Despite the news, the team, believing that the hospital was finding a place in the community, expressed "a strong concern that the hospital should not be abandoned." Doris Woodward was among those who offered to remain until the following March in the hope that a qualified physician could be found as superintendent for the hospital.[57] But once the majority of the team pulled out in March, "it [was] a losing game," because "the FAU team [was] so small it [did] not hold the whip hand ... the local committee is romping off on its own ways. Politics and selfish interest bog the whole thing down."[58] By the time the final FAUer left, UNRRA had sent a doctor and nurse for a year, but beyond that the hospital's future remained uncertain.

But what was team life like for Doris Woodward during this trying period? Just prior to leaving for Qujing to marry Harriet Brown, hospital manager Walter Alexander wrote to his sister, "You would enjoy meeting everyone on the team." In particular, he described Doris as "extremely conscientious – too much so but not unhappily so." She would, he said, "do anything asked, and gladly, full of fun, can have a sharp tongue but very sensitive to others."[59]

Edwin Abbott replaced Walter Alexander in early December 1945. As he described the rump FAU team, it was "very short of nurses. Doris Woodward (FAU) and a YBH nurse (Miss Wong) are the only grads. However there are several grand kids acting as 'undergrad nurses.'"[60] FAU officials had been at many meetings in Kunming with the parents of Elizabeth Hsu Kwang-hsin and Constance Shen Ming-chen before they consented to allow their daughters to work with the FAU as stepping stone to studying in the United States to become physicians. These university girls had the "kind of background and intelligence necessary for good training and were quick to catch on." Equally important, they filled a critical gap when the Burmese student nurses "took it into their heads to take off for home despite their promise to remain for a year."[61] Constance, who had volunteered just two months before her graduation from the high school,[62] "proved herself to be highly intelligent and has tackled unfamiliar work in conditions of some hardship with excellent spirit."[63] After only six months, the seventeen-year-old assumed charge of the operating theatre in Tengyue.

Abbott worked hard, helping out in civilian clinics, covering nursing shifts on the wards, and giving public health lectures. Reading his letters, however, leaves a strong impression that team life more than compensated for the administrative headaches and long hours. "The people here," he wrote, are "a grand group. It is refreshing to come to a group that has their [Quaker] worship meetings each morning."[64] Doris, a regular participant at their Wednesday evening devotionals, "gave us a very uplifting message on loving deep and wide." Afterwards the team and several guests from town lingered for a hymn sing and conversation.[65] When the rest of team pulled out in March, Abbott wrote: "I hated to see them all go. The two girls [Constance and Elizabeth] were such a bright spot in the daily routine – always anxious to help and always cheerful ... The four of us were all who have been meeting for morning meditation and now I expect there will be just me."[66]

The team's complex relationships come alive as his letters, intended only for his future wife's eyes, forthrightly shared his temptations, revelries, frustrations, and accomplishments during his five months there. On his birthday, the "kids had a special meal ... with a big cake Doris made" and presents wrapped in red paper – "a razor blade, a feather, a flower, a pair of earrings and yolks found inside the chicken done up in a box." Of course, Ed was "thrilled and showed it by going around the table and kissing each of them for which [he] got a face slap and one of the yolks in [his] hair. [Then they] played some card games together that goes by the distinctive name of Hell."[67] He recounted another social outing:

> After the feast [later in February] there was a dragon dance in a neighboring village and Doris Woodward and I decided to satisfy our curiosity ... so we went along in the dragon procession to the village and were given seats of honour. Tea, nuts, cigarettes and wine were put in front of us. We were the cynosure of the neighboring eyes and I think more of an attraction than the dragon.[68]

Here at least, Doris was portrayed as an integral part of the FAU family that cut across racial lines.

In March 1946, while travelling to Henan with K.B. Soon, with whom she had become romantically involved, Doris was thrown from the top of an FAU truck when it plunged thirty feet down the side of a steep hill into the river: "What Doris thought [the driver] said was, 'I can't stop. I am going down. Here we go!' ... She suddenly felt the truck tip over to the left and the next moment she was flying through the air. She landed on something ... Then things went black."[69] Doris's recovery took longer than expected. At the end of April, the *Newsletter* reported that she had "got over her fractured ribs but can't get up anyway because she has amoebic dysentery instead."[70] She continued to experience bouts of poor health that necessitated her hospitalization with a lung infection in Shanghai in June. Reporting on the mixed news from Shanghai, the *Newsletter* simply announced without its traditional fanfare: "Doris, now much better, and K.B. [Soon] proudly announce their engagement; on the other hand the doctors have announced that Doris must go home."[71] Waiting for her condition to stabilize enough to make travel arrangements meant that she did not arrive in England until mid-September. Afterwards, she wrote about how she "missed the company the FAU afforded"[72] and wanted to return. But this was not to be.

FAU women who diverged from the path of feminine respectability risked being ostracized or barred from future work with the China Convoy. Two years later, Robert McClure vetoed Doris Woodward's return. Having "followed her from the time she landed in China until she returned home," there was no doubt in his mind about her qualifications or record of service. Professionally, he wrote, she "is well-trained in nursing and has a nice way with her pupils. She had no colour prejudice at all and works well with her colleagues. She is quite a pusher at getting things done without appearing to be so. She gets things done without irritating people about it." He also praised her as "a hard worker, starts early and works late." He did note, however, that she "is not a good administrator."[73]

Despite her professional suitability, Doris had two difficulties that precluded her reappointment, in McClure's opinion. "Psychologically," he claimed, "she is self-contained in a group. She does not pal up with the other girls nor does she 'loosen up' in a group to talk about her work, herself, her ambitions, or her thoughts. One has the impression that at times, is a bit subject to a persecution complex, and certainly felt that others were 'down on her.'" This behaviour was not the primary consideration that blocked her readmission, however. McClure disapproved of her promiscuous behaviour. "Sexually," he contended,

she is a menace of the first order ... she is hypersexed and takes on one man at a time. Just how far each man goes with her is up to the man, I believe.

When her appointment to "go anywhere, do anything" shifted her position again, she seemed with little difficulty to take on a new man in her new position. Naturally this upset the work of those who were found moping around waiting for darkness to fall. She directs her attention to the new men rather than the type to which she is accustomed and in this way had quite an inning.

While McClure admitted that her behaviour changed after she meet K.B. Soon, and was willing to make allowances for the fact that the "excitement of war" may have influenced her sexual conduct, "this side of her behaviour in my mind disqualifies her from coming back into the Unit."[74] Other FAUers concurred that Doris Woodward "would not be useful to the unit work ... in a nutshell, she is a girl who will always, repeat always, make for the first thing in trousers and hangs on until the victim shakes loose if he can."[75] Women were expected to live the hard life at the front on the same basis as men but retain their feminine chaste virtue. It is highly unlikely that either would have similarly censored the "hypersexed" boys of the Cockloft. On the basis of these evaluations, the FSU Council did "not recommend the re-appointment of Doris Woodward."[76] Women's roles and sexuality, whether married or not, continued to be an equally "vexing" question as the FAU prepared to transition towards long-term humanitarian development and relief work.

The experiences of Harriet Brown and Doris Woodward highlight the difficulties of building sustainable health services in conflicted areas, even when local groups were consulted and involved in administration. Divergent political agendas could not always be brokered. While the two nurses expressed a common sense of professional identity complemented by Christian notions of service that bound them to the Unit's shared sense of mission in China, they differed in their perceptions of the nursing service applicable in China. In common with FAU nurses who served on the Salween front, their Western notions of safe, competent, and ethical nursing practice were challenged. While Harriet questioned the feasibility of applying Western standards in a top-down fashion, in Doris's view Western standards were key to modernizing and improving patient care. Nonetheless, as we shall see, whatever her personal reservations, Harriet Brown would be expected to raise the standard of nursing care in Henan's mission hospitals along Western lines.

Volunteering with the FAU simultaneously recast and constrained Chinese and Western women's gendered and professional roles. All six of the Chinese "Kunming girls" were well regarded within the FAU community and valued their time with the Convoy.[77] Juliet Chiu (T'ing-hsien), who had been mentored by Harriet Brown in Liuzhou, had been a wartime refugee before returning to complete her university studies in Beijing with fond memories: "My golden age when I stayed with the Unit has past and never return to me again."[78] For others, joining the Unit opened new medical careers and matrimonial opportunities. All received financial support to further their education or assistance to find permanent employment. After completing an FAU laboratory course, May Mei (Tsu-t'ung) was placed in charge of the laboratory at the Huei Tien Hospital, left the FAU to join UNRRA, and later wed fellow Convoy member William Emslie. Doris Woodward's protégés, Elizabeth Hsu (Kwang-hsin) and Constance Shen (Ming-chen), both received a sponsorship in the form of summer employment with the American Friends Service Committee and financial assistance to cover travel costs to study in the United States.[79] After her marriage, Elizabeth had a long and distinguished career as the head of the microbiology lab and senior researcher at the University of Michigan hospitals. An expert in fungal infections, she was part of the team that discovered Legionnaires' disease.[80] Like Doris Wu, Sheila Iu, and Jane Wong, these young women made valuable contributions to the work and life of the Convoy. All were active agents in determining their careers and life choices.

All of the women's experiences, but particularly Doris Woodward's, demonstrated that women were expected to take on more risks and responsibilities but not demonstrate the unseemly sexual behaviour associated with men in war. Their decision to act as providers of humanitarian relief moved beyond nursing's traditional missionary or military roles. Harriet Brown, Doris Woodward, and the Kunming nurses chose an alternative to wartime service that aligned with their Christian views, future ambitions, and civic responsibilities during wartime. Their decision stemmed from a mix of commitment and naïveté. Few anticipated the dangers and professional or personal costs involved in Convoy life. For all, it was a journey of self-discovery, fraught with tensions, as they attempted to reconcile how they imagined humanitarian nursing with the stark realities of wartime China. Harriet Brown, in particular, epitomized the struggle of many Western FAUers to define what it meant to be a Christian pacifist humanitarian in practice, often forced to operate within the parameters set by the Unit's ability to negotiate the conditions under which it worked.

The stories of Harriet Brown and Doris Woodward reveal the hurdles the FAU experienced in transferring Western nursing practice and hospital administration that would survive devolution to Chinese staff at a turning point for the Convoy. The FAU's contested experience in its main task of devolving FAU hospitals in southwestern China contributed to the decision to relocate to Henan. As traditionally recounted, Henan desperately needed immediate medical and famine relief and long-term reconstruction. Certainly, McClure was eager to return to his stomping ground, where "I carry some weight in that area and I do know it best."[81] He wanted to reassert the authority of missionary societies before the Nationalist Chinese army occupied the mission hospitals. But the Unit's difficulties with UNRRA, more especially CNRRA, and the Chinese National Health Administration figured more prominently in determining its future direction than previously suggested.

Recognizing that its success in rehabilitating the Henan mission hospitals would depend "on the way we manage to devolve such schemes into permanent Chinese bodies," the Unit hoped to learn from its experiences in handing over the Tengyue, Nantan, and Liuzhou hospitals.[82] First, the complete lack of coordination between the NHA, UNRRA, and CNRRA in undertaking medical relief and rehabilitation work, in McClure's view, was symptomatic of what could be expected if the Unit remained in western China. There were "no reasons why [a] similar mix-up should not occur in the future." His response was to negotiate permission with the NHA and UNRRA to undertake an integrated area project in Henan. In short, the Unit took the friendly advice offered by the CNRRA and other aid agencies "that we should leap frog from this province and its complicated situations and set up elsewhere with a freer hand."[83] Its experience also reaffirmed the need for more predictable financial support and assurance that properly trained Chinese personnel would carry on once the Unit left. In Henan, the mission societies, as well as the UNRRA/CNRRA, could be tapped to underwrite the cost of rebuilding hospitals and to provide Western-trained staff to carry on the work started by the FAU teams in training local personnel.

Having identified new opportunities that offered more autonomy and a more stable financial footing, it remained to be seen whether relocating could mitigate the perils of humanitarian work in a country where war never abated.

7 Henan
Hope and Despair, 1945–47

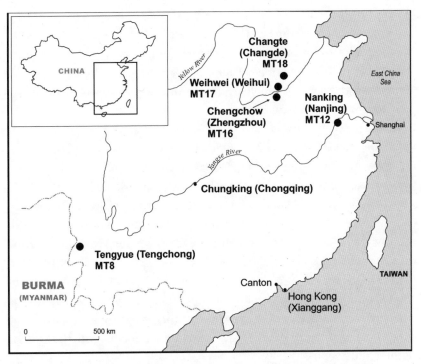

Map 8 Friends Ambulance Unit Teams in Honan (Henan), 1945–47

Little McC
Little McC
Sat on his be
Feeding on readers' Di
He hatched up a plan
To develop Honan
And said: "What a good boy am I!"

– *NEWSLETTER* 181, 27 OCTOBER 1945

Reflecting the sentiment expressed in the poem, the new American recruit Taber Jenkins wrote home that it was Robert McClure "who got the Unit to move up here to Honan [Henan] much to the disgust of many. He is perpetually taking up jobs we are not equipped to do, thus forcing us to blunder through or give it up with apologies."[1] Only time would tell whether Jenkins's assessment would prove correct.

Robert McClure had identified the American Baptist hospital in Zhengzhou (designated MT16 in Map 8), then being used as the Japanese headquarters, as a base from which to launch an ambitious area project. It was a race to beat the Generalissimo's men there. McClure wanted to strike before the Chinese army could move in and use the facilities for barracks. If the mission hospitals were not protected and rehabilitated until they could be handed back to the missionary societies, McClure foresaw a "long continuing period of misery and suffering for the general populace." Rehabilitating the hospitals was only the first step. The Friends Ambulance Unit's long-term plans included projects on public health and sanitation, agriculture, and industrial cooperatives. It still hoped "to show in a sort of model way what can be done to get badly war-damaged areas back onto its feet, working with the Chinese leaders and people."[2]

Rehabilitating the mission hospital buildings whose Western personnel had been forced to withdraw during the Japanese occupation meant negotiating their handover from the Japanese. It involved securing funding and supplies abroad and from the warring Chinese Nationalist and Communist relief agencies operating within the fledgling United Nations Relief and Rehabilitation Administration. It required recruiting and reorganizing staff, and rebuilding nursing programs from the ground up – all complicated by runaway inflation, civil war, and thousands of returning destitute refugees.

McClure remained at the heart of negotiations to establish the terms under which the FAU would rehabilitate and devolve the Henan mission societies' hospitals. In light of the Unit's previous difficulties rehabilitating and devolving hospitals, he took steps to coordinate interagency and government relief throughout the province and with Chinese National Relief and Rehabilitation Administration and UNRRA. At the local level, he helped establish the Honan International Relief Committee (HIRC) and ensured that FAU personnel held key positions and served as the first FAU medical representative. But here as elsewhere, the Unit's work depended on supplies and funding provided by the UNRRA/CNRRA and other international aid agencies. Relations with the CNRRA and UNRRA "had been a thorny problem," but at the end of the month (March 1946), an agreement with the head of the Henan CNRRA for two FAU men to work inside the CNRAA "suggests that the worst was past and that their Trojan diplomacy might succeed where other attempts had failed."[3] Despite the leadership's effort to coordinate the Unit's work with other relief agencies and the returning missionary societies, the nurses' testimonies attest that politics and personalities consistently coloured the humanitarian exchanges of the FAU and the Friends Service Unit at all levels in Henan. Although some negotiations with the missionary societies were straightforward, others encountered unexpected roadblocks.

In 1946, Elizabeth Hughes, a recently married British surgical nurse, and Margaret Stanley and Joan Kennedy, both single American public health nurses, eagerly anticipated their two-year nursing assignments with the celebrated China Convoy. All promised to adhere to the GADA principle and to "share the burden of suffering." In so doing, they were cast into an adventure punctuated by danger and characterized by unremitting demands to care under chaotic circumstances, along with three very different love stories. They were the only FAU nurses who witnessed the birth of modern China from both sides of the conflict; for two of them, it meant serving beyond their original contracts. Joan Kennedy would return home early. All worked in the Western-style mission hospitals being rehabilitated as part of the Henan project, then under Nationalist control, before joining Medical Team 19 (MT19) deep in Communist-held territory "during the intensity of battles and bombing."[4] Their experiences illuminate the barriers that the Convoy confronted in grounding humanitarian action in a few basic principles: independence, neutrality, and impartiality caught in the cross-fire of civil war. Equally important, when put to the test, they developed different methods to reconcile their personalities and identities as Western nurses and soldiers of peace with prevailing views on how respectable Western Christian women should behave. As apt foils to each other, they foreshadowed the complex personal and professional entanglements of humanitarian nursing within intrastate conflict zones.

As before, the decision to volunteer offered opportunities for exotic travel, adventure, new professional horizons, and an opportunity for service, but the roads that led Elizabeth Hughes, Margaret Stanley, and Joan Kennedy to China differed significantly.

Although raised in a middle-class, nominally Congregationalist family, Elizabeth Webb Hughes absorbed her early Christian pacifist views from an uncle who had been imprisoned as a conscientious objector during the First World War: "His principles sort of unnoticeably filtered through to me. And I really sort of accepted them as the norm." Only later did she realize "that Christians were not necessarily pacifists because to me the Christian message is so utterly pacifist ... It's love thy neighbour and do good to those who spitefully use you." As war approached, she remembered wrestling with her pacifist beliefs: "Really only by going and living on a desert island and being utterly self-sufficient could you separate yourself from the war." Never a strong academic, Elizabeth intended to be a fashion buyer but decided that being a "properly trained nurse" was a more "practical" alternative in wartime. In 1944, she completed a four-year nursing program at Queen Elizabeth Hospital in Birmingham, a "very peculiar hospital" where the clinical training was highly specialized, focusing on surgery. Viewing overseas relief work as more adventurous than hospital nursing, she immediately volunteered with the FAU. Also citing her desire to atone for the damages of war, Elizabeth "just got on with it because it obviously needed doing."[5] However, the "small bright woman" was initially turned down for China, the result of "an impression she gave of emotional instability."[6] Instead, she was assigned to FAU teams working in the eastern Mediterranean, although there was no indication why the Mediterranean war theatre would be a more appropriate placement for someone who seemed unstable. Her highly transitory experience working with refugees in several countries there reinforced her common-sense approach to nurses' work in conflict-ridden China.

Elizabeth Hughes joined the China Convoy via a marriage certificate. While working with the FAU, she met her future husband, Eric, who had always dreamed of serving in China. She had been granted permission to return to England to marry Eric, who was originally scheduled to go to China with a British Red Cross team. When the British Red Cross decided against sending further teams, FAU London headquarters determined that sending the couple to reinforce the Convoy's medical staff made the most sense. But doubts still lingered about Elizabeth's suitability for China.[7] London headquarters therefore carefully verified her service record and personal character to ensure that she would "fit into community life" before approving her application, making it clear, however, that Elizabeth was joining the Convoy as a fully qualified nurse in her own right and should not expect to be at Eric's side. Thinking that China "sounded tremendously romantic" and unaware that China was embroiled in a bitter civil war, she quickly agreed.[8]

Margaret Stanley's background was quite different. Raised in a devout Midwestern American Quaker family, she had graduated from Friends University in Wichita, Kansas, in 1942 with a premed major. She then worked as a secretary to finance her lifelong ambition to study nursing. After earning a master's degree at Western Reserve University in 1945, she briefly worked in Cleveland's Visiting Nursing Association before volunteering. The outbreak of war tested Margaret's pacifist convictions. Erroneously believing that the wartime grant for nurse cadets obligated her to perform military service after graduation, she had refused federal financial aid while at Western Reserve University. Increasingly identifying with close Quaker friends who had chosen jail over military service, she too "wanted to try to relieve some suffering" and to live "in such a way as to do away with the cause of war." Like Elizabeth Hughes, Margaret "did not picture [China] realistically ... [but I] had no question in my mind at all about [my] assignment."[9]

Like Margaret Stanley, Joan Kennedy was a well-educated public health nurse. Tragic circumstances led to her choice of nursing as a vocation. Her mother died before she entered Florida State College for Women intending to major in chemistry. After her father's unexpected death in 1941, during her final year in college, she was steered towards a nursing degree as a means of securing a respectable livelihood. She completed her basic nursing training at the Presbyterian Hospital School of Nursing in Charlotte, North Carolina, in 1944, before completing a BS in public health and psychiatry nursing from Columbia University. After a brief stint at Bellevue Hospital, she joined the Henry Street Visiting Nurses Services in 1944, where she remained until she volunteered to go to China. Although born into the Presbyterian manse, she was listed as a "nominal" member of the Presbyterian Church on her application form. However, she had been attending Quaker meetings in New York before applying to the American Friends Service Committee. Sometime while studying in New York, she became acquainted with some of the conscientious objectors working as orderlies in the hospital. Their friendship grew as they invited her to folk dancing evenings and, ultimately, to Quaker meetings. She had continued attending meetings after her graduation. What is clear is that she had a prior offer from the UNRRA "but turned it down and likes the AFSC approach better." She had been "sold" on exotic China over Europe by Ted Mills, a British China Convoy member.[10] According to her personnel file, while at Bellevue she was involved in investigating the psychiatric effects of malaria drugs. This knowledge would have been highly valued given the suicide of one FAU physician due to atropine (a commonly used drug) poisoning. Unlike Margaret Stanley, Joan had some experience in obstetrical work. Like Margaret, she received the "usual Pendle Hill orientation (2 months)," including "a start on Chinese." Unlike in the case of Harriet Brown, Pendle Hill did not afford either Margaret or Joan the opportunity to forge strong ties of friendship within a group that would become their supportive China family, buffering the cultural and professional shock. By the time they attended, there were few other recruits. Although interested primarily in public health, psychiatry, and teaching, Joan made it clear that she was willing to work in a hospital but had no interest in theatre work: "She likes the sound of the village schemes, Kala Azar work etc."[11]

Margaret Stanley arrived at the Hwa Mei Hospital in Zhengzhou (MT16) on 31 March 1946, and Elizabeth and Eric Hughes arrived shortly afterwards, Elizabeth having had two months' orientation to medical work in China in Qujing. By the time Joan Kennedy arrived in late November 1946, circumstances had changed at the base hospital. Despite her interest in public health work, Unit leaders believed she needed to be oriented to medical work in an FAU-run hospital. The question was where. The single foreign personnel who remained during Hwa Mei's devolution was British physician Peter Early. Given his busy caseload, he would have had only limited time to help Joan adjust to Chinese medical conditions. Unit leaders at Hwa Mei Hospital hesitated to send additional Western staff to mission hospitals where the FAU was trying to hand off responsibility to Chinese nurses. The United Church of Canada North China Mission's hospital at Weihui seemed preferable, because since Elizabeth and Margaret had already been transferred there, Joan would "be able to catch on to the routine and have an excellent opportunity of learning medical Chinese language."[12]

Working in the Henan mission hospitals was a period of transition, "of being betwixt and between cultures" that daily tested all three nurses' perception of what it meant to be a Western-trained nurse working within a pacifist relief agency.[13] Like their FAU predecessors, none of the three foresaw the degree of personal or professional adaptation that humanitarian work in China would require. China's poverty and filth was a rude shock to them, challenging their Western notions of civility and hygiene. Recalling her initial impression of Chinese society, Elizabeth "thought how terribly, terribly dirty and dusty everything was and how I would never be clean again. I felt thoroughly bewildered."[14] Margaret, too, was taken aback by "sounds, sights, and smells I had never come across before."[15] Negotiating the professional, cultural, and political differences within FAU medical projects changed her perception of herself, transforming her from a Western nurse to a pacifist one enchanted by China and its people. For Elizabeth and Joan, the Henan interlude had less impact.

By the time Margaret Stanley arrived, the Hwa Mei Hospital was in full swing with a heavy patient load. Assigned to take over from Margaret Briggs, who was preparing to leave immediately after her upcoming marriage, her days at Hwa Mei "were busy and long" as she coped with new and unexpected duties.[16] Along with office work, she learned to administer spinal anesthesia so that she could be part of the surgical team on call day or night. Expected to supervise and teach the more experienced returning Chinese staff, she instead learned "a great deal from her students," including how to diagnose cholera by smell. She could not have predicted that a chauffeured car would regularly roll up to the hospital entrance to whisk her off to the Chinese officers' quarters to teach English, or that she would be feted at their "glamorous feasts." For the most part, however, she preferred to spend her leisure time with her Chinese nursing friends, eagerly exchanging language lessons while sharing simple pleasures such as riding bikes or hiking through the sugar cane fields.[17]

Transferred to MT17 at the United Church of Canada's Kwang Sheng Hospital in Changde, 3,200 kilometres north of Zhengzhou, Margaret found herself working in "a little island of Nationalist control in a sea of Communism."[18] The FAU team encountered a "picture of filth and desolation difficult to describe" when it arrived.[19] Even when fighting came within a few kilometres, the team carried on with rehabilitating the hospital. Staff cared for most battle casualties in the region and handled major non-trauma surgeries. Normal hospital routines "were set aside as the patients' relatives would come in and sleep under the bed ... and they all have something to say."[20] The frequent changes among FAU personnel, often inexperienced and still struggling with the language, exacerbated the difficulties of providing patient care. In the first year, there were six different Western nurses, sometimes two at a time but often just one.[21] By June, McClure reported that the team was functioning with a sixty-bed hospital, but its future remained uncertain. UNRRA had withdrawn its doctor because the fighting was close by, and lack of supplies forced the closure of the kala-azar clinic.

More immediately, contending with professional and personal ties where interracial relationships were cautiously accepted at best and frowned on at worst increasingly occupied Margaret's thoughts and feelings. Some colleagues felt fortunate in having her join them there. "Her competence and genuineness and good spirits are refreshing and much appreciated."[22] Here, as before, she was reported to be "enjoying the close fellowship" with her Chinese ward staff.[23] The initial field reports concealed the mushrooming tensions that disrupted team unity.

Quietly nurturing these friendships with the Chinese nurses, Stanley took pride in her reputation for "being the most uncooperative member" of the hospital team because she was determined to fight for better living and working conditions for the Chinese staff.[24] Park Woodrow, the hospital manager, was exasperated by her. Describing the friction within the team, he claimed that "the Unit here continues its knife in the back tactics. Sometime I would like to get together with you and try to find out who threw the first knife – Margaret or the other side. I am making a historical survey for posterity – 'How to Live Most Uncooperatively.'" Learning of Margaret's proposed transfer to the hospital at Weihui, Woodrow, normally a quiet, reticent man, was determined to arrange the hospital's affairs "so that she will not have to come back."[25]

Margaret's diary, however, recorded her struggle to reconcile her Quaker dedication to forging a brotherly community with the FAU's expectations that she maintain a professional distance and authority required to improve nursing standards. She recorded "crack[ing] down" on the Chinese nurses: "I am working everybody at top speed. If anyone gets a bedsore or maggots – NO DAYS OFF!"[26] In part, she may have been responding to criticism of her performance. As one member recounted, "There has been some criticism of her ability as a nurse, which so far I find, is completely unfounded. The criticism has come from her attitude towards the Chinese. According to some she is not strict enough with them and doesn't give them a lacing when they need it."[27]

Ignoring any veiled disapproval of interracial courtships, Margaret became increasingly fond of a young Chinese physician, James Chai (En-chung), or Jay, as she called him: "Although I told myself that I could not let personal feelings get in the way of work I was there to do, [we] were drawn together more and more."[28] Her diary includes the description of a memorable August evening when Jay "took my willing hand and we walked to the compound wall ... Moonlight filtered into dancing patterns all about. From this vantage point we could view two worlds – one inside and one outside the compound ... I would have sat there on the wall with Jay into the night, but ... I knew the work of the hospital demanded our best energies."[29] Despite her mixed emotions about leaving Jay, Margaret looked forward to her transfer to Weihui rather than remain where the goal was "to make an efficient medical machine [without] attending to the thing for which we came – friendship with the Chinese."[30]

Elizabeth Hughes arrived at Hui Min Hospital in Weihui in the first week of September, followed a few days later by Margaret Stanley. Joan Kennedy soon joined them. As Stanley recalled:

> Our work was not part of a blueprint that we laid out; but worked out with the actual foreign owners of the hospital and depending on local needs and with local people, whoever they were. The fact that we could go in and do what we could without a long-term commitment to carry on put us in a very unusual position.[31]

It did not, however, protect the team from becoming entangled in Church politics. The hospital was rife with professional and racial tension that extended beyond its relations with the Chinese staff. The hospital administrator summed up the Convoy's quandary thus: "We are in the midst of a difficult political situation, which if not handled wisely (and for the most part it must be handled by the Mission staff and the Chinese members of the Synod of the CCC [China Christian Council]) could speedily end our activities here."[32]

When the FAU initially agreed to meet the North Synod of the Church of Christ in China's request to rehabilitate the hospital, FAUers assumed that they would work with the existing hospital and mission staff.[33] The team's initial empathy with the hospital staff's predicament during the Japanese occupation quickly dissipated. The team arrived on 5 July 1946 and five days later assumed control of the hospital. "Dr. Tuan, two nurses and all the business staff were invited to turn in their resignations." Mission officials had locked horns with Tuan,[34] who had kept the hospital running but allowed it fall into disrepair during the Japanese occupation. Walter Alexander, the FAU business manager at the hospital, spelled out the situation:

> 190 persons were attending a daily Kala Azar clinic and receiving half or less of the usual dosage so that the treatment was from 25 to 35 days; all of the post-operative cases were septic and since three nurses were required for the Kala Azar clinic only 2 were working on the wards most of the time; over 40 or more patients ... [we] found possible and necessary to discharge immediately.[35]

The FAU argued that it had little choice but "to rely on the advice of the Synod and Mission personnel as to who should be kept and who should be paid off."[36] Other factors were clearly at play behind the scenes, however.

Robert McClure had strong ties to the hospital: "The Weihwei [Weihui] hospital, that pioneer of 'modern hospitals' in Central China had been built by his father's successors, Drs. Struthers and Auld." After Pearl Harbor, the hospital's administration had been entrusted to the Chinese church. According to McClure's biographer, it was unclear whether "the compound itself was the responsibility of the church but the hospital was the responsibility of its Chief, Dr. Tuan."[37] Accusations surrounding his corruption and fraternization during the Japanese occupation further tarnished his reputation.[38] Mission officials increasingly regarded Tuan as a "trouble-maker," and their mediation efforts collapsed because of "a fundamental difference in ideology," his outrageous salary demands, and his lack of deference to mission authority.[39] As McClure explained, "for the good of the hospital it is best that we let him go. I still had hoped ... that it would be possible to rehabilitate Dr. Tuan and, with patience." McClure had not persuaded him "that the rules of the game have been changed and that we saw no reason why he should not be able to play an effective game."[40] In response, the hospital board lowered Tuan's salary, then attempted to compromise when they found that other Chinese physicians received higher salaries. Presented with an ultimatum to either accept his resignation or agree to his salary, the hospital board chose the first option: "To take any other course would seem to leave absolute authority in Dr. Tuan's hands."[41] Moreover, Tuan's departure would "help to clear the present political situation," opening the door for a physician chosen by the FAU to resume control.[42] The local political struggle, however, was temporarily complicated when Tuan resigned but agreed to remain without pay until his replacement arrived. Normally no Chinese physician would come while he remained. In short, the FAU was hardly a disinterested, neutral party at any level.

In August, Walter Alexander contended that his wife, Harriet (Brown), had to take control because the head nurses were "not capable of carrying on their jobs." He complained that "the one four-year graduate and the male nurse each knows more than the two [head nurses] put together," and that "the drag of four grads and 10 students who have been trained under the old system to be lazy and generally slack is a terrific burden for foreign nurses ... And to allow the school of nursing to go as it has under Miss Li [Shuying] would be a waste of time and the lives of the students."[43] Although Liu Tse[44] had initially been invited to stay, he "decided to leave and on the whole we feel that he is the loser and the situation will be made easier by his leaving."[45] Alexander reported that "so far as the staff is concerned, we have concluded that it would be easier to start with no staff and build them up than to try to retain staff who have worked under bad conditions for many years."[46] Others had a more empathetic view of Liu, who " had been carrying the whole load" and carried on "right through an attack of malaria, though headaches and nausea constantly bothered him." He was, in the FAU lab technician's opinion, "a swell guy."[47]

Walter Alexander acknowledged: "Nursing is our bottle neck at present. Though the wards are ready for 25–35 patients, the OPD is going full blast, we have to limit our patients to the nursing staff."[48] Claiming that the Chinese ward nurse had "forgotten all she ever knew about nursing," Harriet was expected to cover the OPD, wards, and administration.[49] Overworked and pregnant, she contracted malaria, forcing the couple's repatriation in early September. A new head nurse was needed. That appointment reveals much about the Unit's priorities and the two contenders: Elizabeth Hughes and Margaret Stanley.

Alexander had identified a nurse in Changde who he thought "would fill the bill with the nursing school."[50] In August, he wrote: "We could not trust anyone who has trained in [the Weihui] hospital for many months ... you can see what I mean about the need for Elizabeth [Hughes],"[51] but Kathleen Stokes, the medical secretary at Zhengzhou, initially identified a different nurse for the job.[52] Stanley had already received a letter requesting her transfer to Weihui: a head nurse was required "whose compatibility with the native nurses is a strong point."[53] While Stanley's value as a peacemaker was recognized, skepticism remained about her administrative abilities:

> With the relations between the Chinese and the foreigners what it is there, Margaret will do a lot to improve things. She is still spoken of in Chengchow [Zhengzhou] as the best nurse these girls have over them. She does lack administration and routine knowledge and for that reason I suggest that Liz be responsible for the whole kit and kaboodle.[54]

The die had been cast. Margaret Stanley would be the conciliator and Elizabeth Hughes the taskmaster.[55]

Not all FAU members either understood or condoned the FAU's course of action that might "do as much damage as good if we have just taken over." They had a more positive view of the Chinese head nurses' "courageous" wartime role and questioned the hospital's future sustainability once the FAU team withdrew.[56] They wondered, "How do you expect Margaret Stanley to do a better job than Miss Long, [Li Shuying] an excellent Christian who has stood the test of the war and kept things going [and] who knows the language and the ways of her people?"[57] Nurse Stanley had been warned that her new assignment "will be tough."[58] Initially, she appeared complacent, perhaps underestimating just how "tough" it would be "firing people and rebuilding it all."[59] Instead she viewed her transfer to Weihui as "a good thing at present ... my feeling is that experience in Chengchow [Zhengzhou] and Changte [Changde] has been for the most part on the receiving end. Now there may be an opportunity to do a bit of giving." She remained "confident" that the relationship between the hospital staff and FAU here "will surely improve."[60] By early October she was "beginning to feel a bit of friendliness" from the Chinese hospital staff "who are reputedly 'agin' us."[61] But she could not say the same about her FAU colleagues.

"The Margaret-Elizabeth relationship," according to the hospital manager, Jack Norton, could "not be discussed right now." He refrained from writing a confidential letter to the Unit's medical secretary, for fear "that anything said right now might do more harm than good." It was, he said, nothing to "fuss about" in the sense that they "both are conscious that they have to make themselves agree."[62] Objecting to Hughes's rigid administrative approach, which precluded collaborative information sharing and problem solving, Stanley complained that "Elizabeth takes over the Nursing Situation en force

– this and that are now thus and so and everybody is expected to believe it. I think our presumptuousness is a bit much."[63] Joan Kennedy's brief stay before being transferred to Changde did little to improve the collegiality among the FAU's nursing staff; Joan, in Margaret's opinion, was a "self-willed creature."[64] The two nurses had decidedly different personalities. Margaret was a woman of strong opinions and conviction; Joan was more reticent and disliked confrontation. She preferred to form her own opinions rather than having them orchestrated by Margaret. It is clear that neither Elizabeth nor Margaret would become a trusted confidante for the young American woman far from home and with little family support. It was with relief that Margaret accepted reassignment back to Changde: "Old Friends there. It is the life I love." Significantly, she resolved "to stay even if Elizabeth Hughes comes [to Changde]."[65]

By November, the FAU team at Changde was "feeling very dissatisfied with the work we are doing in the hospital ... the FAU has done all that it is likely to do that is constructive in the hospital. It is very clear that the Mission are only waiting for the FAU to go, so that they can change back to their previous arrangements in many details of Hospital Administration." The "particular point that is being harped on ... almost daily is the most rigid segregation of the sexes." Mission staff "clearly regarded it as highly immoral when I told [them] that male and female patients were interviewed in the *same* consulting rooms at *different* times." Then a dispute over Chinese staff salary levels brought "matters to a head." The mission staff, unhappy with the decision to raise staff salaries to accommodate inflation, asked the FAU Changde section leader to intervene as arbitrator. The FAU staff concluded that, with this lack of confidence between the two groups, "it was best for us to leave as soon as possible."[66] It was agreed that control would revert to the synod at the end of November.

Stanley's return to Changde coincided with a significant turnover in staff. Seconded nurse Elvira Lehman rejoined the Mennonite group in Kaifeng. Joan Kennedy departed to join the Yan'an team (MT19). New Zealanders Bunny and Heath Thompson would shortly be seconded to the Union Hospital in Hankou. Moreover, fighting had moved closer, increasing the workload in all departments of the Changde hospital: "Operations all day. Finished the day schedule as the day ended – Midnight." As they juggled the delivery of babies amid gunshot surgeries, the respect of Margaret and others for the Chinese nurses only grew: "O.R. [operating room] people, Miss O.R. Yang, Lui Sung May and Su Chou Fu all tired but they keep at it automatically. Miss

O.R. Yang is the best nurse I know." Although she recorded that she, too, "worked up so much momentum I can't slow down; don't feel tired am energetic always," tempers did fray, including hers, under the stress.[67] Stanley's hard work led to her appointment as superintendent of nurses, but it was the prospect for improvement rather than the title that mattered: "On the verge of accomplishing something each day in the hospital. Supplies to distribute, all the CD's [contagious diseases] in one room. All women in labour in by night and home by day."[68]

Occasionally there was a respite: the OR tables were covered, and Margaret joined the men for a game of poker. More frequently, she found quiet refuge from her gruelling workdays in the FAU's daily silent worship or in reading the Bengali poet Rabindranath Tagore in the sunshine.[69] Jay's return to work by her side and his approval – "that things in the hospital seem to be better co-ordinated"[70] – contributed strongly to her happiness. As she confided in her diary, he "makes living worthwhile in all respects."[71] And her growing ability to converse about everyday happenings with the Chinese nursing staff strengthened female friendships outside work. Sometimes these ties meant that she willingly faced ostracism from "our good FAU family," for example, "by accepting May's, Yang's, and Miss Chang's invitation to have supper [on a festival day] ... And the Col. and Capt. coming to dinner. My My!"[72]

Both Elizabeth Hughes and Margaret Stanley disapproved of the Henan missionaries' lavish lifestyles and discriminatory treatment of the Chinese nurses. Elizabeth disliked the fact that the mission staff lived in "large western style houses with central heating" but considered it quite "normal" that the Chinese nurses were "expected to live in these huts with dirt floors." After all, "many [of them] were very well qualified people." It "seemed ridiculous. Not a Christian attitude at all."[73] Critical of the mission staff's behaviour, Margaret distanced the Quakers from Henan missionaries, saying, "I was not a missionary. The Friends were known not to be missionaries and to live in some ways a much different kind of life." She perceived her "very purpose to fit in ... regardless of the politics, regardless of religious background. Our one tie was a commitment to our dedication of trying out ways of living in peace together."[74] Despite their protests, however, both Margaret and Elizabeth lived in the Western-style housing in Henan.

Balancing professional responsibilities with personal happiness remained a challenge for both women. As a married woman, often separated from her husband for long periods, Hughes gave priority to her new marriage but her professional and social contacts remained circumscribed for other reasons.

Language was key to developing cross-cultural ties. "A bit saturated" by the futile language training on her previous FAU assignments, she did not have "the incentive to persevere with [another] difficult language."[75] Stanley, in contrast, immersed herself in Chinese language and culture and carefully cultivated close personal and professional ties with her Chinese colleagues and patients. She experienced stronger emotions in attempting to deal with unremitting demands to care that could never be met. She coped by reaching out to comfort the children in her care, even sharing her room with a paralyzed little girl so that she could receive treatment. It was typical of her that the highlight of a lavish Thanksgiving feast thrown by the local American military was the gifts of oranges and apples she received. Sharing them with her little patients on the porch "made [her] happier than the whole feast."[76]

Little was recorded about Joan Kennedy's adjustment to Convoy life, except that she had become romantically involved while at Changde with Park Woodrow, the hospital manager. Her selection for the Yan'an team was most likely determined by the desire to avoid a repeat of the Elizabeth-Margaret situation, rather than being based on an endorsement of her professional competence, resilience, or previous field experience, such as Elizabeth had acquired in the Middle East.

Stanley and Hughes had already begun to adopt distinct personal and professional coping strategies. Personal traits, training, previous experience, personal faith, and gender expectations all factored into their adjustment. They had different perceptions of what it meant to be a humanitarian nurse in practice. Working mainly in operating theatres, already familiar professional terrain, Elizabeth Hughes perceived her role as that of a vital "bridge," interpreting the wishes of the English-speaking doctors more efficiently than the Chinese-speaking nurses could.[77] Although a public health nurse, Margaret Stanley was expected to be a nurse educator, nurse anesthetist, and administrator. Pushed to expand her professional horizons, she perceived her role as more akin to that of a cross-cultural broker facilitating knowledge flows. She freely admitted her limitations and observed that her "respect increased daily for our medical staff as I watched them make do with what they had while administering medical care of high standards."[78] Her "faith that we could find ways to help people had been sustained during my [time] in Honan [Henan], where I was one of many taking on more responsibility than we dreamed we were capable of and doing things we had never expected to do. We learned every day from each other, from our Chinese colleagues, from our interpreters and from our patients. We would continue learning in the field."[79] That said, her unbridled enthusiasm to find ways to work, live, and learn alongside her Chinese colleagues still had to accommodate the fact, as she herself acknowledged, that the overall medical care in the Henan hospitals had been set up on Western standards patterned after such institutes as the Peking Union Medical College, and that the buildings were of Western design.[80] As Stanley learned, regardless of her own views, FAU nurses who veered from expected professional behaviour risked rebuke.

Stanley was prepared, however, to breach traditional professional boundaries and/or societal expectations that contravened her Quaker belief that her prime task was to advance global fraternity while relieving human suffering – a pattern that would precipitate tensions when, in March 1947, she unexpectedly joined Elizabeth Hughes, already assigned since late November to MT19. In March the following year, she would replace Joan Kennedy at the International Peace Hospital (IPH) in Yan'an, deep within Communist territory. Hughes welcomed the opportunity to work and live with her husband more permanently. As for Margaret Stanley, it meant severing the important female and romantic relationships that had mitigated her loneliness and professional adjustment since arriving in China. Despite the stern warning of colleagues (including Chinese members) to proceed with caution in her relationship, she had formed a deep attachment with James Chai and had shared a deeply moving visit with his family before joining MT19.[81] There would be many times in the months to come that she would long to have him by her side.

8 "Early Team"
Guerrilla Warfare Nursing, 1946–47

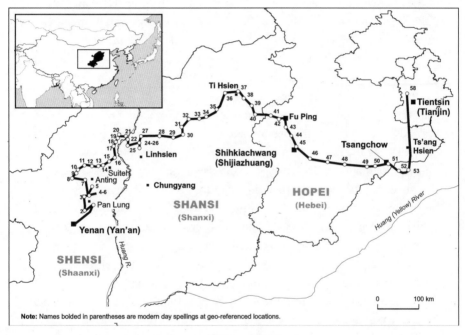

Note: Names bolded in parentheses are modern day spellings at geo-referenced locations.

Map 9 Margaret Stanley and Frank Miles's trek from Yan'an to Tianjin, 1948

> [We] had become convinced of the desperate need of the people
> in that area, not as Communists, but simply as human beings cut
> off from any medical services, from any drugs and who had little
> medical personnel to help them in fighting against the many
> diseases in that area.
>
> – BRONSON CLARK

Providing aid on both sides of the Chinese civil war had long been a goal of the Friends Ambulance Unit. As the civil war heated up, it became more difficult but increasingly important for the Unit to visibly assert its impartiality and neutrality. After earlier attempts to work in Communist-held areas in Henan petered out, new avenues were explored that led to the arrival of Medical Team 19 at the International Peace Hospital (IPH) in Yan'an, the Communist capital, in December 1946. The use of "Early Team" and "Earlyland" as code names when communicating to or about MT19 revealed the FAU's growing circumspection about its links across the political lines on both sides and its desire to guard its reputation as a neutral and impartial humanitarian agency. In retrospect, the use of code names and the belief that, because its humanitarian aid was directed at the people regardless of political allegiances, the FAU's humanitarian action could be divorced from politics appears naïve. In the end, the personal intervention of General George C. Marshall would be required to ensure safe passage and transport of MT19 to the IPH in Yan'an. American air crews associated with Marshall's peace initiative flew the team, accompanied by tons of medical supplies, just as his peace team stationed there began to withdraw, signalling the final breakdown of negotiations for a political settlement to the civil war.

On the eve of the team's departure from Chengchow, Bronson Clark, a key player in the tangled negotiations with British, American, and Communist authorities, accounted for his actions from the time he fortuitously secured a ride from Henan to Beijing aboard the plane of Isobel Cripps, president of the British United Aid to China Fund, to MT19's departure only a few weeks later. Once Clark was in Beijing, Michael Harris, secretary of the Fund and a former FAU member, helped him secure permission from General Thomas Timberman, director of operations at the executive headquarters of Marshall's truce mission, to fly to Yan'an on 6 November 1946. Once in Yan'an, Clark spent a week surveying the medical facilities and discussing what medical supplies were needed. Despite listening politely to his "proposal in which I asked them to feel free to make use of the team in any way they saw fit," he felt "all during my week's visit that the Communists never believed the team or the supplies would be able to get into Yan'an."[1] As his colourful account indicates, skill, connections, tenacity, and a modicum of luck all figured in the story.

On his arrival back in Beijing, he wrote:

> My problem was to secure an interview with Lt. General [Alvan Cullom] Gillem, who is the Commander of all US troops in China. This was a task. After all, he had three stars, while I had only one! By carrying a personal letter to him from Lady Cripps, I did manage to see him and I requested air transport for the team and supplies. He said my proposal was a fine idea but that I would have to secure permission and approval from Nanking [Nanjing] (i.e., General Marshall).

Undaunted by this "no for a beginner," Clark "decided it was time to bring up reinforcements." Lewis Hoskins, "who had met the American Ambassador twice and knew him quite well," readily agreed to the Nanjing trip to approach Marshall. Learning that the ambassador had just left for Beijing for three days, Hoskins and Clark went to see Wilma Fairbanks, who was in charge of cultural relations at the American embassy and an old acquaintance from Chongqing. She readily consented to help them by contacting the secretary of Ambassador Leighton Stuart. Then they "witnessed what had been true for the whole trip." When she readily agreed to help them, "red tape was slashed and people everywhere gave us number one priority." When Ambassador Stuart returned, "before he had even time to greet his staff, his secretary ushered us in to see him! He was enthusiastic about the proposal and agreed to present the request personally to General George C. Marshall. Somewhere along the line our request had jumped from one plane to two!" Once General Marshall stated his approval, all that was required was confirmation from Yan'an. "The Communist representative in Nanking [Nanjing] was contacted by radio and the confirmation came promptly through."[2] They flew directly back to Shanghai, where the real work lay ahead.

The FAU had "no supplies, no medical team and no trucks," but Clark knew that this might be the only opportunity to take badly needed supplies to the Communist areas. Trucks were borrowed from the British Red Cross, and teams of two were sent out to scrounge for supplies, armed only with their own audacity.[3] What followed was a frantic and often humorous race against the clock because each day news of a complete breakdown of the talks between the Communists and Nationalists was expected, which would mean that the US Army could have flown no more planes. A general meeting of the Shanghai Section was called.

> We therefore set our goal of assembling 7,500 pounds of medical supplies within forty-eight hours! Monday morning the office was packed with people. They disbanded and then the phones began ringing. Lewis [Hoskins] stood behind his desk holding the phone like the commander on the bridge, taking down items and weights. Within four hours we were offered 25,000 pounds! ... The American Red Cross had already allocated all the supplies, but they cancelled all that and offered us anything we wanted. We took a list down to their godown [warehouse] where we were informed it would take at least a week to fill. We informed that the stuff had to be in our godown that night and it was! ... The man in the CNRRA godown stood amazed as FAU men entered the place, tore open cases, took out stuff – without so much as a delivery order! "How do you guys do this?" was all he could say.[4]

The incident attests to the fact that, although the Unit remained determined to preserve its institutional integrity and autonomy to determine where it worked, in practice compromise and collaboration remained integral to gaining the access and supplies that were central to its humanitarian work.

The original team in Yan'an had six members: Douglas Clifford and Peter Early, doctors; Elizabeth Hughes and Joan Kennedy, nurses; Jack Dodds, laboratory technician; and Eric Hughes, radiologist. During the first year, three members left: Kennedy departed in January, Dodds in July, and Early in September 1947. Margaret Stanley, who replaced Kennedy, arrived along with Frank Miles, a medical mechanic, in March 1947, and remained until mid-February 1948. Elizabeth and Eric Hughes and Douglas Clifford stayed until late summer 1948, when the IPH was reorganized as the civil war rapidly shifted southward.

Life in the Yan'an cave villages was tough and unforgiving for the new arrivals. All initially experienced profound cultural and professional shock. They found it difficult to accept that they could not fully utilize their professional skills to save lives and relieve suffering.[5] Eventually, however, most found satisfaction in working with like-minded people "who were making every effort to build up a hospital under circumstances which were difficult"[6] or in believing "that if we had not been there the outcome would have been quite different."[7]

By March 1947, MT19 at the IPH was a melting pot representing five nationalities that had coalesced into a team. Given their distinctive personalities, motivations, field experience, and perceptions of their responsibilities as providers of humanitarian aid, the journey had a few rough patches. With little choice but to care for and depend on each other, strong ties formed. New Zealander Douglas Clifford, who had only recently qualified as a surgeon, had worked at the Hwa Mei Hospital in Zhengzhou for nine months.[8] A quiet, thoughtful man, he had been drawn to service with the FAU to "justify" his stance as a conscientious objector on religious grounds and "to demonstrate that he was not a shirker or a coward."[9] Peter Early and the Hugheses had already become acquainted while working with the FAU in the Middle East before coming to China.[10] Frank Miles was a birthright Quaker whose father had volunteered with the American Friends Service Committee in France as a conscientious objector during the First World War. Miles had served with the Civilian Public Service (CPS) as a conscientious objector during the Second World War before volunteering to serve in China as a medical mechanic in 1946. He explained his motivation thus: "I was still finding it difficult to re-enter normal society ... I continued to feel that I had done nothing that involved real risk or was comparable to what my friends did in the military service."[11] Others might have disagreed. During his CPS stint, Miles cut trails in the Great Smoky Mountains National Park, served as a "guinea pig" for jaundice experiments at the University of Pennsylvania, and spent time as an attendant in both the State Mental Hospital in Trenton, New Jersey, and the psychiatric clinic of the Duke University Medical School in North Carolina. For Miles, the simple act of helping had its own rewards. It offered a sense of purpose, a respite from materialism, and a sense of belonging. As he later recalled, "I wanted to do something which left a physical something there that Frank Miles had contributed, whether a building, wiring in a building or the plowing of a field."[12] Working with MT19 in a remote and militarily unsettled part of China appeared to meet all of Miles's expectations.

Jack Dodds first encountered the Quaker Peace Testimony as a teenager in the Toronto Friends' Boys Club. As a conscientious objector, Dodds, unlike his physician teammates, had been forced to abandon his university studies and was exiled to a rugged work camp in Banff, Alberta, before being transferred to the Banting Institute's penicillin plant following a brief stint with Canada Steamship Lines.[13] Once in China, he earned a reputation as an affable and resourceful jack of all trades for the FAU in southwestern China and Henan. He drove trucks carrying refugees, oversaw hospital construction, undertook lab work during cholera epidemics and in a leper colony, then joined a kala-azar team in Henan.

The American public health nurse Joan Kennedy was the reserved raw recruit who had still not taken China in her stride.

Douglas Clifford observed that MT19 "did not have all the training it could have wished for to manage all the problems that it encountered."[14] However, lack of training cannot entirely account for the differences in individuals' ability to cope with working and living in the caves and villages of Yan'an over the next eighteen months. The personality traits and professional perspectives that shaped acculturation come alive in Miles's letters home:

> The two doctors ... about as fine choices as could have been made for people to work here ... are both quiet, patient, unassuming, and very capable guys. Peter, as well as having a great fund of medical information, is a literal storehouse of musical knowledge ... Doug is a painstaking and technically perfect worker; he can't be hurried but you can always be sure his work is as nearly perfect as circumstances permit ...
>
> Eric is what we term a wag, he has a great sense of humor which often sends the crowd into roars of laughter ... Liz is a whiz in the theater, she is well trained and efficient. While the rather easy going way of the Chinese disturbs her at times, more than it does others, I think she has enjoyed her work here very much ... Jack Dodds, of Canada and our lab technician, is the "Old China Hand" of the group. He has many stories to tell of West China days, when, we are all lead [*sic*] to believe, life was amazingly carefree and exciting ... Margaret Stanley ... does some supervision of the wards and a good deal of teaching of nursing technique. Her Chinese is especially good; she has lived with a group of 4 or 5 nurses most of the time, which has given her plenty of opportunities for using it.[15]

The original MT19 team arrived knowing "that the military situation was pretty unstable." While it "was a foregone conclusion that we would stay,"[16] they had months to reappraise that decision before evacuating with the hospital in March. Conversely, Margaret Stanley discovered that "I was halfway around the world from home, ready to begin nursing the sick but [found] myself in an isolated group of foreigners I scarcely knew, thrust together by circumstances to work in a hospital that was packing up to remove itself from the scene of potential battles and without a clue as to where we would go."[17] Right from the beginning, she intellectualized the physical, spiritual, and emotional aspects of her Yan'an odyssey:

> I must think about this. It's a new feeling ... Reality. FAU in padded clothes ... crazy Eric and "positively I am always right Elizabeth." Humorous Jack. Slow Doug. Quiet Peter ... Read Pygmalion and wonder if I am playing a part sometimes. How can I have been so much a part of Jim's [James Chai's] life and still seem unconcerned and happy here.[18]

In contrast, Elizabeth Hughes took a more matter-of-fact approach, focusing on nursing and family life.

Prior to the arrival of Margaret Stanley and Frank Miles, work at the hospital was light, as staff and patients had been evacuated in anticipation that Yan'an would come under attack and began to return only gradually. At the IPH, as "honoured guests," team members were quartered in a spacious guesthouse, complete with a cook and two "little devils" (teenage assistants) to prepare their three daily meals. Elizabeth recalled their first few months at the IPH: "We were welcomed; we were feted, we had very interesting conversations with very high people including Zhou Enlai and we attended a dinner with [Mao Zedong]."[19] The team was regularly invited to local theatre productions and splendid feasts, sometimes to discuss improvements to hospital medical services, other times to be politically courted by high-ranking Chinese government officials, including Mao and Zhou. Given the resident entourage of Western press attached to the peace mission, MT19 was the ideal propaganda weapon to enhance the Communist regime's legitimacy in Western circles. The Communists "would say, 'We have the FAU medical team working at the IPH, you should come interview them.'"[20] There were plenty of opportunities for social diversions as long as the American peace team was quartered nearby. Douglas Clifford described a typical week: "Things go on pretty slowly, much as usual; some work in the hospital, a couple of feasts, a trip down to the [American] Liaison Group Compound one evening to see a couple of films, a dance on Friday night."[21] At future family gatherings, Joan Kennedy would relish describing dancing with Zhou Enlai, although her memories of attending never-ending political rallies were far less fond.

The expectation that MT19 would improve the hospital's medical services and teaching programs along Western lines was unfulfilled.[22] As Mao abandoned traditional military tactics geared towards holding cities in favour of full-scale guerrilla warfare, his revolutionary forces abandoned their wartime capital, and Chiang Kai-shek's forces captured it on 19 March 1947.[23] As one of four mobile hospitals with Mao's 8th Route Army on the retreat from Yan'an, the team moved twenty times from village to village as dictated by the military situation, treating villagers and military casualties en route.[24] Covering a distance of 1,600 *li*, the IPH staff and patients travelled on foot and by donkey over mountain footpaths, often at night to avoid being detected when the fighting was close by. After one night march, dawn arrived before they reached their destination. A weary Margaret Stanley "quickly perked up," however, when word came down the line "to cover anything which might reflect a glint of sunlight thereby giving bomber pilots the target they were seeking." As the first morning planes roared overhead, she scrambled to a nearby field, and "laid face down under a stack of young wheat" until it was safe to continue.[25] In August, MT19 made a perilous raft crossing over the Yellow River into Shaanxi Province before finally establishing a more permanent base in Shaanxi Province.[26]

Even before the team evacuated the IPH, it was clear that Chinese and Western cultures would clash as the medical staff worked out how to get along. While this interaction afforded opportunities to learn from each other and develop new perspectives about other people and cultures, some did not rise to the challenge.

A fair assessment of Joan Kennedy's short time in Yan'an is difficult; her response to the arduous practice setting can be gleaned only from cursory references in official records or colleagues' private letters home. According to her teammates, she was simply unable to adjust. As Douglas Clifford saw it, "she could not take it here, I am afraid & didn't try much, complained about the food (which most of us think is quite good), the cold, the people, the introspection, so we weren't very sorry to see her go. As Eric Hughes candidly puts it, 'We are now in the second wave of liberation!'"[27] Jack Dodds hoped that her replacement would not be "such a flop,"[28] but Margaret Stanley always cited Joan's ill health as the prime reason for being sent to replace her. Joan suffered from chronic bronchitis, aggravated by the cold, damp conditions of cave living during Yan'an's bitter winters. Of course, as events would show, part of her behaviour while in Yan'an was attributable to the extraordinary stress that she felt unable to share with anyone.

The circumstances surrounding her unexpected departure in early March remained veiled from FAU staff. "We hear that she had flown to Beijing from Yan'an, something was wrong, and then [FAU chairman] Griff [Levering] flew up there and the next thing we heard was a cable from Griff saying that Joan and Park Woodrow had been married."[29] When Philadelphia inquired why it was not briefed in detail about the circumstances triggering the Woodrows' sudden return,[30] the apologetic reply was simply, "You no doubt understand by now why a great deal was not said."[31] Decades later, a franker yet respectful explanation of Joan's "health problems" was given by Frank Miles. "Joan," he explained, "had decided to make a start on her family."[32] Given the societal censoring of unmarried mothers and Joan's lack of family support, marriage appeared the best option. Once back home, it became obvious that the marriage lacked a strong foundation and the couple divorced within two years. Joan, as a single mother with a limited personal support network, returned to nursing to support her young son. This experience tainted her memories of China, but she retained ties with valued colleagues such as Spence Coxe and Chris Evans, attending and co-hosting their New Year's gatherings. She raised her son in Quaker circles.[33]

Although Elizabeth Hughes and Margaret Stanley confronted difficult personal and professional circumstances, they remained. Both coped with serious physical conditions. Margaret underwent a tonsillectomy with only a modicum of anesthetic; a pregnant Elizabeth had to be carried by stretcher for part of their journey when she spiked a fever triggered by a septic finger.

Hughes described their working conditions in western China and Henan as fairly similar to what they had experienced in the Middle East. In contrast, the IPH was unlike anything that she could have imagined in England. It "was far more primitive than any hospital I had previously seen, including the ... dreadful [Chinese] cholera hospital" in Henan.[34] In Yan'an, "we had to do the best we could with what was offered to us ... We were often extremely short of drugs. You couldn't get at patients properly because they had to be nursed in awkward places." Water had to be carried several kilometres. Special diets were quite unobtainable, and dressings "had to be reused in a way entirely un-hygienic. So really it was a question of adapting, going back to first principles and deciding what was essential and what could go by the board. We were down absolutely to bare essentials."[35]

Hughes' report, covering the period before the hospital's evacuation, chronicled her struggle to carve out professional space that adapted Western nursing knowledge and standards to local needs, resources, and practice:

> The IPH had been functioning for some years before I arrived and many systems and routines established, many of which were not clear or explained to us at first. For instance, nurses graduate in time to become interns and later doctors ... interns do things that would normally be done by nurses. Not fully understanding many of these things, and not knowing exactly what position or authority I was to have in the hospital, I did not have an easy time settling down.

She found herself an unwanted Western interloper in the operating theatre: "There were so many theatre staff, that there was no need for me to help [to clean up]." Applying Western surgical standards, she initially "found that the staff seemed very slow and unmethodical in these tasks. When I offered to help, they ... refused so vigorously that it seemed futile to insist." Believing that the operating room staff is "too large for effective work" and that its "attention to aseptic technique was erratic," she was taken aback that the surgical nurses "did not take any of the hints that I threw out about being ready for emergencies or ways of improving techniques." Dismayed by her inability to create an orderly and efficient operating theatre, she lamented, "They were used to one system and any attempts to alter this, even in a small degree, met with little enthusiasm." Similarly, in the wards, her attempts to introduce admissions procedures that included delousing and routine bathing "met with only partial success." She was shocked that patients who could not provide a change of bedding were left to lie in their own filth. It took time for her to realize "how poor the district is and how expensive soap, cloth and everyday things are."[36] She failed to appreciate that her Western standards, prioritizing efficiency and standardized nursing techniques, often conflicted with local needs, resources, or priorities. Her recommendations, for example, to reduce the OR team size conflicted directly with the IPH officials' desire to maximize the numbers trained. Most IPH nurses received only enough training to get by.

After evacuating Yan'an, a Chinese nurse rather than Hughes was appointed head surgical nurse for the mobile hospital. As conditions became more chaotic, she developed a greater respect for and collegiality with her

Chinese counterparts, whose aptitude for "overcoming the difficulties associated with the lack of proper buildings, equipment, facilities ... would have stumped us foreigners." They began "learning each other's reasons for our methods." She introduced the Chinese nurses to intravenous therapy techniques and assembled all the apparatus necessary for it; in turn, Hughes learned to sterilize dressings in a bread steamer. Despite her contention that "it has been possible to adapt the Chinese nurses' methods and ours fairly satisfactorily to suit the circumstances of situation, supplies and doctors' wishes," she remained perturbed by her continued inability to get "the nurses to see the reasons for my methods or to make changes or improvements in the things that I have criticized."[37] It took Elizabeth Hughes time to accept the limitations of her role. It also speaks to the Chinese nurses' agency and ability to incorporate both Western and Chinese methods into the Chinese healthcare system. They adopted Western nursing practices selectively, according to their own perceptions of what was needed and feasible.

Despite her later accounts, Margaret Stanley experienced similar difficulties adjusting to the unpredictable rhythms of a mobile medical unit constantly moving to be closer to the battlefront but still out of harm's way. Often patients arrived before the team had set up in its new location. Casualties, often with maggot-infested wounds, arrived after being carried for several days. Gangrene developed following inadequate first aid, and tetanus took its toll. Gunshot patients also suffered from anemia, tuberculosis, malnutrition, or venereal diseases.[38] When such grievously ill patients arrived in overwhelming numbers, Stanley's priority, to bathe each patient, was vetoed. "All available labour was used in converting local [cave] homes into wards." She was soon "too busy dressing wounds after the doctors examined them to worry long about ... patients' [comfort]."[39] Over time, she learned that her skills complemented the local nurses' knowledge, and she better understood the importance of acknowledging their contribution. As she explained, "the problems were ... unique to that area and the learning process was different. It was a learning process for us all."[40] Over time, their shared learning and collaboration forged closer personal and professional ties.

Still struggling to overcome the language barrier and understand the local customs and medical practices, Margaret Stanley, like Elizabeth Hughes, was astounded and sometimes disappointed by the tensions and misunderstanding associated with her well-meaning efforts. Nurse Stanley discovered that "convincing patients to accept treatment was a great big problem. In the first place, we were foreign devils. But even with the best of translations and Chinese staff working with the patients over a long period of time, it could be difficult for a patient to accept that he had to have an amputation for example."[41] Moreover, once again civilian patients frequently came to the hospital only as a last resort, having exhausted traditional Chinese remedies.

Similarly, when relapsing fever struck a family of villagers living next to their cave and a student nurse contracted typhus, Stanley initiated a delousing campaign: "cutting hair, searching clothes and bedding and killing the lice found, bathing the patient and sprinkling clothing with DDT." Instead of becoming accepted nursing routine, "it seemed to be looked upon as some special order from the doctor. And no matter how many classes we conducted, or how many examples we could show to be the result of carelessness in personal hygiene, illness was taken as a matter of course and accepted by the staff." In this instance, Margaret was not looking at the situation through Western eyes that equated cleanliness with civility and citizenship. Rather, the public health nurse viewed personal hygiene as one of the few weapons in her arsenal readily available against disease, and initially found it difficult "to sympathize with this seeming lassitude" of the IPH nurses. After suffering a diarrhea attack, however, she "could understand that one's heart is not in one's work when ascaris [small intestinal roundworm] is playing tag in the stomach and intestines."[42] It took time before Margaret Stanley could stand in the shoes of her Chinese nursing staff, whose diet certainly was not as good as hers.

Stanley's 1948 description of setting up makeshift cave hospital wards at each of the stops on their journey illustrates the bonds of friendship formed while practising a kind of health care that "was quite different from anything I have read in textbooks or heard from teachers of public health back home":[43]

We spent days sweeping out the caves ... with brooms made of brush. We numbered the caves in Arabic numerals and the built-in beds that usually take up one-half of each cave were spread with straw. Fireplaces were built of mud and straw ... Native cotton was rolled into bandages ... We made woven fly-swatters from cornstalks peelings with twigs for handles. We used local pork fat in making ointments, sulphur and sulphanilamide. We used up our small supply of DDT and in vain we tried to catch up with an epidemic of relapsing fever ... We felt frustrated because we had nothing with which to fight the flies.[44]

Front-line nursing meant accepting that "we could do nothing to help," because medical supplies either were not available or were reserved for patients who had a good chance of surviving.[45] Like her Chinese counterparts, Margaret focused increasingly on how nursing care could improve patient comfort rather than on its limitations. She "vividly" remembered witnessing "lots of patients in pain" undergo surgical procedures with little medication: "We knew it. They knew it. But the nurses were often right there; their physical presence and their concern perhaps understood by the patients to such a degree that this was a help." Capturing the essence of compassionate care, she recalled: "One phrase the Chinese nurses often used for people, 'Bieh K'u' (don't cry, don't cry) ... The nurses and the patients and the doctors were all right in there together."[46]

In a 1950 article for the *American Journal of Nursing*, Stanley recounted her own efforts to provide compassionate care in a cave and how it was received. After brushing the daily accumulation of clay dust from the rush mat on the *kang* (a waist-high stone bed), she placed the sacking, the piece of sheeting, and the cotton ring on which the patient's injured hip would soon rest. "At the head of the bed I placed his bundle of clothing. The versatile and ever present comforter, pretty well blackened around the edges, was spread on top of all of this ... But he was happy; this was his bed, a place to sleep and rest – he asked for nothing more."[47] While she conceded the difficulties of squatting on a *kang* to tend to a patient, she claimed, "From the moment of my arrival in China I never really longed for the gadgets of a more complicated civilization." She found satisfaction in knowing that even though "his bed was a kang in a dirty, draughty, vermin ridden cave, [she] could still help him recover from his illness or injury."[48] Nursing in northern China stripped away the luxuries of Western nursing, leaving Margaret Stanley looking to her Chinese counterparts to learn "how to make the best of the situation in which we found ourselves."[49]

During their trek, Elizabeth Hughes managed differently. She again navigated the professional frontiers by limiting her work to assisting the FAU doctors in the operating theatre: "I knew their likes and dislikes and their methods – many of which were revolutionary to the Chinese nurses." She sought emotional refuge within her marriage and first pregnancy. She later admitted, "I feel the psychological effect of pregnancy made me unaware of difficulties and I really lived in a dream world."[50] While both Elizabeth and Margaret felt uncomfortable that they had better and more frequent meals, warmer clothes, and better accommodations than their Chinese colleagues,

Elizabeth in particular felt guilty about her special treatment during her pregnancy. She had talked with many Chinese nurse soldiers and medical colleagues who had endured repeated abortions or had been forced to abandon their children. After her son David's birth, she stopped nursing until she left in late summer. Elizabeth had sought to create a sense of professional order and normal family life in the midst of chaos, but she also been willing to accept considerable personal risk, uncertainties, and hardships to respond to the humanitarian imperative. Her transition home, while financially difficult, was a welcome return to family life.[51] Her time with MT19 remained a cherished memory. The return of Elizabeth and Eric drew a lot of media attention, most of which focused on stories of the "cave baby." When asked whether she would continue nursing, she said, "I hope not. I got a baby now."[52] But she left regretting that she had not made a significant difference in the way that Margaret Stanley had.

Both women created a sense of home during their nomadic life of nursing with the China Convoy, but in very different ways. Stanley's open-mindedness, humility, and genuine desire to accompany the Chinese in friendship fostered strong personal and professional cross-cultural ties. Sharing her cave dormitory-style with the female Chinese nurses, she believed, made "it easier for us to work together in the hospital."[53] In particular, she fondly remembered her friendship with Nurse Wu during their long and sometimes dangerous treks between cave villages:

> Wu's generous, tireless nursing, her lovely voice and her sweet temperament sustained patients and co-workers. The closer I worked with her, the more I grew to depend on her as a companion and colleague. She demonstrated an inexhaustible supply of bonhomie. We were often busy at the beginning or end of the day but the two of us rolled out our sleeping blankets and slept on the same kang at night.[54]

Even when Wu was reassigned, the two would trek many kilometres between villages to visit for a few precious hours; on the final visit before her departure, the two friends exchanged touching gifts.

Margaret Stanley's diary, however, alludes to several dark periods, especially when she succumbed to frequent bouts of tonsillitis, before she became acclimatized to team life. As a latecomer on MT19, she needed time to feel accepted by her teammates: "Letters come from Irene Li and Judith Yen Chung give me heart. I seem to have found a place among the Chinese but not among my own kind. Not surprised."[55] She felt that her teammates did not always approve of her living with her Chinese colleagues. By the time they crossed the Yellow River, she was adapting to the transitory rhythm of Chinese workdays, nursing in caves with patients and FAU colleagues who did not always behave as she would have liked:

> There is a Powerful Magnetism here attuned to myself in something that makes for Peace in my Soul in spite of the things that would be irritations if one let them. Yen Ching, the dispenser responsible for medicine, labeled 20% AgNo3 as 2% ... [The] absence of someone of my own, patients who leave their caves after breakfast and can not be found for Rx, their everlasting request for me to sing so that they can laugh at my two-song repertoire, their stubborn refusal to change nursing procedures, emphasis on the "English way." Li Shing Mei's busybodyness even to preventing me from sleeping on our roof because she fears wolves. Mr. Chang's incorrect translations, changing almost daily of nurses' duties so that they don't seem to accumulate experience ... In spite [of all this] – I find happiness here in China which I have had no other place.[56]

Caring for each other on the long marches or when each fell ill strengthened friendships within the team over time so that by late summer her diary stated simply: "D[ouglas] C[lifford], Liz, Frank, and I are getting on admirably."[57]

She also attributed her happiness in part to the "progress of [my] students."[58] One group, a class of middle-school boys, arrived after walking for two weeks, surviving by catching and eating tadpoles. At night, she regularly accompanied these teenage nurses and took her turn to fetch more supplies as they made night rounds from cave to cave. Initially daunted by the prospect of teaching "little students, who didn't know why we boiled our forceps, and couldn't understand why we asked them not to blow their noses onto the ward floors," she later acknowledged that "if it hadn't been for those devoted teenagers doing the work of nurses in war-torn China, many patients would have gone unattended."[59] She unravelled her favourite red sweater to make them all mittens to wear on night rounds.

Margaret Stanley's commitment to building strong personal ties and working according to local partners' pace and priorities strengthened over time. Her relationship with her Chinese Communist colleagues was one of friendship, mutual respect, and a shared learning underpinned by common goals. Modestly, she acknowledged: "They may have learned a little from such instruction as I have attempted. But I have certainly learned a great deal from them."[60] She recorded feeling "ever more comfortable" with her Chinese colleagues, who called her "comrade" in the spirit of its literal meaning, "one with the same goal. Our common goal was better health. I discerned ever more clearly, that the apprentice system of learning-on-the-job in our hospital met the desperate needs for health workers and included strong concerns and feelings for health in general."[61] She accepted that after three years of experience, talented nurses would be trained as China's future "barefoot doctors." She had left Yan'an determined to impress on the Chinese Nurses' Association that Chinese nurses should not be sent to America to study: "American nurses should go into the situation to teach practically, thereby omitting the confusion of American contraptions and customs irrelevant to the home needs."[62]

Margaret Stanley's resolute adherence to Quakers' ethics provided an important grounding for her approach to life and work in the China Convoy. The core of her faith was her living relationship with and obedience to God. For her, the team's daily silent meetings, always alive with the possibility of prophecy, were central to her spiritual quest to understand and practise Quaker values in her daily work and relationships:

> We sat quietly, meditating, worshiping, thinking thoughts that have no words, reaching out in silence to find strength together from the Source of all strength – awed, too, by the magnitude of nature's magnificence on the mountaintop. Peter paraphrased a familiar quotation, "What are we, that Thou art mindful of us?" In a manner of Friends worship that query seemed to speak to my condition. What could be the meaning of my life to the Creator of all life? As a Quaker willing to give my life trying to follow God's guidance, I had joined others in living our conviction, trying the way of peace in the midst of war. I wanted to understand just what purpose my day-to-day life was serving ... After something less than an hour we rose and descended the hill, yet the mood of the meeting stayed with me and gave me strength to meet whatever lay ahead.[63]

Her diary described quiet meditation as "moments of utter aliveness when awareness was at a peak, mind clear, filled with ineffable longing to face with inner peace whatever that day had in store."[64] Her commitment to living a life that outwardly attests to this inward experience also helped her reconcile personal desires with her need to alleviate the suffering of others:

> This is life that should be intensely satisfying. But in human fashion I say, if only Jay [James Chai] were here it would be. Now it is my duty to make myself contented ... [I] am beholden to God for his great generosity in general. It continues to be that if I spent the rest of my life doing for others, I would never make up for what they have done for me.[65]

After fourteen months with MT19, Margaret decided it was time to return home. As the team's patient load decreased, she no longer felt "essential" there.[66] Her nursing staff exercised more control daily, and the hospital administration "made decisions at meetings in which I was not included and which sometimes took precedence over scheduled classes."[67] Other considerations figured in her growing restlessness. Unable "to shake off the mood of sadness" after witnessing a Chinese mother die unnecessarily in childbirth after days of prolonged labour, she realized her need for midwifery training "in order to do something about it, wherever I might be." She remained conflicted, however. Should she pursue midwifery or get a job to help support her parents? And what would become of her "unrealized dream of having a family and home of my own?"[68]

From 12 February until 13 March 1948, Margaret, accompanied by the team's medical mechanic, Frank Miles, and a Chinese interpreter travelled over 1,260 *li* during their ten-week trek by cart, mule, and foot from their hillside cave home across Shaanxi to Shijiazhuang in Hebei Province and then on to Tianjin. They "walked into Chinese paintings, black rocky mountains piled up high one on top of the other, the morning mist and our frost breath softening the rugged scene." They were "always graciously cared for" in the homes of the local people.[69] But images of ruined villages, caravans carrying captured Canadian and American military supplies, and unnecessary suffering punctuated her diary accounts.

As always, public health provided a critical lens for Margaret Stanley's observations of the villagers' terrible suffering associated with protracted war and poverty. The "most moving experience in [her] life" came while accompanying Miss Lin, a public health nurse from the Isabella Fisher Hospital in Tianjin on her home calls, "with ten patients impromptu for every one scheduled." It made Stanley want "to start my visiting nursing again right then and there."[70] At every opportunity, she stressed the importance of public health education.[71] It was, as she said, "a matter of life and death."[72] This was never clearer than during one gut-wrenching stopover. Before Margaret "could catch [her] breath from astonishment and think of a reply," a young Chinese mother drew aside her worn tunic-jacket, revealing the "wizened, limp, dry skin" of a naked child. Immediately, she knew, "I was looking at a classic case of marasmus [severe malnourishment]." The mother begged her to take her child: "You eat well. You dress well. You can take care of it better than I." For Margaret,

> it was a bolt of lightning, burning deep, searing the very core of my being with what I was seeing and feeling – electrifyingly activating a despair that had been accumulating under the surface of my China experience ... I must not only refuse to take the baby but refuse to believe what was happening. How could I bear it? ... Either I would have to take the baby and all the others offered me and embrace their crying need, and the misery I had seen, or reject it ... If I were to embrace it all, I would surely stretch arms and spirits to the bursting point.[73]

The kaleidoscope of accompanying emotions forced Margaret to acknowledge the limits of her personal humanitarian capacity and, conversely, the resilience and agency of the Chinese people.

For but a brief moment, the two travelling companions' journey allowed them time to ponder their shared Quaker ideals, aspirations, and vision of a future, regardless of the state of the external world. Neither anticipated the new feelings that intruded on their friendship as a consequence. Their China interlude had been a time of spiritual introspection for them. Like Margaret, Frank had "been trying to make [his] life conform to the inner knowledge of good which is in each of us."[74] For Margaret, her deeply held Quaker beliefs of simplicity, integrity, community, and equality coalesced into abiding commitment to service as a way of life rather than an interesting sojourn abroad. Frank, too, believed that service was a cardinal tenet of a meaningful life. He had already decided to remain for another year: "This is a highly important time to spread the message of love, here as in every other part of the world ... And lastly, I would like to feel that I have given more of myself in this sort of effort before I leave China."[75] Both, equally quick to chastise their own failure to live up to Quaker ideals, always believed that they had gained more than they had given in service to the Chinese people. Both had an intellectual turn of mind and savoured quiet evenings reading and discussing the insights of Tolstoy on war and peace. Inevitably they "opened their hearts to each other" concerning their discomfort with the opulence, materialism, and misguided energies that they observed among Westerners, only to discover that "we see clearly, face to face, shall we say that [these] people ... are not happy."[76] Their common quest for a sense of purpose that gave real meaning to their lives forged emotional ties that deepened into respectful love.

Although physically attracted to Margaret, who "has no need of cosmetics to bring out her beauty and charm,"[77] Miles had decided "that [he] should make no advances towards anyone till I get out of the L.A.s [liberated areas] at least ... because it would not be fair to either of us. But I'll be darned if I can make myself really want to."[78] After much internal debate, he broached the topic of their future with Margaret:

It does seem that there is no way for things to work as I would like to have them. Last year when M. went to Yenan [Yan'an] she was quite certain that Jim was the man, though no promise was made. Now I have disturbed the picture and she is betwixt and between – but I am quite sure she still feels that if she were away from me for a while, the choice would go in Jim's direction. So it would appear that I should extricate myself from the picture, if the happiest solution for M is to be made ... I find it terribly difficult to say to myself: "This can't be." But I'm afraid that's what must be said.[79]

Although Margaret went on ahead by plane from Beijing to FAU head-quarters in Shanghai, she remained conflicted: "Hope Frank comes soon because I feel inadequate by myself."[80] After his arrival, Margaret wrote: "A glorious day on which I found that Frank's and my lives are inextricably intertwined. May I know what is wisest."[81] At the time, both planned to re-main with the Unit at Zhongmou, but events over the next few days left Margaret determined to return home in mid-June. When Frank Miles raised the subject again, it became evident that Margaret "didn't know where she stood and she was still going to visit Nanjing with similar feelings for Jim."[82] But James Chai's unexpected arrival the next day crystallized the situa-tion: Margaret experienced "an at home feeling at once – the calm which is the Peace." When Frank left alone for Zhongmou, he gave Margaret "his beloved Peking platter and [she found] it difficult to say goodbye to Brother

Frank – Comrade Miles."[83] Working side by side would have been unfair for all parties involved, Margaret knew. She would return home to study midwifery but hoped to rejoin Chai and build a life together.

For Margaret, as a young Quaker woman trying to follow her heart without hurting others, the decision of whom to marry was not straightforward. Both societal norms and parents' expectations were at play. Even before her arrival in Shanghai, she had learned that her father, unable to receive adequate assurance from the American Friends Service Committee about his daughter's safety, had arrived unannounced at Friends Service Unit headquarters three weeks earlier. Margaret's premonition that he had travelled to China to bring her home to settle down proved correct. Her uneasiness grew when they met. Although they spoke of Jay only "indirectly," her parents' views were made explicitly clear: it "was a mistake to marry into a different culture because of the resulting problems, especially for the children."[84]

Margaret Stanley's China years broadened her world view and provided an alternative lens through which to re-examine her childhood beliefs and Western civil society. During her cultural adaptation in Yan'an, a new situational identity had emerged that was intersecting with and antagonistic to the culture into which she had been born and in which she had socialized.[85] The unexpected meeting with her father in Shanghai epitomized her cultural no man's land. As they conversed, Margaret realized, as had many other Convoy members:

> I had changed in many more ways than my accent. How could I convey to my father what changes had occurred? Since leaving home in 1946, I had gone places I had not known existed until I saw them. I had been in places no American had seen before. I had learned a new language and had become steeped in a different culture. I had learned that pain and suffering are the same in any language. Having required a different way of looking at life, I could not return to my former way of thinking. Could I expect people to understand?[86]

Although excited that Jim had given her a ring on their final visit in Nanjing, "a promise of a future interminably, irretrievably intertwined,"[87] she deliberately concealed their engagement: "People ask me, 'Am I coming back to China?' I say, of course, but fear their repulsion so don't mention why I am coming back."[88] When Margaret and Jim parted company for the last time on 15 June, she "went with him in a sense, yearning, feeling that a part of me was gone. Leaving him and leaving China were somehow required of me though I didn't know why." "At the last, his 'Tsai-Chien' [until I see you again] and my 'Goodbye' were all we could say." She did not want "to say anything, wanting only to wrap myself in some kind of insulating cocoon to keep away the reality."[89]

Margaret Stanley remembered little of the voyage home. She "floated timeless and effortless between two worlds." "How could it be," she wondered, "that both tides and events were carrying me back home, yet they were taking away from what had become home to me?"[90] Her departure seemed like a divorce, leaving her feeling vulnerable and alone. She had changed but remained uncertain how she would connect to the outside world with her new insights. Margaret straddled two cultures, more easily leaving behind the "trappings" of modern nursing and Western-style hospitals, but still she belonged to neither.

Back home, Margaret experienced what is now termed "reverse culture shock" as she compared the stark differences between China and opulent Western societies. She was "distressed by evidence of waste, disposable household and hospital goods ... being thrown out instead of being put to good use. Conversations with friends drifted to niceties and to generalities. My feet hurt in leather shoes walking on concrete ... With no one to talk to about China, I felt isolated and very much alone."[91] Both Margaret Stanley and Elizabeth Hughes returned less willing to accept the Cold War stereotypes of either the Chinese Nationalists or Communists.[92] When Margaret received a lukewarm response to her offer to present slide shows based on her China experiences, she abandoned the project until the 1970s, when the political climate proved more receptive. For the rest of her life, according to her family, she remained a sojourner between two worlds.[93]

Other ex-China Convoy members reported experiencing similar difficulties as they tried to "fit into the pattern of life here at home." Many yearned to "get back to the life they had left ... to re-live their experiences in China, even if it included all the many frustrations and drawbacks." Their response could not be explained merely by the "glamour attached to work in China" but rather by a compelling combination of factors. "The feeling of being really needed in China no matter what qualification one possesses" was cited as an important consideration. In addition, there was a "feeling of unity which has led to deeper relationships as well as a common interest in and sympathy for the activities of other sections." Perhaps the point that took precedence was the "simplicity and sense of purpose about Chinese life which compares so favourably with our bustling mechanical civilization whose ends seem to have so little direct relation to people."[94] For them it was not the amount of the help but the friendships formed with the Chinese people that mattered.

It was impossible to walk away from MT19 unchanged.

Nursing in the China Convoy changed both Margaret and Elizabeth. Both shared a deep respect and affection for the Chinese people. Witnessing their suffering challenged their beliefs about how the world should work. Both wished they could have done more to alleviate the effects of war and its aftermath. Both nurses hoped that health could be a tool of reconciliation and peace building. But for Margaret, as a Quaker, this weighed more heavily on her mind. For her, to "realize that the few precious supplies that we had were going to mending and healing wounds that had been made from military supplies from my own country, too, was perhaps the hardest thing for me to bear."[95] She was keenly aware of her tenuous position as a cultural outsider and the limits of her personal humanitarian efforts, particularly as an American. She learned that "I could never learn enough because the culture was really obscure to me ... you need to be part of it and grow up in it so that, I as foreigner, could only see it as a foreigner."[96]

Although their pacifist and religious views differed, Margaret and Elizabeth both believed that the humanitarian imperative was paramount and that nothing should override it. While they were not oblivious to the Communists' flaws, they regarded political affiliation as irrelevant to their mandate of helping people in need. However, as Margaret later observed, humanitarian work could never "be totally divorced from political attitudes, social concerns and religious movements."[97] Differences in their perception of how pacifism translated to their work within these common boundaries, however, may partially explain how each interpreted and negotiated new professional and cultural frontiers. Margaret's perception, in keeping with other North American recruits discussed earlier, was shaped by the social gospel movement. When expressing this progressive tradition, she later claimed:

My interest was in helping alleviate people's problems but not necessarily in a medical setting, such as hospital nursing ... my interest was in the whole person and not just in their physical problems. So the kind of work that appealed to me was some kind of work that followed that philosophy. I believe Friends have to try, not only take care of people who suffer in some physical way but also try to cope with social problems, war related problems. I wanted to work with others who have this kind of philosophy.[98]

In practice, as she later acknowledged, they "were so caught up in the daily tragedy of trying to patch up people's sick bodies and coping with disease and illness in ourselves as well as others; just absorbing all the facets of life that impinged upon us," that there was little time for theorizing.[99] Despite the limitations of MT19's humanitarian work, Margaret Stanley believed that her endeavour was taken for what it was – "a human effort to live, people to people in friendship, doing what we could." In the process, she "learned so much about other ways of life than my own" and developed a deep respect for "Chinese endurance, vitality and coping with hardships."[100] Simultaneously, MT19 enabled her to work in a Quakerly way, honouring not only its peace testimony but respectful of the cardinal importance Quakers placed on personal relationships. Humanitarian nursing for Margaret was an opportunity to gain emotional, spiritual, and professional satisfaction by understanding the kinship that bound humankind across borders.

Elizabeth Hughes's broadly based Christian pacifism and pragmatic nature predisposed her to emphasize the Unit's medical or "work" side. Margaret Stanley's strong Quaker beliefs, placing greater stress on the ethics of how humanitarian aid and global fraternity was delivered, placed her squarely on the "faith" side.[101] As it was for the majority of the China Convoy, her purpose was plainly not evangelism: "Overall most Unit members agreed that it was their responsibility to practice Christian compassion and tolerance rather than to preach such virtues."[102] As she said, "the compassion for the people that took us there in the first place, carried us through experiences we might never have thought we had the strength to cope with – there was so little that we could do to help improve the lives of the people."[103]

Personality and different pacifists' backgrounds may only partially explain Margaret's more compelling desire to accompany her Chinese colleagues on their terms and her deeper thirst to understand and learn from them. Did their educational backgrounds make a difference in their professional acclimatization? Students, such as Elizabeth, who graduated from the hospital apprentice system learned by rote and were exposed to a culture of submission, precision, routine, duty, and strict accountability when they provided service in the wards. In contrast, public health nursing attracted women seeking greater professional autonomy. Stanley and her fellow public health nurses were encouraged to take a preventive perspective that looked at the underlying socio-economic determinants of health and favoured considering the patient's whole situation rather than focusing on the disease or technique. Perhaps this view predisposed Margaret Stanley to grasp more quickly that improving health care could not be separated from a willingness to learn from and listen to those she came to support. A broader sampling of humanitarian nurses' educational background and relative effectiveness as cross-cultural brokers than can be provided by this study would be needed, however, before any correlation can be substantiated conclusively. As Joan Kennedy illustrates, training alone cannot account for the differences. Margaret's personality and intellectual curiosity, as much as anything she had been taught, brought her to China and determined her lifelong fascination with its history and people.

Agency, assimilation, and accommodation coloured the acculturation of the Western nurses to China. Elizabeth Hughes and Margaret Stanley initially perceived nursing with the China Convoy as an opportunity for both adventure in an exotic location and, at the same time, humanitarian service that incorporated scientific standards of nursing. While responding to human suffering, they found that Western nursing, based on hygiene and notions of efficiency, strict hospital routines, and careful patient observation and recording, collided with the realities of mobile warfare cut off from supplies. They had to accept that hospital routines and classes were constantly rescheduled for political rallies. In MT19, as for their predecessors, their Chinese colleagues not only taught them the art of making do but also helped them accept the limits of their personal diplomacy in a nation undergoing radical transformation. While Chinese nurses adopted and adapted structures and traditions of modern Western nursing, their practice was different, dictated by necessity and political objectives. The most striking example was the inclusion of male nurses throughout China and the Chinese Communists' use of the nursing profession as a stepping stone in the education of physicians. Barefoot doctors provided visible evidence of the Communist Party's determination to improve health care for the common people.

The cross-cultural experiences of Margaret Stanley and Elizabeth Hughes argue against a monolithic portrait of Convoy nurses' humanitarian work in China. Acculturation occurs differently for everyone. Differences in their personality, pacifist perspectives, faith, personal circumstances, and nursing education sculpted their distinct responses to living and working in China. As important, by moving beyond the cloistered communities associated with the Henan mission hospitals to work and live as non-combatants with the Communist troops engaged in highly mobile guerrilla warfare, the two women were forerunners of nurses without borders. The experiences that

MT19 nurses faced were in some respects exceptional among Western Convoy nurses. Their friendships and contacts gave them an opportunity to understand what Chinese civilians and soldiers lived through on a daily basis. But even then they still had a more privileged lifestyle. As Margaret confessed, the "hard part" was living with my friends the Chinese nurses in a cave, "myself with a mosquito net and the rest without nets; I would escape malaria ... more readily than they." She had soap while they used water that was run through ashes or soda. The comparison of Elizabeth's healthy baby with village children, whose mothers took it "for granted that a certain percentage of their children would die," provides a striking example of MT19's continued status as "honoured guests." Their new awareness of this privileged status "working among underprivileged for whom you can sometimes do nothing" shaped a more positive view of Chinese communist society and helped team members reconcile the choices made.[104] Here, as team members recognized and accepted, negotiating humanitarian space to gain access to patients compromised the team's autonomy and risked its neutrality and professional standards.[105]

MT19's experiences foreshadowed the fact that, in such conflict zones, neutrality, autonomy, and impartiality would be constantly negotiated in specific contexts. After 1947, nursing on new FSU teams, spawned amid the deepening civil war, would again highlight the fact that the ability to negotiate in an impartial and neutral manner with all actors in conflict situations is essential for humanitarian assistance and the protection of staff. Equally, the narratives of MT19 nurses reaffirm that war conditions served to reify certain gender roles while challenging others. Moreover, for all of MT19 medical staff, balancing their Western expertise with respect for the agency of local actors remained a crucial goal. As the participation of local actors continued to be a key strategy for the China Convoy's development work after 1947, the tensions over participation mounted.

PART 3

Unwelcome Visitors: Negotiating Access with the Communists, 1947–51

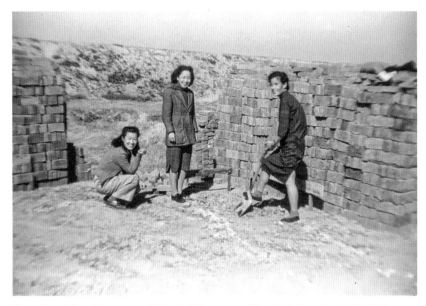

First shovel; breaking ground for the Zhongmou Hospital, October 1947. *Left to right:* Doris Wu, Marina King, Jean Liu. *Source:* Mark and Mardy Shaw Collection

Traction equipment made by FAU medical mechanics from airplane wreckage. *Source:* Lindsay Crozier Collection

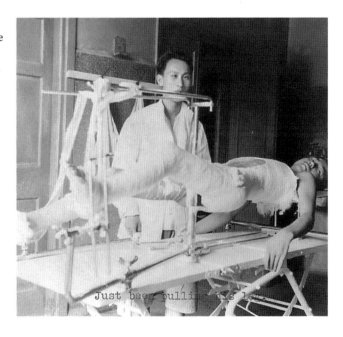

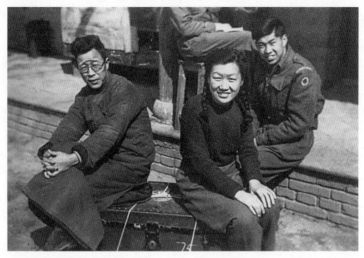

John Brown and Jean Liu, Zhungmou. *Source:* American Friends Service
Committee Archives

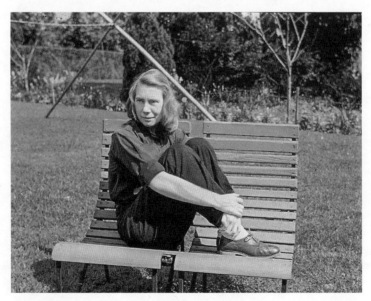

Elizabeth File in garden at Shanghai Hostel. *Source:* American Friends
Service Committee Archives

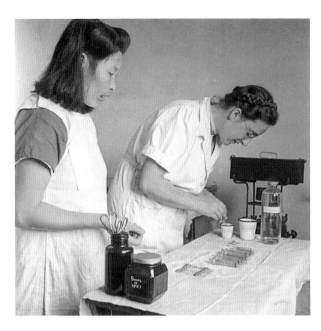

Gladys Saint with Chinese nursing student at Zhungmou. Formal pictures depicting Western standards were used for publicity and fundraising. *Source:* American Friends Service Committee Archives

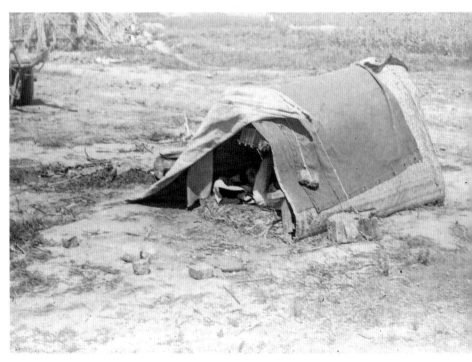

Temporary shelter for kala-azar outpatients at Zhongmou hospital. *Source:* Mark and Mardy Shaw Collection

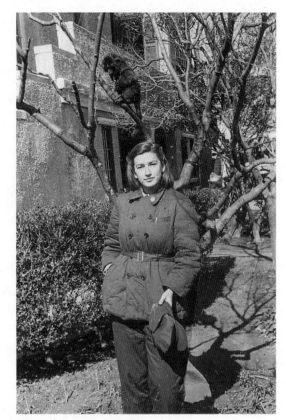

American physician
Shirley Gage.
Source: Douglas
Clifford Collection

Shirley Gage and her
"hut boys," Zhongmou.
Source: American Friends
Service Committee
Archives

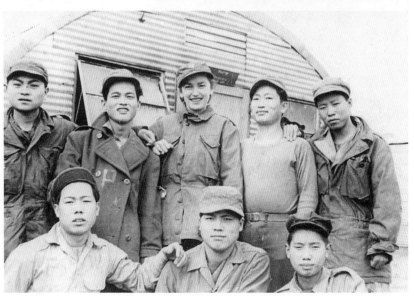

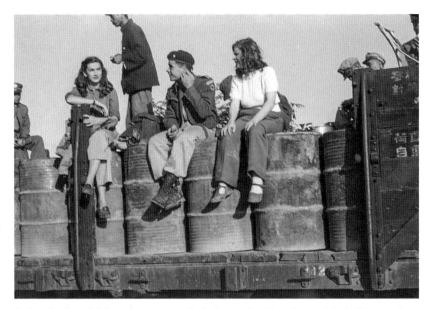

Riding "yellow fish" on the train roofs. *Left to right:* Mary Jones, Mark Shaw, and Shirley Gage, Zhongmou. *Source:* Mark and Mardy Shaw Collection

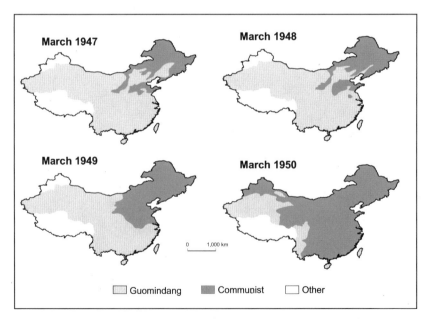

Map 10   Communist-held areas, 1947–50

March 31st 1947
Ring out, wild bells to China's sky
The flying cloud, the frost light
The Convoy's pegging out tonight
Ring out wild bells and let it die!
...

The time has come to drink the cup
Down with short-term project life
Each member will have a wife
Though the Budget's cut, the Pool is up!
Ring in the valiant Coxe so free!
The lengthy scarf, the weepy voice!
Lift up your hearts and cry Rejoice!
The FSU is about to be!

– DBS, *FSU CHRONICLE* 1, 5 APRIL 1947

Headquartered in the Friends Hostel, Shanghai, the Friends Service Unit (FSU) officially took over administrative responsibility from the Friends Ambulance Unit (FAU) on 31 March 1947. The poem in the epigraph, at once mournful and irreverent, reflected the uncertainty and conflicting emotions surrounding the FSU's inauguration under the administrative auspices of the American Friends Service Committee (AFSC). Could American Spencer Coxe, a relative newcomer, named chairman in January 1947, rein in the China Convoy boys, who his predecessor found had always "been extremely jealous of [the Unit's] democratic rights" but who "possibly lack[ed] a full appreciation of its democratic responsibilities"?[1] Most of the ninety Chinese, Canadian, American, New Zealander, and British FAU members transferred to the FSU. Although membership remained restricted to those who supported the Quaker views on peace and personal relationships – as the practical demonstration of the transforming power of love to overcome violence and injustice, growing shadings of belief would prove divisive.

The FSU, intended to be smaller than the FAU, would focus on "long-term projects of social betterment."[2] To avoid setting up as "a sort of group of benevolent colonialists," however, the FSU aimed "to give the local population the right to be responsible in their own way for the conduct of the project."[3] The new Unit placed increasing emphasis on enabling self-help as a pillar of its long-term humanitarian and developmental work, but its members still demanded the flexibility to undertake emergency relief work. As always, newcomers would bring their own ideas of what it meant to be a pacifist humanitarian organization amid the mounting political and military turmoil. The Unit remained doggedly determined to carry out these twin humanitarian goals even as civil war spread like wildfire throughout the country. Could the FSU redefine its pacifist witness as the Communists gained strength from 1947 to 1949 and the Cold War reconfigured Western-driven humanitarianism?

The FSU's humanitarian endeavours cannot be evaluated without analyzing the struggle of the major powers for peace and security as a response to their perceived diplomatic failures. In many ways, the Truman Doctrine marked the formal declaration of the Cold War between the United States and the Soviet Union. Announcing on 12 March 1947 that the United States would provide political, military, and economic assistance to support democratic regimes under threat from internal or external authoritarian forces, it solidified the US position on containment that spilled over into American aid for China.

American leaders preferred a Guomindang victory and certainly did not want to be charged by domestic critics with facilitating the "loss" of China to communism. However, General Marshall, who had led the unsuccessful attempt to unite the Communists and Guomindang into a democratic government as a bulwark against Russia, contended that the United States could not afford to invest large sums of money or use millions of American soldiers in an area of secondary concern in the confrontation with the Soviet Union. Although Washington's financial and material support for the Guomindang was limited, it was sufficient to intensify anti-American feeling among the Communists. Throughout 1948, it became increasingly clear that US economic and military aid could not turn the Communist tide. On 2 June 1949, there was a domestic backlash when the US government, attempting to wash its hands of the corrupt and militarily inept Chiang Kai-shek regime, failed to extend the China Aid Act in support of the Guomindang. Accordingly, in August 1949, the Truman administration published *The China White Paper* to exonerate the United States for the loss of China to the Communists and silence its domestic critics by showing that "they had done everything to support Chiang, that it was not our fault that the Communists were winning. It was Chiang's own fault."[4] The *White Paper* did neither. Instead, it provided Mao Zedong with ammunition to stir up even more fervent anti-Americanism in China. The Communists "made the White Paper the centre of their first mass anti-American campaign," the first step of an orchestrated plan "to eliminate Western influence in China."[5] That same year, the Communists won the war and the Nationalists fled to Taiwan.

When Mao proclaimed the creation of the People's Republic of China (PRC) on 1 October, there was little doubt that he would align his country with the Soviets. With Democrats fearing a backlash in the 1950 mid-term elections if the US abandonment of Chiang was perceived to have precipitated final his defeat, Truman delayed recognition of the People's Republic, assuming that the Communists would invade Taiwan in the summer of 1950 and easily prevail over the Nationalist forces. With Chiang defeated and the elections over, the thinking went, the administration could move towards recognition of Communist China before the end of 1950. However, war broke out in Korea in June 1950, eventually pitting the United States against the People's Republic and closing the door on any potential accommodation between the two countries. Truman's desire to contain the spread of communism led to the US policy of protecting Chiang's government in Taiwan, and recognition of Communist China was delayed for nearly thirty years. The impact of these events on the FSU in China was tremendous; it became impossible to maintain the distinction between the well-intended actions of Americans employed by the FSU and the direct acts of their government against the Chinese government.

Not only was China in turmoil, but the FSU was beset by personnel and financial challenges that raised doubts about whether "Spencer's organization,"[6] as it had been dubbed in the *FSU Chronicle*, the new Unit newsletter, would survive its first year. Changes in its size, composition, and experience fed the perception that the FSU had abandoned FAU traditions and its pacifist ethos. As the Unit's membership declined from 101 in January to 75 by May, the FSU became more and more American in composition.[7] Dissident voices claimed:

> The smaller Unit is not a closer Unit. The spirit of adventure that kept the Convoy alive has not enthused the Unit. We feel more of an offshoot of the AFSC and not such an important offshoot at that. Some of us, too, feel that the Unit is becoming more missionary in its outlook, and that membership is now almost synonymous with membership, or at least attendership of the Society [of Friends].[8]

The apparent lack of direction in the first four months of 1947 led to growing uneasiness within the FSU rank and file. The uncertain future of the Unit was further complicated by the fact that its rehabilitation work ended as the final Henan mission hospital devolved in the spring of 1947.

Every aspect of the FSU's future activities and community life were hotly debated among the Hankou, Zhengzhou, Zhongmou, Shanghai, and Chongqing sections. Members' witty, heated barbs, sometimes verging on personal attacks, peppered the *FSU Chronicle*.

Although they were initially welcomed in the new Unit to improve the prospects of longer-term service commitments, women became a source of contention as the budget tightened.[9] Even the sacrosanct GADA principle came under attack. Coxe entered the fray in August. In his view, one school of thought held that the Unit should "be a small group of skilled and 'mature' people, engaged in fairly long-term projects of a stable nature. This school in general believes that we should have closer ties with the home committees." The opposing school "favours the rough-and-ready, Jack-of-all-Trades type of Unit, prepared to undertake emergency tasks. These people are jealous of the Unit's autonomy and look askance at our becoming too closely aligned with the home committees. In general they feel GADA is a GOOD THING." Coxe believed that the FAU spirit could be maintained by having core permanent projects determined by "greatest need and where we can make our pacifist witness to best advantage," while keeping sufficient personnel for emergency assistance. He had little patience for the "foolish talk" of either side. Coxe's view was "not only that we hold the Quaker pacifist attitude to war and peace, but also that we are part of the Friends' tradition of disinterested service to people in want, motivated by a desire to express the power of Love in a world full of hate." Accordingly, Coxe argued that GADA "implies a willingness to go anywhere and do anything, not a policy of flitting about for its own sake."[10] Understandably, as he scrambled to stave off financial collapse, "anything else seemed frivolous."[11]

The new Unit had been dealt a deadly blow. When its anticipated funding failed to materialize, it became impossible to set a clear direction for programming priorities until well into August 1947. Indeed, the inaugural *FSU Chronicle* painted "a pretty grim picture" of its financial position. As the editor put it, "if typewriters could shed tears, this newspaper would be wet." It announced that the FSU would not receive "at least 50% of our USC [United Service to China, known from 1941 to 1946 as United China Relief Incorporated] budget and in fact are in danger of losing more."[12] It appeared to

Convoy pundits that Americans were unwilling to send money for "a country, which is exhausting itself in civil strife, coupled with an uncertainty of their own future and an increasing apathy towards foreign affairs now that the emergency is ended and an attention is focused on Russia."[13] Coxe aptly summed up the predicament: "We are in the soup indeed, for we have virtually no funds (except for Kala-azar, which the Canadian Aid to China will support), and will have to repatriate everybody that cannot be put on a Kala-azar or self-supporting team."[14] Throughout the summer, the FSU received assurances that its programs and staff levels would be supported until the next budget cycle. When the FSU submitted a budget to the AFSC to fund its program from 1 October 1947 for a year, Coxe received assurance of financial support for a minimum program, but "just how minimum remains to be seen."[15]

In the interim, "reduction, retrenchment and repatriation" became the new mantra at Shanghai headquarters, while Zhongmou, kala-azar, and the Yan'an team remained the core of the Unit's reduced projects.[16] Faced with diminishing financial resources, Spencer Coxe looked for self-supporting projects to keep other FSU personnel fully occupied. His attempts frequently proved divisive, however, such as when, following FAU precedents, he negotiated with the United Nations Relief and Rehabilitation Administration (UNRRA) to fund the FSU team assigned to transport work in the Shandong Communist area. While some viewed it as financially advantageous, "without any strings attached," others contended that it jeopardized the Unit's "voluntary nature" and would "give rise to misunderstandings"[17] or could compromise the Unit's "outward identity."[18] Ironically, few protested when the Chinese National Relief and Rehabilitation Administration (CNRRA) funded the construction and initial running of the Zhongmou twenty-five-bed hospital without any guarantee that funding for its long-term operation could be secured.

Throughout 1948–49, the Unit still hoped to promote reconciliation by ensuring that its medical work in Henan covered both Nationalist- and Communist-held areas.[19] Accordingly, British physician Emmanuel Tuckman led a small team (MT22) across no man's land to deal with an epidemic of kala-azar in the border regions of the "liberated areas," as Communist-held territories were then commonly called. There, four doctors, graduates of Yan'an Medical College, and twelve student teams joined them to set up four more mobile teams. Here as elsewhere, indigenous enterprise was crucial in the FSU's translation of Western medical knowledge within local communities. Kala-azar work provided Tuckman with the opportunity to contrast life under the Communist regime with the corruption and economic degradation of the Chinese peasantry that had witnessed in Henan under the Guomindang. As had been the case with MT19 in Yan'an, his favourable representation of the Communist regime's improvements in medical services especially and in land reforms indicated his openness to the idea that the Chinese people had the right to make political choices that were different from those of Westerners in order to improve their lives.[20] His attitude also reflected growing realization within FSU ranks that "the long-term solution of China's health problems depends on raising the standard of living of the whole population, on developing education and on bettering social and economic conditions."[21] MT22 would ultimately have a checkered career, however. A serious illness necessitated Tuckman's repatriation to England, leaving only two FAU-trained lay medical personnel, John Emery Rue and John Fu, to carry on without adequate support from Shanghai. But the FSU open-mindedness towards life under the Communist regime, typified by Tuckman, remained a defining characteristic of the FSU.

While the FSU repeatedly attempted to work on both sides of the conflict and ensure that both understood its neutrality, it had a vested interest in fostering contacts with the Communist regime. Even before the Communists appeared at Zhongmou, the FSU – fearing that its machinery, hospital equipment, and supplies would be attractive to Communist forces – attempted to negotiate a way to protect FSU property and personnel. Timothy Hayworth, director of the Zhongmou project, accompanied an UNRRA convoy taking equipment to Communist headquarters 150 kilometres southeast of Kaifeng in order to obtain a guarantee that troops entering Zhongmou would leave the FSU cooperative projects and hospital alone and its staff free to work.

When these oral guarantees proved inadequate after the Zhongmou area was occupied briefly in December 1947, FSU chairman Lewis Hoskins determined that written agreements should be negotiated to protect the Unit's personnel and property. In 1948, Hoskins led a team "considerably beyond Hantan [Handan]," criss-crossing Nationalist/Communist lines and travelling often by night to avoid being strafed by Nationalist planes, to negotiate arrangements with officials of the China Liberated Areas Relief Association (CLARA) for the FSU to work in Communist territories. The agreement protected the Zhongmou project specifically and identified future areas of work: kala-azar work north of the river at Hwai Ching; a new team at "a needier Peace Hospital" at Kwangt'ao (nearer to Zhongmou); and a

Unit-directed hospital at Handan. Hoskins made the Unit's mandate clear to the Communist authorities and obtained permission for the FSU to expand its medical work in Guomindang territories to "maintain the balance."[22]

Reconciling the Unit's desire to run its own show with the desire of the Communist authorities to control all work in "liberated" areas became progressively more challenging. As the next round of negotiations revealed, both sides had to believe that negotiations were not a zero-sum game.

Between the March and October staff meetings in 1948, when he would be appointed FSU Chairman, Frank Miles, spent three and a half months in the "liberated" areas negotiating plans for future work and passes to ensure the safety of FSU personnel. But would the FSU's expansion of humanitarian work to include reconciliation and peace building compromise its neutrality? At the end of July, CLARA chairman Tung Pi-wu warned of the dangers of renewed flooding of the Yellow River if the Guomindang continued its bombing raids, and he requested the Unit to appeal for their cessation on humanitarian grounds. Meanwhile US ambassador J. Leighton Stuart requested that the Unit initiate exploratory talks with the Communist authorities on the possibilities of peace in China. Even though the chances of a "positive result were slight," Miles, accompanied by Charles Cadbury and Henry Yu, made another trip to the "liberated" areas: "This was the most important job and opportunity confronting the Unit at the time, the past seven years of service in China having built to this role." Discussions centred on the potential flooding of the Yellow River and the prospect of a peace overture. Miles reported: "The valuable discussion period had to be cut short, unfortunately, because the arrival of dawn necessitated the removal of the Chairman of CLARA ... to the county where greater safety could be assured from the current bombing raids on the city." While Miles believed that the expedition was "infinitely worthwhile and that it was of great significance that we could sit down with a high official and discuss in practical terms the wisdom and possibilities of peace," he was realistic enough to realize that no "immediate positive result was likely to be forthcoming."[23]

For almost two years, the FSU teams, operating as enclaves cut off from headquarters, attempted to carry on, even as their numbers and funding dwindled and personnel movements were increasingly restricted. By 1949, the Unit's personnel rosters listed forty-five staff (nineteen Chinese, thirteen American, eleven British, one Canadian, and one German), and its financial condition continued to deteriorate as the AFSC anticipated "a drastic shrinkage of funds" that would force cuts to its China program. Medical work, particularly the kala-azar program, viewed as "a cheap program" that carried fewer political strings than hospitals, would be stressed.[24] Moreover, once it became apparent that multilateral aid would not transform the conflict or set the stage for liberal economic or political development, one of the Unit's chief benefactors, UNRRA, wound up its work on 31 March 1949. Accordingly, at the end of August, Philadelphia recommended a three-pronged policy: (1) change Zhongmou to a primarily self-sustaining agricultural program centred on a model farm, with emphasis on education; (2) expand the kala-azar work; and (3) maintain a reservoir of short-term personnel to run emergency projects. As the Communists "liberated" cities, cutting railway lines, FSU staff movements became more dangerous. The Communist armies entered Nanjing on 23 April 1949. By 27 May, Shanghai was a Communist city. In October, Zhongmou, still the centre of the Unit's medical work, was occupied. The FSU's final toehold in Nationalist China, its depot and clinic in Chongqing, was "liberated" on 30 November. Lewis Hoskins's successor, Frank Miles, predicted: "We are not in the homestretch but at the beginning of our most trying period."[25]

Unit members had attempted to stand apart from the political issues in the conflict, still hoping to alternate placement of new teams between Communist- and Guomindang-controlled areas. As the Communists tightened their grip on the country, they no longer valued the legitimizing effects that associating with a Western-based aid organization might lend their regime. The days of knowing someone in the inner circles who could pull strings were disappearing. The FSU's access was increasingly constrained by the new Communist regime's desire to demonstrate its ability to meet everyone's needs. Even when the FSU provided services that would not otherwise be available, it was viewed as a competitor that robbed some of the new regime's glory.[26] Frank Miles conceded that the Communists increasingly held that there was "no partial or non-political position ... people must be completely for them or against them."[27]

The Unit's inability to secure travel permits had already signalled its waning influence. From October 1948 until the following July, there were long intervals between field reports received in Shanghai. Being unable to visit Henan made it impossible for Miles to "understand the problems that members were having, to interpret on-going unit work," or to make long-term plans.[28] Eventually, "after six weeks of extended negotiations," he obtained a travel permit to Henan, but permission was denied for other members to attend the Yearly Meeting in Zhongmou or to go north to take up positions.[29]

The Unit was forced to be patient and take advantage of opportunities as they appeared, a fact that London and Philadelphia seemed unable to fully grasp.[30] By the time American Chris Evans replaced Frank Miles as chairman at the end of November 1949, the scaled-down FSU lacked leverage in its negotiations with the new Communist regime. As the *FSU Chronicle* warned new recruits, GADA had been replaced by "SHDN (Stay Here, Do Nothing)."[31] "Pessimism reached its height in early October" 1949 when Unit thinking tended towards withdrawing. While the staff meeting came to a decision to carry on, no one approached the future optimistically.[32]

In July 1950, the Unit's staff meeting in Shanghai decided against withdrawing, in favour of exploring ways that the FSU could continue to operate, but if new personnel were not recruited, it would be forced to withdraw. In 1951, the last chairman of the FSU, American Robert Reuman, concluded that every possible option had been explored to enable the last handful of foreign members to continue working, but to no avail. It was "almost impossible to continue to live in China and attain any success whatsoever in attempts to increase understanding and goodwill ... One would have to be endowed with superhuman powers and alas we are but common people."[33] Foreigners were unwelcome guests under the new regime, and there was no option but to withdraw. The final FSU council meeting formally disbanded the Unit on 1 March 1951.

The colourful personalities of the China Convoy members, the limitations of personnel and funds, and, more importantly, the changing realities within "liberated" China as the "core of the Unit became enveloped by a Red Skin"[34] would govern the FSU's humanitarian direction and force repeated negotiation of its pacifist imperative to care. The FSU leaders' high-level negotiations, discussed above, disclose only part of its humanitarian record, designed to improve mutual understanding and develop personal relations to promote peace as well as humanitarian access. Recovering the FSU team's stories from the field reveals that the impact of changing perceptions of Western-based aid agencies would be as important as the Convoy's previous record and political connections during the transition of power to the Communist regime. The strength of conviction and fierce democratic spirit of the Unit men and women speaks to the need to also understand their perceptions and contribution to daily work carried out in the field. Few Chinese understood Quaker pacifism or its humanitarian practice. Effective provision of humanitarian assistance would depend on the ability of FSU personnel to engage with local officials across political lines to maximize support for programs and to build partnerships in an increasingly insecure environment. Persuasion and trust building remained the only weapons available to FSU members during these humanitarian negotiations.

The four historical case studies discussed in Chapter 9 examine the implications of personalities, politics, and principles for the FSU's humanitarian work from 1947 to 1951. Several themes are woven throughout the narratives. Against the greatest odds imaginable, these teams struggled to save lives. All are profoundly human illustrations of the simultaneous satisfaction and frustration that FSU field workers confronted working in war-torn China, and illuminate contemporary global challenges. They expand the scholarly debate about the relevance of Western-driven humanitarianism and traditional humanitarian principles, especially in intrastate conflicts. Their experiences in the field expose the ill-defined boundaries between humanitarianism and longer-term development. The FSU never felt comfortable defining itself as a purely medical humanitarian organization. Until the bitter end, the FSU worked with the new Communist regime; indeed, members perceived their humanitarian action as presenting an alternative view to Cold War America's perception of Communist China as a Soviet puppet. But were its goals of economic development, reconciliation, and peacemaking compatible with its humanitarian imperative to relieve wartime suffering impartially, neutrally, and independently?

The stories from ground level that follow examine the multiple identities that both Chinese and Western women negotiated in China. The first case study, of MT20, examines a malaria control project in Yunnan. As much a product of opportunity as of pacifist principles, MT20's humanitarian exchanges expose the antagonism and rivalry between the FSU's Western biomedical approach and the traditional healing systems within rural communities. The FSU's controversial area rehabilitation project and medical work at Zhongmou (MT21) and its splinter all-female emergency team (MT24) sent to establish a hospital on the edge of the battlefield provide the telling second case study that spotlights the gendered and cultural tensions inherent in the FSU's humanitarian work. The key agency of Chinese nurses, especially within such contested sites, was also evident. MT23, a separate spearhead team sent to Nanjing, the third case study, further illuminates the growing political tensions that imbricated the FSU's humanitarianism as the shadow of the Cold War extended across China. MT25, the story of Jack

Jones's fervent campaign to establish the South Bank Clinic in Chongqing, the "joy of [his] life,"[35] is the final case study. Throughout the Convoy's history, men, sometimes trained by the FAU but sometimes self-taught, assumed nursing and other medical tasks that blurred professional boundaries. Jones epitomized the non-conformist jack-of-all-trades Convoy man who was prepared to challenge anyone who opposed his views on the Convoy's humanitarian mandate that shunned evangelicalism. His China odyssey, like that of the founders of the Zhongmou project, reflect individuals' dilemmas in attempting to reconcile personal beliefs with working for a relief organization that is not always consistent with those values.

9 Nursing beyond the Trenches, 1947–50

> It is not easy to work both sides of Civil war, and although the Unit is doing it, the task has called for more than a little courage and more than a little faith. People who think in terms of human need are not easily understood by a world that thinks increasingly in terms of Right and Left. The situation has been a challenge that has not been refused.
>
> – BRITISH FRIENDS SERVICE COUNCIL, *ANNUAL REPORT 1948*

The encroachment of civil war, runaway inflation, and difficulties in finding personnel and funding, right from inception of the Friends Service Unit in 1947, indicated the problems ahead. For the next three years, however, the FSU endeavoured to carry on its medical work in Henan and emergency work wherever needed, to demonstrate "not merely its impartiality but its positive good will to all men, regardless of their politics."[1] Its showcase project remained Zhongmou, where it operated a variety of community medical and educational services and cooperative enterprises. To preserve its institutional integrity, the FSU sought to retain enough flexibility to respond to emergencies without regard to political affiliation.

In 1948, one such request for assistance came from the Church of Christ in China based in Kunming, and the local authorities at Shihping, south of there. Would the FSU send a team to deal with the outbreak of a particularly virulent strain of malaria? Despite its public discourse, this particular decision was equally shaped by far more pragmatic considerations.

Jack Jones, the maverick west China transport director based in Chongqing, travelled to Shihping at the end of April 1948 to investigate. His selection was not accidental. Jones was renowned for his outspoken views on divisive issues within Convoy circles. The son of a Congregationalist minister, Emery Reynolds Jones became acquainted with and accepted Quaker views on pacifism only during the war. In 1940, while attending the Friends Meeting House in Hertfordshire, England, he applied for and was granted an exemption from military service on the condition that he work on the land or join the Friends Ambulance Unit. It was only in 1944, however, that Jack, as he was known to the China Convoy, applied to and was accepted by the FAU. "After sixteen months of work and training in hospitals (where 'FAU' was said to mean Faeces and Urine) and in vehicle maintenance and truck driving," he volunteered for China. With the prospect that returning soldiers would be given preference for already scarce jobs in England, and conscious of his own lack of marketable skills or experience, China "was his chance for a big adventure."[2] In his early thirties, Jones had "been a rolling stone who had done a lot of things but had stuck at nothing." He had worked on a fishing trawler, as a gardener, and in a beet factory, performed as a daredevil speed-way driver, and even composed a book of poems. Despite his restlessness and inexperience, Jones rose quickly within Convoy ranks to become the transport director. Writing under the pseudonym "Home Brew," he was a literary sensation in the Unit's newsletters. Always witty and wry and often controversial, his writings paint a frank portrait of Convoy drivers' rugged life. He wrote colourful accounts of being captured by bandits and of a near-death experience when his truck rolled down a ravine. Others articles, more serious in tone, opposed women in the Convoy as well as the growing schism between the "faith" and "work" factions. An outspoken critic for the small group, predominantly British, who believed that the FSU had been twisted from its course and no longer respected the FAU in aim and spirit, Jones helped compel inclusion of the statement that "non-religious members were welcome" in the FSU in the 1947 Yearly Staff Meeting minutes.[3] He stood squarely with the camp that valued versatility, resilience, and practical know-how rather than spiritual values as the criteria for membership. He remained a fierce proponent of continuing the Convoy's medical transport work and all things west China after the Unit relocated to Henan.

The writings of Home Brew reveal much about the man's passionate, idiosyncratic character that, as we shall see later in this chapter, proved a double-edged sword: it was the source of his deep empathy with the Chinese people and of his inability to accept the limitations of personal humanitarianism.

As Jones recounted, travelling from Chongqing to Kunming over China's "appalling" roads in those days was not for the faint-hearted: "The rest of the day over the endless mountains was superb but spoiled by the frontier guards, who guard all the steep pitches ... and hold you up and demand bak-sheesh [bribe] for protecting you from the bandits." The real trouble began the next morning, when Jones, adhering to FSU policy, refused an officer a lift. "Less than half a mile outside the village we were held up by twelve soldiers drawn up in battle array with levelled guns." As soon as Jones's truck stopped, the soldiers

> made a beeline for [the driver] Chi Hsu Li, tried to drag him from the cab, and when that failed began clubbing and butting him with their rifles. I tried to intervene but was pushed away and kept where I was by two soldiers with levelled guns. So I went to look for my [travel permit]. Meanwhile one soldier removed the bayonet from his gun and jabbed Chi Hsu Lin repeatedly with the muzzle, hurting his arm and ribs.

To Jones's surprise, just as he returned, he spotted the officer whom he had refused a lift. "He was in a towering rage, as it is unthinkable for a company commander to be refused a lift. I was polite and conciliatory, chiefly for Chi Hsu Lin's sake, and in the end we got away with the officer and three soldiers on board." When the officer eventually got out, he and the driver shook hands. When he asked to shake hands with Jones, Jones "told him I would not shake hands with a man who set twelve armed men onto one unarmed driver."[4]

Once in Shihping, Jones reported, he and his travelling companion, British physician Rupert Clark, a malaria expert working with the China Inland Mission, "had a wonderful reception" and "accomplished much," despite the fact that "all the chief people are away combating bandits." Left with no doubt that the epidemic "was as serious as alleged last year," he impetuously charged ahead with local preparations. After arranging for the Unit to use the Li family ancestral shrine with six large rooms and four verandas as team headquarters free of charge for as long as it was needed, and ascertaining that the local hospital had lots of Atabrine, he informed Shanghai headquarters that the rest could be left "to your loving grandfather, Jack."[5]

The malaria team, MT20, consisted of British physician John Woodall and three nurses: Jennifer Woodall; her Chinese counterpart, Lung Chien Wong Hsia Hsin, known as Jean Liu; and Roger Way, an American. Way extended his two-year contract to take on this project. At the end of May 1948, the Woodalls, Liu, and Way travelled from Shanghai to the South Bank garage at Chongqing, where they helped with clinic work until they left for Shihping.

In some respects, the team was thrown together by unanticipated events. The assignment provided Jones with a break from his onerous responsibilities as transport director. Perhaps it was also designed to appease him, as he justifiably felt abandoned by Shanghai. He agreed to accompany the team until it was established but announced that if "I am only in the bloody way ... – I am very sensitive when it comes to feeling that way – I shall pull out as soon as I feel the frost."[6] It was classic Jones. The Woodalls had proven a difficult couple to place. Refusing to abide by the GADA principle, they insisted that mobile kala-azar teams were not appropriate to their situation as a married couple. London had neither told the couple that kala-azar work would involve long periods of separation nor informed Shanghai that Jennifer was pregnant.[7] The only answer appeared to be to secure the couple a self-supporting project. When arrangements to second the Woodalls to the United Church's mission to undertake leprosarium work at the Kwang Chi Hospital fell through, other work had to be found.

One of the longest serving of the Kunming students recruited in 1944, Jean Liu epitomized the GADA nurse. By 1948, she had developed a reputation as a hardworking and enthusiastic member willing to take on new challenges. Whether doing relief work among the Henan refugees or striking out with the Convoy men on a dangerous journey to deliver medical supplies to the starving civilians "deep within Red territory," she had exhibited the toughness and self-assurance to get the job done. This particular deal to deliver medical supplies had been brokered to deliver equal amounts to both sides "as an example of unselfishness." The medical convoy's destination was the besieged city of Yung-nien, where a notorious warlord had taken refuge in the walled city surrounded by a moat. It was, one driver recalled, a "grand gesture, those small boats of brotherhood and mercy crossing the foul waters of hatred, lust, and murder." To Liu and the others, "the whole thing seemed futile as we are probably just prolonging the starvation period of our fellow men. On the other hand, we had come to help them and their enemies." In contrast to the Communist village where they had stayed the previous night, in Yung-nien "an atmosphere of death hung about the place." The team quickly concluded that they could be of little use in a city where "the people were starving in an orderly fashion, with the poor going first and the property owners hanging on according to the amount of their possessions."[8] The team quickly departed, but the contrast between Communists' and Nationalists' treatment of villagers lingered long afterwards.

Jean was remembered as providing an important link with the Chinese community from the time she arrived in Henan. A close colleague who worked with her on several assignments recalled her as open, friendly, totally reliable, and trustworthy. She seemed more at ease with foreigners and did not retreat behind cultural barriers as other Chinese members often did.[9] For Jean, the physical hardships associated with the austere Convoy life in Zhongmou, with its accompanying dangers, pestilence, and floods, were offset by her inclusion within a community engaged in challenging and important work. Despite the shortage of nurses, Jean took charge of the textile cooperatives in Shih Li T'ou, near Zhongmou. Her business background, language skills, and availability all factored into her appointment. When the Communists briefly occupied the village in December 1948, all of her personal clothing and the cotton needed for the textile project were looted. Despite this set-back, Jean remained an ardent supporter of adult education programs for Chinese women.

Understandably, Jean Liu left Zhongmou to join MT20 with mixed memories of Convoy life. At times the work was exhilarating, at other moments disheartening. Romance that should have brought happiness instead unleashed outrage within the local Chinese community. A young Chinese nurse who had tried to commit suicide in the aftermath of a marriage proposal from a Convoy man, was taken to Zhengzhou to be hospitalized. The affair "assumed major proportions in the eyes of some people whose feelings are dead set against a Chinese girl marrying a foreigner, and felt that it was responsible for her death, which according to rumours, had already happened," reported the newly arrived hospital manager, Mark Shaw. The rumours triggered an anti-foreigner demonstration. "All the workers had gone on strike and nothing was getting done. After two days of not working, word got back that the girl really was all right and work resumed." But the incident did not end here. Forgetting about the earlier affair, public attention now shifted to Jean Liu. Posters condemning her relationship with a British member "as anything from illicit love to marriage" appeared everywhere, and the townspeople boycotted the Unit compound. The smear campaign, Shaw believed, was driven by two factors: in carrying out their administrative duties, the couple had "rubbed some others the wrong way," and there was "general dissatisfaction of working under foreigners."[10]

Shaw's letter to his future wife provides a riveting account of the town meeting called to "get things straightened out." A Chinese FAU doctor from Zhengzhou very quietly explained the situation. But then "one of the Chinese members who had been suspected of causing much of the trouble and getting everyone excited about things, got into an argument with several people trying to talk himself out of the spot he was in." Tensions grew when someone mentioned that the troublemaker had taken pictures of the rather obscene posters. A fight almost broke out when he was asked to return the film, but eventually the camera was retrieved and "presented to the head of the meeting to get the film developed and check on the pictures. (What was said on the posters was bad enough to want the section to keep them from being circulated by a person known to have a grudge against the unit.)" The Chinese photographer appeared to change his mind and "made a dive for the camera" intending to destroy the film. "Things [became] a bit dramatic at this point" as the discussion heated up yet again. Ultimately, tempers cooled and the unhappy Chinese employee left by train the next day. As Shaw commented, "life here, whatever it may be is not dull."[11] Seventy years later, the British member involved regretted ending his relationship with Jean: "I was not indeed someone to cut their ties with home and set out untrained but with attachments, in the wide-open world. Not my greatest moment."[12] Given the heightened emotions surrounding their courtship, his decision to bow to convention, although regrettable, becomes more understandable. Racism manifested itself in complex and unexpected ways as it had for Chinese FAU nurses who aligned their fortunes with a Western aid organization.

Immediately after arriving in Shihping, the team met to define where and how it would work and coordinate its activities with the anti-malaria program of the Yunnan Provincial Health Administration (YPHA). They met with the *hsien chang* (local official), whom Jones characterized as "a reasonable sort of chap and certainly not obstructionist," to establish a work plan. Despite warnings of bandit attacks in the surrounding countryside, the team decided to include nearby islands as well as village schools in its coverage area. The agreement negotiated with YPHA head Dr. Wu reflected the team's desire "to have a well-defined place" within the YPHA's scheme to cover the whole district. John Woodall wanted to be "in complete charge of any department of work he undertakes." Given that the YPHA was working on such a large scale, he feared that he "was not going to be able to attain any degree of autonomy unless he had definite small fields assigned to him."[13] Personalities and the desire to maintain the Unit's institutional integrity shaped MT20's humanitarian negotiations with local authorities.

Duties were quickly decided at another team meeting that was conducted Jones-style, "not the sort that sends out minutes." John took charge of the clinic and Jennifer of the laboratory work, Roger and Jean formed the mobile team covering the schools and islands, and Jean functioned as the team's pinch hitter. "Jean will be the laboratory assistant, chief popular educator at the shrine [clinic], accountant, translator, record keeper etc." John also planned to hand over routine clinic work to her so that he could carry out field research into the mosquito populations.[14] In Jack Jones's opinion, the team would have "[to] work like hell to justify the confidence shown them and not to let anyone down."[15] Hard work alone, however, could not mitigate the unexpected resistance within local communities to MT20's malaria work.

MT20 encountered ongoing challenges. In the outpatient clinic, Jean Liu took patient histories, "a difficult and exasperating job when everyone speaks a weird dialect, is shy about telling his name, doesn't know his age, and thinks that all that business is irrelevant." When the patient had "no roof to her mouth the difficulties are compounded." Jack Jones characterized the attitude of most patients as "gimme some pills and let's get the hell out of here."[16] Despite these hurdles, Liu let few non-malaria patients slip by her. In order for the schoolchildren to receive their medication after their first meal, the team had to adopt the Chinese custom of eating two meals, at 10 a.m. and 5 p.m. Ultimately, the school program faltered over the holiday session because students failed to show up twice weekly to receive their medication. Building trust and understanding, here as elsewhere within the larger community, could not simply be sorted out but required nurturing over time.

The islanders, Jones reported, scorned the team's anti-malaria public health education campaign that identified mosquitoes as carriers of malaria. They "got together in a corner and after a discussion came to the conclusion that it was the biggest bit of baloney they had heard in their lives. Everyone knows that malaria is caused by devils, mosquitoes have nothing whatever to do with it."[17] Roger Way confirmed MT20's "poor reception" among the islanders. No one "would bring their drinking water to be tested and few came to be treated. By the team's fifth and sixth visits," he continued, "we could not even get anyone to get in his boat and paddle out to get us. So we gave up." He admitted that "if it were not for the big island, we would consider this phase of our work was almost a failure."[18] Moreover, while the number of clinic patients in town rose steadily throughout August, completion of their course of treatment "was disgustingly low." Finding it difficult to understand why anyone had to die of malaria when "all they need to do is come and take a few pills," he attributed the behaviour here, as elsewhere, to "the power of apathy and contentment with one's lot [which] is even greater than the fear of death."[19] Like FAU teams before it, MT20 failed to anticipate the stubborn resistance to Western medicine within rural Chinese communities wedded to very different perceptions of health and death.

Other issues compounded the team's problems. Although Jennifer Woodall oversaw the laboratory work, Jean Liu became a proficient assistant, and when John Woodall became ill, she examined the patients. In response to their continued poor health, the Woodalls were released from their contract and repatriated in November 1948. In the meantime, Jean received news that she had been awarded a partial scholarship to St. Francis Xavier University in Nova Scotia. Regarding her as a "valuable member," everyone was "sorry to see her leave" but knew it would "be a great experience for her."[20] Nursing was not Jean's chosen course of study; she entered a specialized program designed to manage cooperative enterprises. Before joining the Unit, she had studied economics at the United College of Yan'an and had intended to pursue a career in financial planning. Nursing had been a stopgap measure through the war years rather than a chosen vocation.[21] She later married fellow Unit member Peter Verrall, who was also a student at St. Francis Xavier University. The couple happily raised two sons until her premature death in 1969.

Even as the FSU attempted to meet requests for new teams, it struggled to maintain enough staff for the expanded medical programming begun by the FAU and centred in Zhongmou. The project signalled the realization that rehabilitating the mission hospitals in an area was only the first step. Before the war with Japan, Zhongmou, just south of the Yellow River, had been a thriving market town on the railway from the coast of Shandong to Xi'an and Pachi. Now the devastation of the Japanese war and the flooding of the Yellow River when the dikes were broken scarred every village. Henan refugees walked thousands of kilometres returning to their land where "all signs of the former habitation have been completely obliterated." The local farmers "are digging down four or five feet to recover the timber from the roofs of their old houses, but they make a joke out of it. Any other people would indulge in mass suicide if they had the hardships of these people."[22] In an effort to meet the desperate needs of refugees flooding into the area without adequate sanitation facilities, food, or shelter, the FAU started an emergency feeding station, opened two small clinics, and started epidemic control during a cholera outbreak. To provide livelihood opportunities, the Unit also opened a small school and established textile, brick-making, and agricultural cooperatives. Farmers were given loans to purchase seeds, animals, and equipment on the condition that they formed an agricultural cooperative. Challenging poverty-producing conditions and walking alongside the Chinese on their terms as an integral part of their daily struggles remained integral to the Unit's witness for peace.

Although the FSU continued the initiatives for an additional two years, the project never became self-sustaining and the cooperative projects were discontinued in February 1949.[23] The entire Zhongmou project, "originally thought of as the centre of Unit work," chairman Frank Miles concluded, developed primarily because "windfalls came in our direction. Most of the expansion came without sufficient thought being given to the goals we are striving for in the rehabilitation project and also how the various additions to the project fit into the achievement of these goals."[24] This was particularly true of its medical work.

The FSU had inherited a project with a conflicted past. The tension between secular and religious orientations that characterized the FAU's humanitarian practice in Henan formed the backdrop for the Unit's work in the hamlet of Shih Li T'ou, near Zhongmou. The project was intended to quell dissent among a splinter group who sought a closer Christian relationship with the Chinese people. Canadian Al Dobson, representative of the "faith group," struggled to reconcile the Unit's work with his personal spiritual journey. In his opinion, there were "so many things [in the Unit's work] that could have been done differently and in a more Christian spirit." He freely confessed that "the sight of so many people dying and in the conditions that they breathe their last – in dirt, loneliness and pain – was disheartening."[25] Dobson determined that it was time "to work in one place so we can carry out our proposal, which includes working with people who are primarily interested in the Unit and its work, not just the Unit's money ... Primarily we want to speak about Christianity." He believed that it "was fruitless when recovering patients live in the same old way and same old conditions." He longed not only to heal their bodies but their souls with the "life giving words of Christianity."[26] Those views set him in conflict with the overwhelming majority of members, who opposed direct proselytization.[27]

Dobson's time at Shih Li T'ou substantiates the observation by Canadian Jack Dodds that in the Unit "[we] tried our hand at everything from midwivery to reviving drowning people."[28] Although assigned as quartermaster at Shih Li T'ou, Dobson described in his letters back home "how the theory in our First Aid and Nursing training" was put into practice on days when no doctor was available. Unit members treated dislocated shoulders and examined "cataracts in eyes, old wounds covered with black looking patches put on by local quacks, heard pains in various parts ... and counselled them that injections are no good for these ailments, they must come back when the doctor is there."[29] Years later, British member Doug Turner recalled the beginnings of the Shih Li T'ou makeshift clinic and its legacies:

> We spent many long hours [during the cholera epidemic] sitting up late into the night with patients being brought in; we dealt with many hundreds of cases. Following on from that we soon had a very healthy little clinic going in Chungmou [Zhongmou] with four peasant nurses. They were very good and showed themselves capable of coping with all sorts of emergencies. We employed two local doctors and instituted a very rigorous barefoot doctor campaign for many, many miles around.[30]

While the passage of time embellished Turner's account of the Unit's contribution to the barefoot doctor movement, the Unit did make modest attempts to train Chinese kala-azar workers and nurses to continue its community public health programs.

Dobson and Turner found the frugal communal lifestyle closer to the fellowship with the Chinese that they had long sought. Although their simple life, living in mud huts, was difficult at times, fond memories of a shared closeness would later bring Dobson and the others back to China.[31] Believing that they could not recapture the China they had known and loved, Turner chose never to return:

> I remember doing surgeries with the Chinese, and although I could ask the questions in Chinese, I had to have an interpreter with me, who could ask the identical question, to get an answer, because I was so strange to them that they couldn't hear what I said. It's helped me to understand that hearing is not always a simple thing about words.
>
> Looking back, I feel I lived at the end of an era, and perhaps that's one reason why I have talked little about my time there. I put leeches in suppurating wounds and they healed; I anaesthetised people dripping ether onto a face mask with no oxygen cylinder in sight; I spent nights working with a charcoal fire and a still, preparing intravenous fluid for our cholera patients; I saw the sower sowing his seed the Bible way; by the Yellow River it was like building the Pyramids as they tried to repair the banks – thousands of

men trundling wheelbarrows, squeaking as solid wooden wheels turned on wooden axles and not a machine in sight; I sat by the house built on sand in Chungmou [Zhongmou] as the river in turbulence ate into the sand about a yard every ten minutes and we looked at each other and wondered, and then suddenly the turbulence ceased and the river ran powerfully on another course; and above all living in Shih Li T'ou, a village outside Chungmou – probably the village unchanged for thousands of years, and we the first white people that ever lived there, and now all gone, all different ... we lived at the end of an era.[32]

From these humble beginnings, the Unit built the Zhongmou hospital, with the Chinese National Relief and Rehabilitation Administration covering its construction and initial operation. The hospital was completed in July 1948. As the mission societies resumed control of their Henan hospitals, the FSU's medical work continued here and, with it, the hope that Zhongmou would become a base from which to train recruits and launch other projects to meet emergencies.

While the FSU medical facilities improved, the Zhongmou section lacked the camaraderie and closeness of earlier FAU staff. In April 1948, the Zhongmou team reported that "the atmosphere is heavy with ... disintegration. Everything seems to be collapsing. Businesses closing, beggars increasing, refugees. Everyone is disillusioned ... here it is aggravating because we have neither the people nor the money to do the things we would like to."[33] Staff were being repatriated or reassigned. Doris and John Wilks left in early 1948, increasingly uncomfortable at the prospect of working under a Communist regime. By April, Jean Liu had transferred to malaria work.

Fortunately, just as the Zhongmou hospital neared completion, Mardy Dearden, a birthright Quaker, came to China to join her fiancé, Mark Shaw, when he extended his contract for a further two years. After their marriage at Zhongmou, she continued to act as warden. Prepared to be "any kind of helper that I could be," Mardy was taught to give injections to the young patients in the kala-azar clinic and assumed more and more responsibilities in the hospital, because both were short of nurses. Knowing that kala-azar was almost always fatal if not treated, she found this work far more satisfying than taking care of the section's clothing allocations and meals.[34] As civil war intensified around Zhongmou, the couple would be a steadying force through difficult times as new staff arrived.

With the growing workload, the arrival of two British nurses strongly recommended by London – Mary Jones and Gladys Saint – and American physician Shirley Gage was eagerly anticipated. Instead, their failure to "keep on an even keel" and their "emotional outbursts" were viewed as an "upsetting factor in the hospital work." Despite acknowledging the arduous conditions Convoy women faced, Frank Miles concluded that men "usually come around when approached straightforwardly on problems of emotional adjustment." Accordingly, he recommended screening women more carefully and "trying to spread them more thinly around and keep the proportionate number of men high."[35] Despite London's efforts to vet candidates, it remained difficult to predict anyone's reaction to China or their long-term resilience in the field. Personalities, the isolated geographical setting, team dynamics, and gendered norms coloured the three women's acculturation to Convoy life in very different ways.

Neither nurse had much surgical experience[36] or preparation for her China assignment. London regretted that there had been inadequate "time to prime Saint on all things she ought to know about China or the Unit," but felt confident that "she seems a very cool and capable person" who would catch on.[37] As reported, Gladys Saint "was well introduced with little preparation during her first two months to many of the items that fall under the DA [Do Anything] of GADA" in conditions unlike anything she had ever experienced.[38] Saint arrived at Zhongmou when the hospital was "flourishing with new and old registrations averaging over 200 per day" at the morning clinic. Staff then saw over 200 patients at afternoon kala-azar and syphilis clinics before starting daily operations that often lasted well into the evening. The overflow of patients attending the kala-azar clinic meant that several hundred Chinese squatted on the hospital lawns with totally inadequate sanitation facilities. The hospital also coped with scores of battle casualties, Communist and Guomindang, who arrived from the fighting in nearby Kaifeng from May to July 1948.

Mary Jones, regarded as a competent nurse, initially earned praise as "a jewel" who got along with everyone and had "worked a much needed revolution in ward routines." Gladys presented "more of a problem." She had not "settled very well into China and the frustrations that she feels have interfered with her effectiveness."[39] Described as "a very different kind of personality, extremely rigid and uncompromising," Saint was not fitting in either socially or professionally. Rather than seeking to make gradual improvements, "she tried to shove people and things around into the order she wanted."[40] Mardy Dearden's letters home vividly detailed why Gladys "might have to be sent back to Jolly Old England." One "short resume" depicts Saint's less than tactful handling of a young Chinese nurse who spent more time charting than caring for the patients. Saint "has less patience than some people, and had a severe talk with her and told her that she'd have to do things our way." During evening shift change, the Chinese nurse shared "her woes (tearfully) [with another Chinese nurse] and they both decided not to work any longer that minute." In fact, Saint "got into so many difficulties with the Chinese nurses and caused so much bitterness that they took her out of the hospital and put her on full-time Chinese lessons."[41]

Another letter explains "the boys' disappointment" and why they "haven't gotten over groaning yet." Gladys "wears her hair pulled straight back from a rather round face and the back part braided tightly and pinned across the back. She is short but weighs nearly as much as Mark does ... I don't think they would be nearly so worried by her appearance if she weren't rather conservative in her approach and also rather set in her ways and having quite such a hard time adjusting." She balked at the communal meals served Chinese-style with big bowls in the middle of the table. "Meals in China are not a social affair and so people eat as fast as they can and leave ... Well for several weeks Gladys wouldn't eat at all because she said she wouldn't 'fight' for her food." Hard-working and devout, Saint continued to be "disappointed by what she feels is a low moral tone at Chungmou [Zhongmou]."[42] Plans for her transfer were rescinded as she appeared to settle down. Despite her "valiant effort to keep herself in hand," however, the combination of being at "opposite poles from Shirley" and "continued difficulties with employees" meant that quite a "few crises" lay ahead.[43] And Gladys did "not hit it off" at all with the vivacious American physician Shirley Gage on several counts.

A recent surgical graduate, Gage was identified by Miles as "act[ing] the least judiciously"[44] and as being the ignition point for most of the turmoil. Her "guinea pig" surgery was only one area of concern. Equally important from the point of view of Saint and others, she was "too much of a party girl, accustomed to social life to be completely happy in drab little Chungmou [Zhongmou]." There was little expectation that she would leave "it drab indefinitely," but FSU chairman Lewis Hoskins hoped "that she doesn't paint it too red" by lending "her influence to the minority of folks there who find recreation and release from their dreary existence and tensions in a party of which drinking is the prime entertainment."[45] Hoskins had already taken up this issue directly with Gage by letter. She was reminded that as a member of "an organization and a religious group ... what we do cannot help but reflect upon these people" and that "the tendency of some members in Chungmou to be a bit free and easy on the matter of drink" had been detrimental to the FSU's relations with local officials. Advised to exercise "sufficient restraint to avoid disappointing our friends or handicapping our relationships with the community and future work," perhaps Gage would take this "in the kind of spirit that it was intended to be given and think that the general community spirit and team work of the group in Chungmou is more important than personal pleasure."[46] There is no record that male members whose conduct appeared to jeopardize the Unit's work received letters of reprimand.

That view did not capture either the complexity of Gage's character or the professional quagmire that China presented to an unseasoned surgeon. A deeply committed birthright Quaker, Gage placed great reliance on individual conscience as the driving force governing her behaviour rather than accepting the perceptions or expectations of others as validation. Her audacity, passion, and altruism served as a wellspring of life's motives and impulses. Unbridled compassion, however, proved her Achilles heel. When, as an unmarried woman, her desire to adopt British war orphans had been frustrated by her mother, she left Smith College without completing her studies, which seemed increasingly irrelevant to the real world. Travel provided the antidote. Defying social conventions, she delighted in travelling by tramp steamer to explore the Amazon basin. While in Brazil, she met and married a wealthy American expatriate, Seymour Marvin, in 1942. After her brother joined the American forces, she wanted to care for "other young men caught up in the terrible war." When Marvin opposed her decision to study medicine, she had the marriage amicably annulled and entered and graduated from Albany Medical College. Serving with the FSU in war-torn China offered an exciting opportunity to relieve human suffering without violating her pacifist principles.[47]

In early 1949, Mark Shaw offered a more empathetic picture of Gage's efforts to cope with the overwhelming caseload that saw patients beyond the two hundred treated daily being regularly turned away for lack of space and staff.[48] Originally constructed as a twenty-five-bed hospital serving a hundred-kilometre area, by early 1949 the hospital had expanded to forty beds to deal with patient overflow. "All of the wards are open and they are full. The OPD [outpatient department] has been going full blast to boots so that Shirley has been terribly busy." He believed that Gage was "doing a grand job, but is tired, and frankly unable to do the job that needs to be done in the

place for a lack of more than 24 hours in any one day."[49] Attempting to offer
a balanced assessment of Gage, Frank Miles also praised her dedication to
her patients but criticized her lack of collegiality and tendency to want to
run the show, especially as she did "not always organize her work program
very effectively."[50]

Gage's letters to her professor at Albany Medical College a month after
Zhongmou was occupied in 1948 provide a gripping portrait of her isolation
"behind the Iron Curtain." They powerfully document the ethical distress she
experienced. She recounted "doing surgery that I haven't even seen before,
much less tried myself" on the "living cadavers" that arrived at the hospital
from the surrounding villages. "I am in utter despair to think what to do for
them." She admitted that "if I tried at times to stop and think about it, I would
be constantly horrified myself. As it is there no time for anything." Gage "was
really terribly proud of my hospital which though small, is going day and
night." As patients filtered back to their village, the hospital's reputation
grew. Daily, she rigged up new cots as more came "that I can't help admitting." While examining a patient's gunshot wound, she removed his bloody
clothing to discover "the left lung lying on the chest wall." That night, "I got
it back into the chest. I didn't reduce it because it wouldn't 'reduce'; I stuffed
it back under a dash of local anaesthesia, thinking Dear Lord is this surgery."
"Everything," she lamented, "is far advanced and with triple complication and
nothing looks anything they describe in the books ... when you do it for the
first time, with no trained assistant, under open drip ether, without penicillin or streptomycin, and without even a Wangensteen suction, it makes you
grow old very quickly." While she did not "mind so much the mistakes ... since
there is some hope that I will not repeat them ... there is so much I don't know
how to cope with and so much I just can't find in the books, and there just
isn't anyone to ask." Letter writing substituted for the lack of collegial advice
and professional validation: "I have learned volumes in diagnosis ... The facilities are pretty bare and the surroundings pretty gaunt but the medicine
would fill several incarnations. It's worth every hour that I miss" at the Albany
Hospital.[51]

Greater challenges were about to test the resolve of Shirley Gage, Gladys
Saint, and Mary Jones ethically and personally.

Although the Zhongmou team was already stretched to its limits, in
November 1948 an opportunity arose that it could not ignore. After heavy
fighting near Xuzhou, Jiangsu Province, resulted in a major defeat of the

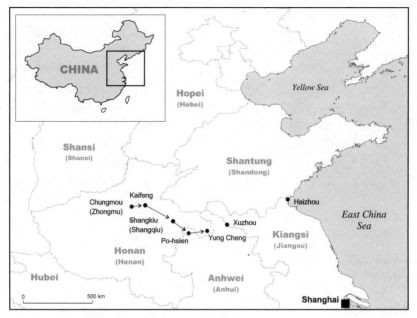

Map 11 Gladys Saint's negotiating trip

Guomindang forces, the Communists occupied a large part of northern Jiangsu as well as Anhui. The China Liberated Areas Relief Association (CLARA) and the Communist commander-in-chief of the Henan, Anhui, and Jiangsu regions repeatedly requested the FSU to dispatch a team to the battle area. The wounded Guomindang soldiers were housed in the surrounding villages without medical attention, and the bodies awaiting burial posed a public health problem. The Communists deftly stressed that the FSU would be providing medical care for Guomindang soldiers as well as civilians.

Zhongmou members "did not feel satisfied at ignoring the request nor did [they] want to rush into anything that might lead to a team being attached to the army."[52] The capacity to do something about suffering associated with the civil war depended on cooperating with the very governments and other actors that created the need for humanitarian action in the first place – not a comfortable position for pacifists wary of associating with army officials. Accordingly, as a first step, the Zhongmou section dispatched Gladys Saint, with C.T. Liu as translator, to investigate conditions in the battle areas surrounding Xuzhou. The first foray of Gladys, and later of Shirley Gage and Mary Jones, into humanitarian diplomacy outside Zhongmou would be a trial by fire that tested their ability to negotiate access at several stages as the project evolved, and then adapt their medical skills to provide care under battlefront conditions.

Gladys's trip was terrifying and exhilarating. On 14 January 1949, she and Liu left Zhongmou for Kaifeng, where her first task was to navigate "the communist propaganda being pumped into us" while convincing Secretary General Lee Huang Wen that an independent inquiry was necessary. Gladys quickly surmised that if the FSU were viewed as being on only one side of the conflict, permission would likely be withheld. After stressing the FSU's intention to launch a training program at Changde once it was "liberated" by the Communists, she argued that an independent FSU report would justify temporarily abandoning that project in favour of this work. After further coaxing during a small feast, their safe passage was arranged. From Kaifeng, they travelled to Shangqui to meet with the local communist commander, then on to Po Hsien, where the next round of negotiations with the deputy regional commander began, to secure transport via horse cart to Yung-cheng.[53]

Saint compared Yung-cheng to "a slum clearance area in a depressed area of China." By daylight, the situation was even more disconcerting. In an area where the death rate and casualties were "so high they couldn't even be numbered or coped with,"[54] the only hospital serving a population of 50,000 had allotted 50 of the 200 beds to civilian cases. Saint's chilling report portrayed the desperate need for medical services and abysmal conditions: "In a room of about 10 x 13, there were about 30 wounded Nationalist soldiers, lying on a straw covered floor, a pathway being defined by a double row of bricks. Their clothing was a filthy battle stained blood-caked uniform, sticking to their various types of wounds." The civilian ward was a smaller room where patients of all ages lay "in stinking filthy straw in true sardine fashion, literally head to tails and all moaning in agony." Injuries had not been dressed. The cries of four apparently healthy children pleading for their dying mother to awaken intermingled with the groans of wounded civilians. The scene "reminded [Gladys] of the distress and despair that [she] witnessed after the big air raids in England."[55]

Warned to flee before the bombing raid began, the group piled into the ancient horse cart. As the "impatient and rough looking soldier whipped the horses into action and kept the pace pretty high all the way," they passed dying or dead soldiers by the roadside, "everyone just glancing at the bodies as they passed by." The horses galloped over "uneven crooked roads ... broken by bombs and trenches" and "plunged through icy covered streets" until they reached local military headquarters in the late afternoon. Feeling "quite tired from the excitement of the day," Gladys recovered when greeted by a "tall, well groomed smart officer ... a perfect host." Over tea, he provided an account of the casualty numbers and how the eighty villages were divided into three groups using military triage principles: scarce resources would be dispensed where the impact would be greatest and to those patients most likely to survive – exactly the opposite of how triage worked in civilian hospitals.[56]

Sleep eluded Gladys that night. Chinese eyes invaded her privacy even as she undressed, and, nearby, gunfire reverberated throughout the night. Next day, she reported, their Communist guides led "our frightened horses through the maze of trenches." "Not being accustomed to horseback," she described her tour of the battlefront "as just a little breath-taking. All along the way firing could be heard ... an explosion occurred about 30 yards from our path." At her final destination, she began a new round of negotiations with Deputy Chief of Staff Suin Chung, and agreement was reached to establish a hospital at Hsuacha (northeast of Yung-cheng).

Saint cited the dire need for medical relief for both civilians and soldiers, stressing that Communist officials claimed they had done all they could but lacked equipment or personnel to care for Guomindang soldiers or civilians. Equally important, her report highlighted the fact that sending a team would demonstrate that Westerners could work and live together with the Chinese people to alleviate trauma and suffering from war, regardless of political affiliations. Saint found the Communist officials' argument that the FSU had been invited to work in the battle area because the Unit "worked for the lao pei hsing just as the People's Army did" particularly alluring. She left feeling that "the reputation of the Unit has attained a high level in the minds of these people – if only we could send a team and quickly."[57]

The appearance of an American medical couple, James and Hazel Lovett, on 13 February made it possible to send a spearhead team, known as MT24. Twenty-four-year-old Hazel, a registered nurse, was described as "stable, well balanced" and "just the type of person the Unit should have." James, described as an "almost nurse," "had made an outstanding record for himself" while imprisoned for three years as a conscientious objector, and consequently was parolled to the Massachusetts General Hospital to undertake nursing training.[58] His continued refusal to register for the draft, however, had threatened to torpedo his chances to go to China. After the American Friends Service Committee intervened on his behalf as a test case, a suspended sentence was negotiated, conditional on two years of service with the AFSC. After the departure of the Shaws to Hong Kong, the Lovetts' presence buffered growing discord within the team, as Zhongmou oscillated between Communist and Nationalist control.

Mary Jones, accompanied by interpreter Lu Hsien Chi and two paid Chinese nurses, Li Pu and Gwo Chi Hung, left Zhongmou in the middle of a snowstorm on 8 February 1949 to establish a clinic in the village of Yan Lo. Shirley Gage followed on 3 April, when her replacement, Douglas Clifford, finally arrived at Zhongmou. She prophetically summed up her feelings about leaving: "Here I go again. Each step seems to take me further back into the dark ages."[59]

Previous experience had prepared neither Mary Jones nor Shirley Gage for the desolate surroundings, eye-opening medical cases, and dire human suffering: "To those who had not tried to practice medicine in the Middle Ages the circumstances under which we worked would not seem believable." The dire physical conditions, cold winter rain, mud, and wind exacerbated "the feeling of desolation and horror which the sight of half buried bodies and scraps of clothing" aroused in them.[60] Despite the makeshift facilities, Mary did an excellent job until Gage joined the team in early April.[61] As reported, she handled debriding of wounds, extracting of bullets, and other minor surgery, but was unable to perform amputations!

Their shock and frustration permeate their reports. They witnessed firsthand the devastating impact of war that continued long after the guns were silent. Battle led to a rise not only in trauma injuries and epidemics but also in collateral casualties requiring treatment. Even as destitute villagers began to rebuild their homes, new dangers awaited. "Live ammunition was scattered everywhere." Sometimes "whole families were brought in covered in jagged wounds, hands blown off and very often blind. Shrapnel wounds, even less severe seemed very shocking and many were dead or died shortly after." On many nights, MT24 awoke to find a wounded patient abandoned on its doorstep. Team members worked for hours, "still in our pyjamas, hurrying around a dark operating room with the flickering oil lamps, trying to get them out of shock, trying to sew up holes in the gut, but [they] lost most of them in the end."[62]

The rigours and unrelenting demands of providing care without water, adequate food, or clean dressings were physically and emotionally draining. Improvisation became the norm; everyone was "pinch hitting back and forth between two or three jobs." Their regular clinic work, "seeing hundreds of patients a day," was as daunting as the casualty cases. Ordinary diseases were compounded by years of medical neglect. "Tumours reached all sorts of bizarre proportions ... [they] took out one ovarian cyst that weighed ninety five (95) pounds." In half-shattered homes, they "found children huddled together for warmth, some of them ill with pneumonia and many with small-pox."[63] Despite their herculean efforts, the mortality rates, especially in the beginning, were overwhelming and difficult to accept.

After negotiating their relocation to better accommodations in a nearby village, they had two small rooms "that we optimistically called wards" for inpatients. Despite improved facilities, the cultural gap between Western practice and Chinese customs added to the strain on team members. When entire families moved in to cook and care for the patients, they recalled, "try-ing to keep any order out of this chaos was a constant thorn in our side." Attempts to control flies in the operating room with DDT resulted in dead flies "dropping into the incision instead of flying in under their own steam."[64] There was enormous frustration until the team gradually adapted to the local culture and conditions.

Throughout its nine-month stay, MT24 steadily strengthened its com-munity outreach to improve continuity of care. Working closely with the local Communist government, the team trained seventeen young health aides. With their help, MT24 launched a mass cholera inoculation program and public health campaign, warning villagers to boil their drinking water. "This happily scotched the outbreak." But when the clinic continued to be overrun with cases of hookworm, dysentery, and typhoid, Mary Jones and Shirley Gage realized that treating the "endless flood of cases without trying to stop the causes seemed a hopeless job." Accordingly, MT24 changed tactics. Recognizing that many Chinese were reluctant to be inoculated until after they fell ill, the team negotiated stringent conditions with local authorities for undertaking epidemic control within the surrounding villages. The local government undertook to see that all villagers were immunized. As well, it launched a public education program on the causes of dysentery, digging several model human waste–disposal pits in the villages. As reported, the efforts of some local householders in this regard "were really imaginative. Though the whole idea was slightly hazy to them, they had really tried to please us." It took several days to treat the whole village, and MT24 left "hoarse from repeating our routine." But in the end, the villagers showed their appreciation by sending them off "in a very fine cart pulled by three donkeys and a bunch of flowers from a local carnation tree." While Mary

Jones and Shirley Gage liked to think that fewer patients from these villages fell ill, they knew that "making a dent in the sanitation problem was not that easy."[65]

Working in arduous conditions, MT24 nurses played a wide variety of roles: triage, critical care, liaison between resources and the community, public health surveillance, screening, and community education. With good reason, MT24 was credited in official reports to London and Philadelphia as having done very good work that was appreciated. During its nine months in the area, it treated more than 35,000 cases and performed more than 1,700 operations.[66] By the end of October 1949, having already extended its stay by three months, the team concluded that the emergency had passed and returned to Zhongmou. It had adapted when the focus shifted from emergency life-saving work to public health, and it delegated care to local volunteers to maximize resources and community outreach. Once again both the FSU's nursing and physician roles were expansive and experimental, going well beyond the traditional clinical one in its home country.

The opportunity to demonstrate its impartiality and neutrality proved alluring, but the Unit overextended its reach at the cost of its staff's well-being. Working in an environment with bewildering healthcare challenges, fragile security, and scarce resources exacted an emotional and physical toll. Even if MT24 members had recognized their physical and mental fatigue, there was little opportunity for downtime. Team members' spartan living conditions offered little privacy or leisure activities at the end of the day. The same hut where they ate and slept was the emergency room and the operating room, designated only by a straw partition. They left depleted.

Within half an hour of arriving back in Zhongmou, Shirley Gage announced that she wanted to leave the Unit. According to Frank Miles, there was "little question that she is in sad physical condition, and probably with a thorough diagnosis it might be found to be serious." Her Zhongmou colleague did not want to accuse her of malingering, but believed that neither the Unit nor difficult conditions in China were totally responsible for her condition: "Whether she admits it or not, she has not been happy about being in China for at least five months ... I think she never should have been appointed for China." Shanghai had again heard rumours that Gage was drinking and had passed out on several occasions. Although Miles doubted that the situation was as serious as reported, "it seems that she will have to be going very soon."[67]

Gage found it difficult to process the seven months she spent with MT24:

I have just come back ... This really seems like relative civilization ... During that time we saw 30,000 patients ... it was pretty rough medicine and the surgery on the same level. I can't describe it, I hardly believe now that I'm away from it. Dysentery, flies, dirt and the weeks of rain until the huts slipped down into heaps of mud – but – always patients ... We were always pressed for time. It had its low spots; as for instance I had infectious hepatitis while operating and seeing a hundred or so patients a day, which is not good for many laughs ... I am sure I inspired great confidence in the patients, lean as a vulture, bad tempered and bright yellow ... The labour-saving devices, the short cuts, of Western ways were absolutely useless.[68]

The complete integration of MT24 into "the narrow, barren, elementary village life" enabled Gage and Mary Jones to evaluate "a great deal of what was good and bad about it." Gage's empathy for the villagers filled her letters. Famine, she wrote, was just another word to Americans, while the Chinese villagers "live with it at their elbow day after day – This is an old story, grown dead with retelling. It's dead to write it dead to read it. But it means something. And that something is so tremendously alive that it's going to shake the complacency of the whole world."[69] The FSU witnessed the growing momentum for change within China that communism addressed.

Shirley Gage was sent to Shanghai to check out a suspicious condition in her left lung. Even when TB was ruled out, she had to remain there for complete rest and additional observation before making plans for her repatriation. Throughout the rest of her life Gage grappled with the limitations of her humanitarian capacity. Her continued yearning to help those caught up in war would take her to Korea with the US military and later lead her to adopt several Chinese children. In Korea, she provided compassionate care for Chinese prisoners of war until she was injured parachuting into forward positions to provide medical care. Her subsequent choice to study psychiatry reflected her own tormented emotional journey; as she confided to her daughter, she remained the typical wounded warrior untreated for post-traumatic stress.[70]

Those remaining in the Zhongmou had little recovery time. From fall until early December 1949, the hospital "was a mad rush, with over 200 patients a day in the OPD," and the unit nurses "had their hands full."[71]

After the "liberation" of Zhongmou on 22 October 1949, the Unit's relations with local Communist authorities became strained. Tempers flared over several issues. How closely could the team associate with the new regime "and still receive the blessing of the donor agencies?"[72] Communist officials "were suspicious of the Unit as foreign (therefore American, therefore reactionary) and they did not approve of the Unit's educational and industrial activities."[73] When new demands were made that preferential treatment be provided to Communist soldiers and officials, opinions differed about how far the team should accommodate the Communist authorities. The situation was defused only when special hours were established for Communist soldiers. Clifford urged explaining honestly and openly who they were and how they worked. If this frank approach failed to protect the safety of its programs and personnel, the FSU, he contended, should withdraw. Nevertheless, despite strained relations with the Communist authorities, the Zhongmou hospital, with the help of Chinese staff, was working relatively efficiently. During the first five months of 1950, it treated an average of 2,647 outpatients per month, an increase of 27 percent over the previous year, and there was always a long waiting list for its forty-two hospital beds.[74]

Despite Clifford's steadying hand and the steady stream of patients, tensions were rife in the dispirited and overworked team. Throughout the remainder of the year, as the Zhongmou team anxiously waited to see how the new Communist regime would affect its work, morale continued to plummet. Miles believed that "the months of isolation, work without breaks, uncertainties of the situation, and many other things have contributed to making strong differences in the group." One person was overheard "to say of her period of service in Chungmou [Zhongmou] that she looks on it as a prison sentence." Moreover, their working environment became more strained as Chinese members were pressured to stop working for the "foreign dogs."[75] Symptomatically, even food became a divisive issue that consumed hours of a section meeting – one group felt that the diet was adequate and that they should eat the same simple food as the Chinese employees; others contended that food was inadequate to maintain health and wanted to set up a separate kitchen.

In a quintessentially Quaker tradition of self-reflection, Miles attempted to gain a deeper appreciation of the team's lack of "a positive sense of direction" or "the spirit of unity" as it strove to carve out a life within the local Chinese community.[76] Thoughtful and introspective, placing great value on relationships in all aspects of the Unit's work, Miles believed that the

Zhongmou team "had been too much separated from the people that they were trying to help and it has resulted in lack of understanding of both the Unit members and the villagers." Reflecting on the acculturation difficulties experienced by raw recruits, who came out on two-year assignments, he observed that they

> feel rather helpless in doing anything but immediate material tasks ... This results in a general feeling of frustration and a feeling that they are not doing the job they came out to do. Add to this the inability to get away from the project for a brief vacation when they could get a renewed outlook on life and the complete isolation from the outside world, and you have a very tough situation.

As the Communists restricted travel for foreign personnel, discontented staff could not be transferred or reinforced, exacerbating "the bickering and personal differences." While on a weekend leave to the Catholic Mission in Xinxiang, Gladys Saint was placed under house arrest for two weeks when her pass issued by the local authorities was questioned.[77] Earlier FAU teams tackled challenges, overcame obstacles, and handled emergencies in an equally difficult and fragile environment, yet they felt a sense of accomplishment. Perhaps one difference was that the FSU members, unlike earlier FAU teams, knew that as expatriates of countries that had supported the Guomindang regime, they were no longer welcome. They had become tainted by their countries' pro-Nationalist diplomatic stance as Cold War attitudes hardened.

In addition to the general malaise within the section, Doug Clifford, Mary Jones, and Gladys Saint offered other reasons for leaving. Continued poor health factored in Gladys's repatriation in February 1950.[78] Clifford's restlessness went beyond his desire to undertake further postgraduate medical studies. According to Frank Miles, Clifford "had felt frustrated in working at Zhongmou because from his point of view the hospital was far ahead of its day in that the community and the Unit was not able to do enough toward training personnel who would be able to take over at some point." For Clifford, building local competency "was the only lasting value of our presence."[79] Mary Jones's contention that she could do more good back home appears unconvincing. More likely, it reflects her professional burnout and changed personal circumstances. With Shirley Gage's help, plans were being made for MT24's young Chinese-German translator, Hubert Huang, to study astrophysics in the United States. He would go on to marry Mary and have a distinguished career.[80]

When Clifford resigned from the Unit in early March 1950, James Chai returned as the Unit medical director and oversaw the hospital until devolution was concluded the following November. Devolution had been a cardinal principle of the FSU but relinquishing control proved more difficult in practice. The Zhongmou section wanted its successors "to run it 'as we have,' pay the same wages, hire the same employees and charge the same way as we have." But as they admitted, there was no way of knowing that this agreement would remain in force.[81] Despite Clifford's pessimism, the hospital would survive to become a well-respected research and teaching hospital: Zhongmou County People's Hospital.

But the Zhongmou projects' shortcomings should not detract from the compassion, courage, and pioneering fortitude that both nurses and Gage demonstrated. They operated and lived under intense pressure. Gladys Saint and Mary Jones were expected to be purveyors of Western medical knowledge and to provide excellent nursing care. Their reports document their anxiety at not being able to provide the care many patients really needed. It was assumed that their training had given them the skills necessary to hit the ground running. But once nurses were in the field, new demands, dangers, diseases, and deprivations posed enormous challenges. The scope of practice changed dramatically. They were required to become community educators, cross-cultural brokers, and humanitarian diplomats as they cultivated the relationships with local communities and military officials necessary for their work to be effective. While living in nerve-wracking conditions, they were expected to work hard, be flexible, and make personal sacrifices. In exchange and driven by necessity, women were given responsibility and authority beyond the traditional gendered professional roles that nurses or female physicians played. Providing humanitarian service during war provided nursing with a veneer of feminine respectability, but gender norms governing feminine respectability and stereotypes of women as distractions in war remained intact. Nursing in the FSU broadened their personal and professional horizons. In sum, it was a beneficial experience for them – albeit with costs – and for all the lives and communities they touched.

Throughout 1949, the Unit clung to the hope that it could work across political lines. As the civil war intensified throughout 1949, Communist forces occupied Nanjing (24 April), Hankou (16–17 May), and Shanghai (25 May). An emergency medical team (MT23) had been sent to Nanjing in the expectation that the city would be "liberated" shortly and that the team would be in place to deal with civilian and military casualties and the thousands of refugees living there in appalling conditions. Instead, its efforts were rebuffed. The experience of MT23 after the city was liberated demonstrated that the Unit was a minute player, indistinguishable from other Western agencies despite its past humanitarian record or political connections with the Communist regime. The subsequent decision to launch a medical clinic, MT25, headed by Jack Jones, reflected the changed realities of the FSU's rump operation; here, pragmatism coloured its apolitical stance.

MT23 was an all-British team led by its physician, Phyllida Thornton. Edna Hadfield, a quiet, thoughtful Christian, proved a very competent and adaptable nurse. Royston (Roy) Mason held a certificate as an assistant nurse. During his six years in the navy, he had trained as a surgical nurse and worked in the Blitz, and later gained eighteen months' experience in Ceylon. He had joined the navy in a non-combatant role, but the experience changed him and he now viewed himself as a pacifist.[82] Their compatriot, Elizabeth File, recruited through the Canadian Friends Service (CFS), was not a fully qualified nurse but had badly needed secretarial skills.[83] After considerable debate with Philadelphia, she was approved as lay medical worker, and later, after time in the field, it was assumed that she could serve as secretary in Shanghai.

The team's work unexpectedly wound down in the wake of the city's "liberation." Foreigners were regarded with growing suspicion. The United Nations Children's Emergency Fund (UNICEF) feeding centre, housed within MT23 facilities, closed in mid-June. Communist authorities refused to release UNICEF's rice supplies for distribution. Not without cause, Communist officials considered food a "political weapon"[84] and did not want UNICEF to distribute it until "the matter had been thoroughly investigated and referred to higher authorities."[85] Only $500,000 of the $6.5 million UNICEF budget had been allocated for areas under Communist control.[86] By fall, Nanjing newspapers were denouncing Truman's *China White Paper* revelations, and Westerners who viewed themselves as friends of China were especially targeted.[87] Given the political climate, the Nanjing Theological Seminary's sudden request that the FSU team evacuate the clinic at the end of June should not have been surprising. The team independently elected not to seek accommodations elsewhere. Still unable to obtain travel permits to Zhongmou for its medical staff after several months, Shanghai recalled the team where members were seconded to other Shanghai relief organizations pending their repatriation or reassignment to the FSU's Shanghai staff.[88]

Despite the uncertainty and anxiety surrounding the Unit's future and, more particularly, Jack Jones's "suitability to represent us in a Friends' enterprise," a new FSU medical project, establishing a clinic in the FSU compound in Chongqing, then still in Nationalist hands, was launched in 1949. Pragmatism and one man's unbridled compassion to help the community he had come to love and respect coalesced. Acknowledging that Jones was "set in his ways" and did not "easily adjust to other ways," some contended that "Jack's lack of religiosity" had been exaggerated. Jack "is a deeply and sincerely motivated worker in the vineyard of the Lord, though he would not phrase it that way."[89] Jones's proposal to expand the depot clinic that he had always run for employees and their extended families to the wider local community received formal approval from Philadelphia. The most recent recruits – British surgeon Mary Mostyn, American lab technician Felda Jones, and American David White, all of whom had been lingering in Hong Kong – could now be sent "to make a hospital out of Father Jones' famed South Bank clinic." There was little choice. It was the only area for which the FSU could get travel permits. From Philadelphia's perspective, it also had the advantage of giving the Unit a "second toehold" in China from which to expand operations if the political situation stabilized.[90] MT25 would be the Unit's final medical project and one of its most tragic stories.

Despite reservations that Mary Mostyn "would overbalance the Unit's medical personnel in the feminine direction," she had been recruited on the basis of her commitment to the Unit's pacifist principles and her stated long-standing desire to "help in building up educational and health services" in China.[91] She was the first to reach Chongqing in mid-November. Arriving alone at the nearby military airstrip, she reluctantly hitched a ride down the hairpin bends in a truck without lights, only to be enlisted to push it when it broke down. Reaching the city after dark, she waited for the first ferry in the morning and then trudged several kilometres to reach the FSU compound long before anyone was awake.[92] Jack Jones's jubilation over the surprise arrival of his long-awaited doctor quickly dissipated.

Mostyn's impulsiveness completely sideswiped Jones. "As father of a section that has usually come to my knees and told too much rather than too little," he struggled to explain what went wrong: "You will all know by now that Mary got here, blew hot and cold on the clinic for ten days, sent a couple of cables [to Hong Kong] that had Felda flummoxed and Mark [Shaw] athematising [sic] my name and all things West China." When she unapologetically announced that she already had her visa for Chengdu and was leaving immediately, he "was quite bowled over" and "rightly or wrongly I let her carry out her plan."[93] As Jones saw it, Mostyn "didn't seem to cotton to our clinic" and remained reluctant to "have a go with the clientele." She appeared "obviously bored with the women and never examined them." Making excuses for her refusal to treat tuberculosis patients, she claimed that "there was nothing she could do, or that she did not have the right medicine."[94] John Peter, who acted as nurse and translator for her in the clinic during her short stay, was equally critical of her lack of professionalism. While she refused soldiers treatment for scabies on the grounds that drug supplies were low, she handed hundreds of vitamin pills to other patients despite being warned that they would sell them on the black market. Quite simply, Mostyn was unwilling to function in a clinic without heat, water, or sewage. Considering herself a free agent, she arranged her secondment to the better-equipped Chengdu hospital and subsequently to the hospital of the West China Union University – acts contravening the GADA principle that went unchallenged by either Jones or Shanghai.

After Mostyn's departure, Jones and John Peter were "a bit cut up at the turn things had taken" but decided they could "not tell people that we can't deal with them and we did our best with everyone that came today. John did most of it, while I examined the gynae cases (chaperoned by Mrs. Yan Chien) in the inner room. Mary never examined one but I had four very interesting ones."[95] By the time Felda Jones sneaked in from Hong Kong on a private plane on 26 November, followed three days later by a newly married couple, the Reumans, Jack Jones and John Peter were seeing fifty patients a day.

The eclectic team renewed Jack Jones's enthusiasm. Chairman Frank Miles wrote him that Felda's training in social welfare and laboratory work, as well as her previous experiences with AFSC, made her an ideal candidate, capable of understanding "the sort of effort we are making to show the spirit of reconciliation through service." There was never a question about her being a "Negro. In fact, it might be a definite asset to a group to have a person from a little different background."[96] Described as a "wonderful mechanic and medical clinic assistant, a veritable artist with his hands," John Peter was recruited in the chaos of getting the last FAU trucks out of Rangoon before it fell. Using the stage name of Daredevil Cryillo, "he had been looping the loop in a rocket car at Burmese fairs when the Japanese took and burned Rangoon; grabbing one of [the FAU] trucks he had driven up the Burma Road into China and into membership in the Unit."[97] The longest-serving China Convoy member, he had a remarkably diverse career, serving as nurse, convoy leader, skilled medical mechanic, and garage manager in the Chongqing depot.

Delighted that all three newcomers agreed to stay, Jack Jones decided to move the clinic into larger quarters in the godown nearest the front gate of the FSU compound, just a day before the Communists arrived. As Dorothy Reuman explained: "[Jones] had been working in a small room (now ours) and wouldn't have given too good an impression of what we're trying to do."[98] As it was, they "had dinner to the music of continuous machine gun fire and explosions and the next morning awoke to find Communist soldiers in the yard."[99] Jones had taken the precaution of painting a big red cross on the door and posting a sign that said, "The FSU Poor People's Clinic." He had made the right call; getting permission for a new clinic would have been impossible after the Communists arrived.

As Jones explained the clinic's operation, the clinic, "like Gaul is divided into three parts: a waiting room, a clinic devoted to abscesses, ears and eyes and a second clinic devoted to gynaecology and anything that the first clinic send through."[100] The Reumans

> dress[ed] most of the sores, after one of the Jones or John [Peter], who is the cheese in our front room, decide whether sulphanilamide powder or zinc oxide or salts is the proper thing. It's an amazingly gratifying thing to watch some of them come in day after day, starting with a terrible sore and seeing it heal up. You come to see how doctors come to be more interested in the disease and curing it than in the patient, and in helping him, though the two can co-exist.[101]

The Reumans were a remarkable young couple whose letters home paint a striking portrait of the clinic's operation and of the enigmatic Jack Jones. One of Dorothy's touching letters conveys her quiet courage, compassion, and anxiety at being obliged to work in conditions that were inadequate or inappropriate:

If we only had a doctor ... but all we have here are Jack, who has had a little
bit of medical training, in preparation for coming out with the Ambulance
Unit, and John, who has picked up a lot of medical experience, Felda,
whose work has been all lab work, never before clinical, and one of the
Chinese members and his wife [Sam Yen and Mrs. Sam], and the two of us
all of whom are all right for following directions, for applying dressings or
giving baths, but that's about all ...

How we've prayed to heaven often for a doctor here, though, when some
of the soldiers come in, for instance, with wounds which have been left for
a number of days, and you thank God for your cold in your nose so that
you can't smell the gangrene so much, and your heart just about breaks for
them, no place to go, no way to get food, no way to rest, no way or money
to get to a hospital where they could have adequate care or treatment ...
Those are the more obvious kinds that they seem so sorry about, but then
there are those who just through neglect sometimes are suffering when they
wouldn't need to, and cleanliness would often heal them up. So we scrub all
the scabies babies, and put on soothing mixtures, and they're better, and
would stay that way if only they were kept clean. What is so encouraging
about this work is that there are never too many that we can't help in some
way, and it's gratifying work. We just wish we were both medically trained,
so that we could do more. Oh, for a doctor![102]

By the end of January, Dorothy was running a scabies clinic in a converted
truck body for the women and children, assisted by Feng Ah Fu and other
garage employees who scrubbed the men.

Tragic but unforeseen circumstances forced Felda to run the clinic. Jack
Jones was hospitalized after a failed suicide attempt. Then John Peter fell ill.
For more than three weeks, Jack claimed, Felda "carried the whole weight of
the clinic with seldom less than 100 patients a day."[103] It was Bob Reuman who
dissected Jack Jones's psychological complexity and fiercely disputed his
portrayal of the clinic's operation in his absence:

Jack Jones is in many ways the most interesting person. His big failing is
women – he has an almost morbid sexual interest in them all, specializes in
women's cases in the clinic and in their structure and relationships in his
writing and when he falls in love, which is frequent, it is with the utmost
infatuation and lack of control. He is Felda's little dog doing her every bidding
now and as before his attempted suicide, and almost detestable in his imbecile

servility ... Almost without a doubt he has an inferiority complex which finds stability in a person of Felda's temperament, yet this is often masked in an apparent self-confidence and dogmatism ...

[H]e claims from his few years of trial and error that he knows more about medicine than Dr. Mostyn, for example, though he would willingly extend it to include most doctors.[104]

On the one hand, Jack Jones could be an irritating, arrogant colleague with a wry, off-colour sense of humour, given to make sexist quips about women. On the other hand, the genuine affection of his patients and his tender, solicitous concern for his female patients bely any simplistic portrait of a misogynist. In a collection of short stories about the clinic, Jack evokes a captivating yet haunting portrait of the pain, poverty, and mistreatment of Chinese women "who have been through hell" during these turbulent years, but refused to be broken.[105]

While Jack found the clinic work gratifying, it never completely filled the vacuum left by the closing of the Chongqing depot in late 1949 – which he had doggedly opposed. He had "kept the show on the road against all odds, earning desperately needed income by operating a fleet of vehicles for the JCRR [Joint Committee for Relief and Rehabilitation] in Chengtu [Chengdu], selling scrap and even selling vehicles on commission for departing missionaries. The transport unit was thus the achievement of his lifetime."[106] The disposal of his beloved trucks and the increasingly acrimonious layoffs of Chinese staff, who challenged the repatriation payments already received and demanded more money, preyed on the mind of this already overworked man. Devoted to the welfare of his patients attending the bustling clinic, he never took his entitled leave. His immense sense of loss during this time tenderly resonates throughout a carthogenic *FSU Chronicle* article, written after his article about his attempted suicide. Describing the final farewell to his Chinese depot employees, he "unashamedly" gave "rein to my sentiment":

And suddenly it hits me right under the belt – God damn it, this is the end! Blame the *huang chiu* if you like – but suddenly I feel as an old broody hen feels when her chicks refuse to nestle under her any more, fly up onto the perch too soon and pneumonic because they aren't fully fledged ... What is this, a sentimental truckdrivers' association? Of course it was. Under the grease and mud and less mentionable kinds of shit, which covered the roadman, there was always a soft heart; in spite of his stern eyes and uncouth blundering ways he loved his children, trucks, his own pup, his boy [charcoal truck boy] the other boys in his convoy, and some of the employees' wives; he could and often did weep like a girl.[107]

By early May, Jack was still only helping out part-time in the clinic; fortunately, a Canadian missionary physician, Clara Nutting, was visiting the clinic weekly to assist him.

By the fall, however, attendance was dropping, as soldiers could now obtain free medical treatment at any hospital, and patients could not afford to buy the medicines required for their treatment in the open market when clinic supplies were exhausted. The death blow came when the local Communist authorities ordered the clinic to close in November 1950. Jack wrote the clinic's epitaph: "This is the way the world ends, not with a bang but a whimper. That is the way the clinic ended too."[108] Then began the labyrinthine process of securing exit permits, being allegedly detained under house arrest, and ultimately contesting outstanding complaints and attempting to secure a local guarantor of any personal liability that might arise. After many delays and hardships en route, Jones and Peter reached Hong Kong on 31 May 1951.

The FSU still placed emphasis on meeting needs ignored by other organizations, and sought to leave a lasting legacy by building local capacity. It honoured the Quaker Peace Testimony and attitudes that prioritize enduring relationships rather than material relief. Its aspirations and foundational pillars were sorely tested, however. Views that favoured long-term development versus emergency medical and transport work coexisted uneasily, especially as funding and new personnel became scarcer. The need to work closely with the military aggravated tensions within the Unit's ranks. The FSU experience illuminates the ethical challenges endemic to humanitarianism at a transformational stage of the postwar humanitarian landscape before many of the contemporary international structures or legal regimes had been built.

The praxis of faith, institutionally and individually, shaped the FSU's humanitarian exchanges. The differences and tensions in Quaker interpretations of pacifism and professionalism highlight how transnational ideals may be refracted in different contexts.[109] The debates within the Unit about faith versus work were constant until it closed its doors. Al Dobson and Jack Jones represented the extreme wings of Unit views on faith versus work. The majority continued to distinguish the Unit from missionaries and sought to express their Christian pacifist ethos through work rather than preaching, evangelism, or doctrine. But the concern that relief be delivered in a Quakerly fashion that prioritized ethics and not merely outcomes remained. By 1949, chairman Frank Miles voiced the concerns of many Quaker members that they and the Unit were not working in accordance with Quaker principles. He maintained that while it would be "unfortunate" if subscribing to the Quaker attitudes towards war and peace were removed as a requirement, convictions about personal relationships should be given greater importance: "We are not involved in a war and fighting but we do have to live together and work together and it is by the effectiveness or ineffectiveness which we do these things that we are judged."[110] His viewpoint had merit, especially as teams became more isolated and lived in close quarters under tough conditions. Difficulties experienced in reconciling individual perspectives with the Unit's Quaker ethos were not a new phenomenon, especially given the ingrained fiercely democratic tradition of both the FAU and the FSU. The independent-minded, non-conformist perspectives that had motivated them to be conscientious objectors continued to govern their behaviour in China.

As they had for the FAU, questions of what constituted the proper domain of its work always accompanied the FSU's humanitarian endeavours. The FSU wanted to provide assistance to anyone who needed it, regardless of political affiliation, but never defined itself as a strictly humanitarian organization. The recognition that relief had to address the underlying causes of poverty and war increasingly underscored the development of FSU projects. Members talked about reconciliation and building local capacity, but in reality the FSU could not move beyond being an emergency medical agency. In the end, events beyond its control – the volatility of the civil war couched within the Cold War – ultimately constrained its humanitarian endeavours and pacifist witness. The FSU entered a humanitarian field replete with internal political relationships and histories with foreign powers from which it could not extricate itself. What had been perceived as a symbiotic relationship had now become a zero-sum situation.

A mixture of angst and self-reproach, combined with considerable pride, continued to characterize the FSU's work. The narratives of its humanitarian endeavours from 1947 to 1951 unmask how personalities, ethical dilemmas, internal dissension, and the shifting strategic interests of the major power brokers pervaded the Unit's tangled humanitarian exchanges and negotiations until it closed its doors. Despite its challenges and setbacks, its concern remained with the Chinese people. How its members grappled with operating in a conflict environment is an intensely human story. The Unit carried out its activities in places that placed its staff in real danger, often without the supplies it needed to implement its humanitarian programs. At times, most strikingly in the case of Jack Jones, concern for others superseded concern for their own well-being. The health of Gladys Saint and Shirley Gage also deteriorated as they cared for others. None could accept the limitations of their personal humanitarianism. Exploring how FSU members navigated China's turbulent humanitarian terrain spotlights an important feature of the current humanitarian dilemma: its long-term effect on and consequences for humanitarian workers. Humanitarian assistance remained a highly political activity. Despite the FSU's pronouncements and practices seeking to ensure that its actions conferred no military advantage on any party and were driven solely by need, the humanitarian principles of neutrality, impartiality, and independence had to be constantly negotiated. As the Cold War deepened, however, the suspicion that humanitarian workers funded by UNRRA, UNICEF, or private American donors had a hidden agenda made them unwanted interlopers under the new regime. Perception proved as important as the FSU's actual relationships.

Conclusion
Nurses without Weapons, 1941–51

I think we all felt that we were doing something useful even though it was on a very small scale in comparison with need. We were ordinary human beings trying to live extraordinary lives in China.

– DAVID MORRIS

Beginning in 1941, well-intentioned Western men and women from all walks of life and different nationalities began a life-changing journey to bear pacifist witness by sharing in China's suffering. In contrast, for many Chinese women, nursing was a wartime refuge that enabled them to serve their country while promising better career opportunities in the future. Even as women choosing a traditionally feminine profession, neither group conformed to social prescription. Western nurses volunteered for myriad reasons that fulfilled their ideals, dreams, and professional aspirations. Some entered nursing because they had few options, but they expanded those options by seeking new opportunities for themselves as women and nurses. Most believed that the China Convoy would offer a very different nursing experience; it was also their first great adventure abroad. For some, humanitarian service offered a socially acceptable opportunity to live atypical lifestyles. But elements of feminine respectability remained crucial aspects of their nursing experience abroad. Moreover, the expectation that Convoy nurses would establish a sense of domesticity remained firmly entrenched.

Most Western nurses departed for China with little understanding of its society, language, or political condition, and, perhaps most strangely, of the fact that civil war was brewing. All struggled to align their professional ethics with the ravages of war. Dealing with the fallout of war would be both exhilarating and horrible. Most embraced the experience; a few fell short. None left unchanged.

No matter how Western nurses imagined what they would experience in China, they quickly confronted the realities of human suffering on a scale unlike anything they had ever encountered. While each nurse underwent an individual wartime experience, there were commonalities shaped by the Convoy's pacifist ethos, nursing itself, and war. This book reveals the complexity of nurses' motivations for joining. It probes how humanitarian nursing within a Quaker-based organization challenged nurses' perception of their role as purveyors of Western-based knowledge and standards, even as they confronted questions of medical ethics and unfamiliar cultural practices. The Gadabout nurses' narratives are not solely about what happened to them and how they reacted to the challenges. Rather, they are about how men and women as categories of identity have been constructed within the gendered mainstream historiography, particularly the international relations discipline.[1] The China Convoy suggests that nurses' voices should be taken more seriously, not only within the scholarly literature but also within the contemporary policy formation process. Nurses have been and will remain key to the delivery of humanitarian assistance. It is my hope that this book will open avenues of scholarly inquiry within the history and practice of humanitarian nursing.

As Convoy members carried out their work, they faced enormous problems and setbacks. China's nested wars defined the boundaries of the Convoy's humanitarian action. In particular, the shifting interests of the warring Chinese regimes and the Cold War rivalry of the Great Powers constrained the Friends Service Unit's humanitarian endeavours after 1947. The Convoy's espousal of impartiality served many purposes as its members worked in such a dangerous and politically volatile environment. Notably, it created negotiating space for discussions with both the Communist and the Guomindang regimes to ensure the teams' safety and continued access to vulnerable populations. On rare occasions, the Convoy acceded to requests to act as an intermediary between the warring factions. As the civil war escalated and the Convoy's resources dwindled, humanitarian negotiations at all levels intensified in an attempt to ensure the Convoy's continued relevance and survival in changed circumstances. Its humanitarian action raises several pointed questions. Did the Convoy cross the fine line between humanitarian action and interventionism? What was its legacy for future Quaker engagement in the world?

Western and Chinese nurses found their way into the Convoy for different reasons. There were some commonalities, however. Both Western and Chinese nurses' motivations reflected their class, education, Christian religious beliefs, and venturesome personalities. The China Convoy provided a respectable vehicle for these well-educated Christian young women to realize their personal and professional aspirations. Financial considerations figured differently but may not have been the deciding factor for either group. Since Western nurses received only maintenance, in addition to a small stipend from the shared pool of private funds, military nursing – or, later, joining the United Nations Relief and Rehabilitation Administration (UNRRA) nursing brigade – would have been far more lucrative for them.[2] Often internally displaced by war, many Chinese nurses joined out of financial necessity, but there were better-paid alternatives open to them in Free China. In fact, some Chinese nurses, such as Doris Wu, left better-paying jobs and subsequently relinquished their modest salaries when they accepted full membership in the Convoy.

In an era when international career opportunities were scarce for Western women, they were pioneering their role as nurses in forward combat areas with a new type of humanitarian agency. Humanitarian work promised adventure, expanded professional opportunities, or a new personal beginning for some. Others were driven by altruistic or pacifist ideals. A sense of patriotic obligation was not a driving force. All opposed war as an instrument of national policy. None of the men and women who provided nursing services described themselves as a representative of their government abroad. In fact, American nurse Margaret Stanley and British nurse Elizabeth Hughes perceived their presence in China as a counterweight to their governments' high diplomacy. Theirs was a practical demonstration that not all Westerners had the same attitudes towards China or its people. A few defined their humanitarian presence in terms of an idealized nursing community that transcended national borders or their pacifist beliefs.

Christian pacifism broadly shaped the decision of most Western nurses to set aside normal career paths and marriage opportunities to help relieve the suffering caused by war. While most such recruits shared or respected the Convoy's Christian pacifist ethos, their decision was not perceived as a matter of charity. Rather, they understood service with the China Convoy as a chance to respond to human misery and protect fundamental human rights that connected all people across borders. Contending that suffering was the same worldwide, Convoy nurses derived emotional satisfaction from understanding the kinship that bound humanity. As Margaret Stanley observed, "when one finds something in common with people of all nationalities and work, which is actually filling a need that otherwise would not be filled, one realizes the universality of our profession."[3] For many nurses, especially those raised and educated in the Quaker faith, serving in the China Convoy epitomized the ideal nursing practice "tied to the causes of humanity and the needs of the collective which were larger than the individual nurse: social causes, peace, and health promotion." Quoting the old Quaker saying, Margaret recalled that they sought to "live in such a way that you can do away with a cause of war."[4]

But the decision of Western nurses to volunteer for service in China equally reflected their youthful desire for exotic yet respectable travel, and their thirst for professional and personal adventure. For nurses such as Margaret Briggs, Connie Bull, Rita Dangerfield, Harriet Brown, Joan Kennedy, and Margaret Stanley, the compassionate practice of humanitarian nursing also "served to quell personal restlessness, to offer individual creativity, and to create a sense of purpose and a personal sense of meaning to their lives."[5] Within the societal limits of their time, both Western and Chinese nurses made deliberate life choices to create meaning within nursing and in their private lives.

Nation building rather than pacifism was a significant factor for Chinese nurses, and allowances were made for all Chinese members in this regard. In the recruitment of Chinese nurses, being Christian was equated with a broad acceptance of the Unit's pacifist beliefs. In sharp contrast, London and Philadelphia set stringent recruitment criteria for Western nurses; ideally, suitable candidates should be fully trained nurses and pacifists. Most Chinese nurses viewed membership as a wartime gateway to a better life. Trained in Western-based training schools and conversant in English, they viewed the Friends Ambulance Unit as an attractive alternative to military nursing. It offered more professional and personal autonomy but still enabled patriotic Chinese nurses to fulfill their national obligations in wartime. For others, often from well-situated Chinese professional families, service was exchanged for Western nursing training. They and their families hoped their FAU service would lay the groundwork for continued nursing or medical training abroad.

Most scholarship on motivational needs presents a strongly Western perspective.[6] Studies of the field marginalize indigenous nurses and risk portraying them as passive or grateful recipients in humanitarian exchanges within a Western-driven organization. The Chinese Gadabout nurses refute this historical portrait, however. They vigorously negotiated their terms of work and protested successfully when contractual promises were not kept. Most either left with a strong recommendation for employment or received support for further educational opportunities in China or abroad. Their choice to seek employment and ultimately membership in the Friends Ambulance Unit or Friends Service Unit speaks to their sense of themselves and, in most cases, their privileged place in Chinese society. Researching motivational factors within different cultural groups will extend our knowledge of the complexities of delivering humanitarian aid, especially recruiting and retaining well-suited local humanitarian staff.

Most FAU/FSU nurses found their China years demanding, rewarding, and humbling. Working in the China Convoy, however, did not always live up to the dreams or expectations of Chinese or Western nurses. They worked where the delivery of humanitarian aid was challenged by systems and expectations beyond their control. At the same time, service with the Convoy offered them unparalleled professional opportunities and extraordinary personal experiences in its multinational teams and its work across cultural and political frontiers. They experienced China as few other Western women had. Nevertheless, their life and work on FAU/FSU teams from 1941 to 1951 varied enormously, depending on location, team size and dynamics, and the shifting political context.

The crucial nurse/physician relationship varied immensely within teams, ranging from paternal or fraternal protection of young nurses' reputations to romantic involvement. An effective nurse/physician partnership was essential to the delivery of effective patient care, especially in the cases of Chinese nurses, who often acted as mediators between an imported medical system and the local context. On the professional side, however, several FAU/FSU nurses found that the exigencies of wartime nursing blurred the lines between physicians and nurses. Some, such as Margaret Briggs, experienced a greater sense of partnership. Rita Dangerfield's references to making an "independent nursing diagnosis" based upon clinical observation confirm that FAU nurses functioned as far more than physicians' handmaidens. Expected to play a wide array of roles outside the scope of their normal professional practice in difficult environments with scarce resources and demanding caseloads, some, such as Mary Jones, functioned as independent health-care providers with minimal support. Convoy nursing broadened the scope of their nursing practice – to act at times as the physician's assistant or offer recommendations for changes in patient or hospital management – well beyond anything available at home. It heightened their professional competence and confidence. Both Chinese and Western nurses moved beyond their traditional bedside roles. Yet nurses, such as Rita Dangerfield or Connie Bull, were caught in the nurse/doctor game, expected to manage the physicians' environment and the team's social life. In many ways nurses' experiences in the China Convoy remained simultaneously liberating and constraining.

Gender, nation, class, and place imbricated the experiences of both men and women nursing with the China Convoy. Race and nation played out in the Convoy's history in unexpected ways. For many Chinese, nursing was not their ultimate career choice but rather a stepping-stone towards medical training or a better life. But this opportunity came with a high price. Chinese nurses were scorned by their compatriots for choosing employment with a Western aid agency or considering Westerners as future husbands. Western nurses' attitudes towards their Chinese counterparts reflected their common Western medical education and backgrounds, for their shared class, educational background, and professional identities blunted racial stereotyping.

Patients or the rural population were more frequently portrayed as being backward and being prevented from accepting Western treatments by superstitious and outmoded cultural beliefs. Resistance to Western-based medicine should not be underestimated, however. Chinese nurses acted as linchpins between imported knowledge and the local context. Following a long tradition, Chinese nurses selectively integrated Western nursing practice to define a national healthcare system tailored to the nation's capacity, resources, and priorities.[7] Moreover, patients were not passive recipients of Western medical practice. Western nurses in the China Convoy struggled to respect local customs and beliefs that frequently clashed with their desire to deliver excellent nursing care. Both Western and Chinese nurses acted as cultural mediators to bridge gender norms that made Chinese women reluctant to seek maternal care from Western male physicians. Most, such as the malaria team, faced other dilemmas in providing health care to communities with a different understanding of health, illness, and death. Local Chinese challenged Western medical professional expertise, and most Convoy nurses experienced the paradoxical effects of trust and suspicion from their patients and the local communities.

Nursing with the China Convoy remained gendered. Wartime service contradicted the image of nursing as a gentle profession, an extension of women's traditional caregiver role. It should be noted, however, that both Chinese and Western nurses performed the historically respectable role of nursing the wounded in wartime regardless of political context. Patriotism gave wartime nursing a veneer of respectability and importance to outsiders. Humanitarian nursing under the umbrella of a Quaker-sponsored organization enabled single nurses to work independently abroad without sacrificing social respectability but often led to matrimony, which ended their nursing careers. Cast as duty-bound to show compassionate care, Convoy nurses were expected to embrace the rugged physical masculine life on the front lines but retain their femininity and respectability. On the one hand, the hard work, skill, and courage of Doris Wu and Margaret So on the front lines during the Salween campaign earned them recognition in the Unit newsletter. On the other hand, the expectation that both women would fulfill their patriotic obligations while retaining their conventional femininity and moral purity exposes the uneasiness within Convoy ranks about subjecting women to the physical and moral treacherousness associated with the violence of combat. Moreover, war placed nurses in leadership positions that challenged perceptions of femininity as requiring supervision and protection in the supposedly masculine domain of combat, although such challenges were contingent on geography and necessity. For example, Margaret Briggs ventured into the world of diplomacy in Henan, albeit at Robert McClure's side, and she made an independent assessment of the area's medical and nursing needs. Necessity opened up new roles in the FSU for women such as Mary Jones, Gladys Saint, and Shirley Gage. But again, when Gage (or Doris Woodward earlier on) exhibited behaviours frequently associated with men in combat zones, their moral conduct was censured. Convoy nurses were expected to embody the gendered values of the Convoy; to do otherwise might jeopardize its image in the field and back home with its donors.

Reflecting contemporary societal norms, Convoy nurses were constructed within letters, reports, or newsletters as embodying heterosexual normalcy within the violent Chinese society at war. They were frequently praised for bringing a feminine touch that went beyond their gendered maternal and caregiving roles. The refusal to allow Doris Woodward to return to China was telling. Nurses were expected to comfort the sick and dying, not use their presence at the front for their own selfish interests, such as finding a husband or engaging in sexual frivolity. At the end of a gruelling workday, however, they were still required to provide companionship and arrange social gatherings and celebrations within the team's household, as they would within familial households. Convoy rhetoric, typical of the era, depicted two types of nurse: the "good nurse," represented by Robert McClure's immortalization of Nurse Li as a self-sacrificing angel, and the "bad nurse," represented by Doris Woodward, a highly sexualized woman with matrimony instead of duty on her mind, who preyed on men.[8] There was no suggestion that men might have equal sexual appetites. For the majority of women, the Unit became a substitute family that oversaw their interests, including their marriage arrangements and sexual conduct.

It is important to remember that men have historically provided nursing services, especially in military settings. Men, both professionally and Unit-trained, made important contributions to the Convoy's medical work. However, there was a distinction between the nursing roles they were assigned. Both men and women were trained to administer anesthesia, but only men did the kala-azar and public health work that involved a more itinerant lifestyle. Necessity dictated the formation of an all-female team assigned to forward positions in the final stages of the civil war.

Men's nursing work was equally gendered. Nursing connoted feminine traits of caring or tenderness that jarred with societal concepts of manhood, especially in wartime. Although heroic tales were told of Convoy drivers, men's nursing work was never immortalized within Unit newsletters, songs, or poetry. As conscientious objectors, often emotionally and socially castrated by society's scorn for failing to carry out their manly responsibilities, there may have been a reluctance to draw attention to Unit men's nursing roles, conventionally perceived as a feminine occupation. There is no suggestion in the extant documents that female nurses perceived male nurses as encroaching on their professional territory. Given the limited number of fully trained nurses, there was little choice. The complicated ways in which gender shaped and was shaped by Convoy nurses' service suggests the need for a deeper understanding of nursing's gendered experience during the Second World War and the turbulent decades that followed.

Long before there were notions of cultural safety, post-traumatic stress, or core competencies for humanitarian nursing, Gadabout nurses worked out their individual coping strategies in the field. The positive aspects of humanitarian nursing coexisted with cultural, environmental, and organizational stressors that threatened the physical or psychological well-being of nurses and other caregivers. Although not all rose to the challenge, the overwhelming majority demonstrated adaptability, self-reliance, courage, and resilience. For those who dared to care, it was often an emotionally turbulent journey of self-discovery, where personalities, personal beliefs, and human needs clashed. Nurses' contemporary accounts in letters, diaries, reports, and newsletters provide an intimate and compelling look into their demanding daily lives. Whether fully qualified or Unit-trained, most found themselves ill-prepared for humanitarian nursing. They faced the stresses of climate, language, limited organizational support, separation from family and friends, and unrelenting exposure to inhumanity and tragedy. Most reported their lack of preparedness for ethical conflict. They anguished over their inability to deliver nursing services because of time constraints, lack of supplies, deficiencies in the Chinese national healthcare system, volume of patients, or being pulled away to deal with other emergencies or projects.

Their testimonies are powerful accounts of extraordinary nursing in extraordinary times and of how the awful human suffering they witnessed touched them. What coping mechanisms were available, and why were some Western nurses more adept in navigating China's turbulent humanitarian terrain? The characteristics that prompted many to volunteer contributed to their resilience, but other factors also came into play, such as nursing's core values and personal faith. Their strong dedication to their profession, along with their pacifist camaraderie, facilitated their adaptation to difficult living conditions and unrelenting work commitments. Compassion had become an expected standard of nursing.[9] Nursing with the China Convoy offered women opportunities for compassionate service and self-development, and a strong sense of purpose and community that crossed national boundaries. For many, nursing in China's volatile environment fostered a sense that they shared a common fate: "There was always sharing and there was always the feeling that we were in things together." Their common bond – stemming from their dedication to relieving the suffering of war victims – forged a kinship among team members from different religious, national, and political backgrounds. Graham Milne's intimate account of Harriet Brown's tender care of a dying cholera patient demonstrated how compassion provided a source of personal strength to carry on. Years later, Margaret Stanley recalled that "the compassion for people that took us there in the first place carried us through experiences we might never have thought we had strength to cope with – there was so little that we could do to improve their lives."[10] The ability of nurses to transcend the limitations that physicians, especially surgeons, experienced with dying patients partially explains why they became acculturated more readily than physicians on the same medical team.[11] FAU physicians complained more frequently about their lack of autonomy in controlling hospital conditions that affected patients' surgical outcomes. In some respects, humanitarian nursing with the China Convoy offered nurses a global equivalent of the American settlement house experience, in that it was concerned with all aspects of human relationships rather than being contextualized within a particular medical setting.

Female physicians and nurses would remember the China years fondly as a foundational moment in their lives that could not be recaptured or fully quantified. Others remained wounded warriors struggling to erase the haunting memories of human or personal suffering. In order to cope, they embraced various self-care and mutual care strategies. Acting as substitute families, teams created their own social outlets, and members cared for each other in sickness or on long treks. Although the overwhelming majority of Convoy nurses took a non-sectarian and non-proselytizing approach in their humanitarian exchanges, faith shaped team life and individual health. Individuals' faith provided an ethical compass and a source of spiritual rejuvenation. Even for non-Quakers, the shared silence of morning meditation enabled team members to gather strength before the day began. This ritual is reminiscent of the contemporary equivalent: the "pause" to honour a patient's passing in critical care units.

Other outlets provided emotional refuge as well. Some adopted destructive coping mechanisms; some cried; some drank; others compartmentalized traumatic experiences. Diaries and private letters functioned as a nurse's trusted confidant far away from home. There, they could share confidences about their work or private life far from the prying eyes of colleagues or family. Given societal norms, few would have admitted being victims of sexual abuse or discussed their professional or marital anxieties for fear of the stigma attached. Both the FAU newsletter in its various incarnations and the *FSU Chronicle* fostered a sense of family and an esprit de corps among the Unit's far-flung membership by celebrating the milestones of individuals' lives and their contribution to the Unit's work. Within these pages, the ribald poetry, satirical but affectionate songs, and even contentious editorial battles functioned as a safety valve, allowing members to vent and live with their differences. It is striking, however, that nurses seldom chose to contribute accounts of their work or poetry. Why their voices remained muted raises more questions than answers. Given that women's roles in Convoy life remained a sensitive subject throughout its existence, they may have wanted to avoid adding fuel to the fire. Did nurses undervalue their work in comparison to the heroism of the Convoy drivers? Did their self-censorship reflect gender expectations of women's role as conciliators rather than as decision makers?

Ultimately, the courage, competence, and cross-cultural agency of professional and Unit-trained nurses underpinned much of the Convoy's medical humanitarianism. The impassioned experience of nursing with the China Convoy was full of contradictions. Nurses shared intimate experiences of providing care, their friendships, and images of China's rugged beauty existed in uneasy juxtaposition with the geography of unremitting human misery and poverty. Western and Chinese nurses' stories from the field testify to the risk of emotional numbing, self-damaging ways of coping, or even emotional breakdown inherent in humanitarian nursing. Some evidence suggests that nurses who identified more closely with the suffering in war-torn China found their transition back to their former lives more difficult. The China Convoy gave them a different lens through which to re-examine Western societies on returning to an abundance of material goods, the lack of which had prevented adequate health care in China. Those, like Margaret Stanley and Elizabeth Hughes, who welcomed the opportunity to share the Communist China they knew as a corrective to Western Cold War perceptions, got quite a shock. Their compatriots and journalists remained largely unreceptive to their accounts, beyond the sensational aspects of their exotic time abroad or personal stories, such as Elizabeth's having given birth to David in a cave. They treated these nurses according to categories that they understood, exaggerating their femininity, courage, or salacious behaviour.

Convoy nurses' humanitarian experiences open new paths for nursing research and scholarship and Quakers' global engagement. For the China Convoy, the selection of personnel on the basis of Quaker beliefs versus technical skills required for medical or development work aboard remained a thorny issue. The issue would be hotly debated as the growing demand for professionalization preoccupied AFSC decision-making circles in the decades to come.[12] The Convoy nurses' narratives reveal that neither their civilian training nor solid Christian pacifist character was sufficient to ensure their personal or professional resilience in the field. More extensive field research on adapting nursing skills and knowledge to the local context and culture remains crucial to ensuring humanitarian action that is both effective and sustainable in today's complex humanitarian crises. Future inquiry may profitably focus not only on how the movement of nurses across borders affects the development of global health but also on how these nurses are changed and on the difficulties engendered by that experience. Equally important, nurses' field narratives highlight another significant but neglected area of research: self-health as a core competency of humanitarian nursing.

Recasting the Gadabouts' humanitarian exchanges also complicates the historical narrative of both Western and Chinese nurses' roles as embodying and presenting Western ideas of modernity and nursing practice. The portrait that emerges is far more complex and contested than previously suggested. Both the FAU and FSU expected their fully trained nurses, Chinese and Western, to implement Western scientific nursing and sanitation to improve nursing standards and patient outcomes. It soon became apparent to most Western nurses that their previous nursing experience was ill-suited to wartime China. Some Western nurses acquired language skills that opened new windows into Chinese life and expanded opportunities for shared learning. Most Western nurses struggled to provide basic patient care, even with the help of a translator, but Chinese nurses struggled with regional dialects as well. Some Western nurses were largely unaware of, and others merely tolerated, traditional healers and the cultural beliefs of their patients. Others wrestled with their personal beliefs when actual practice did not always align with the Quaker organization's stated ethics, which prioritized global fraternity, not Western standards. Faced with myriad personal and professional dilemmas, Convoy nursing exposed the limits of their personal humanitarian capacity.

Acculturation differed for each nurse. Several factors helped most Convoy nurses cope with professional cultural shock. Western-trained Chinese nurses were key to many Western nurses' acclimatization. Their unique background and professional expertise distinguished and empowered their cross-cultural agency. The Western educational and privileged class backgrounds of these Chinese nurses meant that their cross-cultural exchanges differed from the start. They helped their Western counterparts recognize and accept the limits of their humanitarian capacity. They taught Western nurses the art of making do in resource-strapped practice settings. More open-minded Western nurses collaborated with their Chinese counterparts in innovating and adapting nursing practice.

The diversity of nurses' acculturation experiences exposes a broader series of factors at play. A few nurses and female physicians, such as those on MT19 and MT24, gained significant cultural sensitivity. The intensity of Margaret Stanley's and Elizabeth Hughes's cross-cultural humanitarian exchanges on MT19 was unique in many respects. Both teams operated without a strong support network and were more dependent on local villagers to house, clothe, and feed them. Life in the field changed how they delivered health care. Building local partnerships was crucial for MT24 public health work in villages, where they witnessed first-hand the human carnage of war. Travelling across northern China enabled Margaret and Elizabeth to witness early commune life as a response to the devastating human degradation associated with decades of war and poverty. Yet despite the two nurses' shared experiences in Henan and Yan'an, Margaret developed a more nuanced understanding of, and a deeper respect for, Chinese people's socio-economic struggles, compounded by the cataclysmic effects of war. Her strong Quaker ethics and personality influenced her cross-cultural relationships differently. Ties of friendship had brought her to China. Strong female friendships, carefully fostered by Margaret Stanley with her Chinese nurses, forged a shared kinship that gave meaning to her work beyond team life. Conversely, without the presence of Chinese nurses on larger FAU teams until late in the Salween campaign, British FAU nurses at best tolerated differences in medical traditions and healthcare infrastructure that did not jeopardize patient care. On these larger teams, nurses formed collegial relationships with local Chinese counterparts, but their team life remained that of a self-contained community. Nor were they entirely free of a paternalistic mentality towards patients or local staff. These historical case studies also reaffirm the difficulty and necessity of cultural competency in providing sustainable care tailored to local circumstances and priorities.

The narratives of Convoy nurses challenge any monolithic portrayal of Western nurses as agents of Western imperial control or cultural power,[13] or as evangelists within a faith-based humanitarian organization driven and financed by the West. Both FAU and FSU nurses were impatient with the pietistic approach of missionaries. Convoy nurses counted on their skills and scientific knowledge to protect and promote their patients' health. They viewed nursing as a practical humanitarian service to meet basic human needs and protect universal human rights. Understanding the Gadabouts' multiple identities as women and as nurses in a pacifist relief agency within a wider religious and political tradition and world culture offers a more textured understanding of nursing's humanitarian multifarious engagement.

The vagaries of war, organizational opportunity and limitations, personal agendas, and clashes of personalities figured equally in determining the location and duration of their assignments. During the global war, most FAU nurses focused on providing the best possible care on the front lines while working under the Chinese military, and then turned to epidemic control and hospital launching in newly liberated towns. With the move to Henan, nurses' work became more multifaceted and contentious, and consisted primarily of starting nursing training within mission hospitals. Subsequently, nurses supported the FSU's expanded mandate, which prioritized community involvement and preparation of the local Chinese to take over health care and healthcare institutions. As civil war swept through the country, nurses spearheaded teams working across the political divide. Convoy nurses accepted tasks and geographic locations dictated only in part by the Convoy's operational needs. Nursing within a pioneering international non-governmental organization was a facet of global nursing that differed from missionary, military, or colonial service nursing, with which it shared some elements.[14]

For many, the China Convoy's legacy was deeply personal. Images of China – the country's rugged beauty and the resilient faces of its people, chiselled by the degradations of poverty and suffering – became imprinted in their lives. Their affection and admiration created strong ties to China and a continued commitment to pacifism and humanitarian service. After their return, some of the Convoy men and women men studied nursing, medicine, social work, or engineering in preparation for a lifelong career in humanitarian service. They played important roles in the AFSC, Oxfam, and various UN agencies. Teresa Hsu became internationally acclaimed for a life of humanitarian service. Still others, such as Harriet and Walter Alexander, joined cooperative communities. Most retained their pacifist convictions, and many remained engaged in the peace movement or became political activists for social justice. Others fostered continued dialogue and ties of friendship with China.

Among the nurses, only Margaret Stanley completed more advanced nursing education before serving abroad with the AFSC, this time in the Middle East. Like other members, she welcomed the opportunities to foster friendship with Communist China. For many years, however, memories of

China receded as her life followed a more conventional route of family life with intermittent nursing assignments. In 1972, an unexpected invitation to return to China as part of the AFSC delegation opened a new chapter of Margaret's life. Back home, she gave talks across the country comparing China "then and now, 25 years apart," noting the improvements in health care and population health. She wrote articles in *Eastern Horizon* conveying the transformative experience of her work with the International Peace Hospital and witnessing first-hand the idealism that characterized the early commune movements in Yan'an. Together, she and the celebrated author Helen Snow initiated the "Yenan Hui," a list of foreigners who had worked in Communist-controlled areas from 1935 to 1949 and their publications. In the years that followed, she organized several return trips to China. With delight, she received a positive reply from the Chinese government officially inviting MT19 to visit the places where it had worked during the 1940s. In 1981, she joined a group of physicians and nurses eager to see maternal and child health in China. In late 1985, Margaret returned to China to work for the Gung Ho Cooperatives, hoping to retrace her steps through her beloved Yan'an countryside. On her final trip in 1991, she died there while teaching English to medical students. Fittingly, half of her ashes were scattered in China. As she had always hoped, "the original basic purpose of our work in China, to further understanding between peoples of China and the West, lives on."[15] The children and grandchildren of the original China Reunion Group continue meeting and are collecting and preserving documents recording the Convoy's work. David Brough and Cathy Miles Grant, working in close association with Douglas Clifford, have been key in fostering the cultural exchanges that most recently led to the 2017 exhibition in Yan'an. The striking photographic collections of Douglas Clifford, Frank Miles, and Margaret Stanley, capturing the medical work and everyday life of China's rural people, are the heart of the exhibit.

Whatever their individual hopes, ambitions, or motivations, Convoy nurses worked within a pacifist relief agency committed to delivering humanitarian aid in a Quakerly fashion. Their humanitarian engagement suggests that rather than being a top-down process, the FAU/FSU provision of humanitarian assistance was constantly contested and negotiated. To gain access, the FAU had to negotiate and cooperate with warlords, the International Red Cross, Chinese and American military authorities, and, after 1945, other international relief agencies and the missionary societies, each of whom had its own vested interests. Members wrestled with their Quaker beliefs as they worked alongside the troops or collaborated with missionary societies. Both Units struggled to maintain a separate identity and resisted being swallowed up by the army or UNRRA. In practice, impartiality, neutrality, and autonomy – the ethical cornerstones of the humanitarian imperative – were situational, driven by the confluence of a shifting war front, need, and capacity in each location. To evoke the image a "golden age of diplomacy" in which humanitarians carried out their work unfettered is to understate the very real difficulties encountered in the field.

These prickly issues were threshed out in the China Convoy's Yearly Meetings and newsletters until, in a Quakerly fashion, a sense of how to move forward was found. The noticeable absence of nurses' voices during the Sino-Japanese War may in part be attributed to their geographical isolation from headquarters. Only in 1945 was nurse Margaret Briggs chosen as a sectional representative to attend the 1945 Yearly Meeting, where the decision to relocate to Henan was hotly debated by the rank and file. The smaller size of the FSU gave nurses a greater voice in the Yearly Meetings that determined the FSU's devolution policy and closure. Other nurses had opportunities for input in team or sectional meetings that proved equally important. FAU corpsmen contravened orders to remain in Burma. MT19 members on the ground, not FAU/FSU Headquarters, made the decision to function as a mobile hospital unit attached to Communist military forces. Nurse Gladys Saint conducted the field investigation that led to the decision in the Zhongmou section to mobilize MT24 as a forward field hospital in 1948. Jack Jones was the driving force in the creation of MT25.

Other factors shaped the China Convoy's apolitical stance. Although the FAU/FSU scrutinized funding and supply sources, both depended on outside financial assistance from government sources, private donors, and UNRRA that threatened both Units' institutional integrity. To its credit, the FAU drew a line in the sand when the Canadian government made the extraordinary offer to fund its operations as an entirely Canadian agency. The importance that both Units placed on their relationships with the Chinese – on working *with* rather than *for* them, and on helping the Chinese help themselves – enabled them to navigate the compromises inherent in humanitarian work. Just as the divergence of opinions over what compromises were acceptable sparked heated debates throughout the Convoy's history, the ethics of humanitarian aid is constantly re-evaluated within contemporary humanitarian organizations.[16] The Convoy's experiences reveal a more ambiguous and complex picture of humanitarian action in which the ideals of humanitarian principles and humanitarian space were never divorced from political negotiations. The Convoy's application of the humanitarian imperative was situational.

Its humanitarian activities also moved forward or were held back through a series of political transactions that attempted to balance conflicting humanitarian agendas and mitigate power imbalances. In retrospect, the constant negotiations of front-line staff with local authorities were as important as talks held at higher levels in ensuring both access to those most in need and the safety of Convoy staff. In this respect, the Convoy's negotiating leverage was probably greater before VJ day, when Japan was their common enemy from the Chinese perspective. Moreover, the value of its transport work in wartime Free China, as well as its front-line medical work, enhanced the FAU's reputation. The FSU walked an increasingly difficult political tightrope as the Unit became tainted by American Cold War diplomacy. The FAU/FSU remained uncomfortable about defining its role as simply humanitarian and sought to embrace a wider mandate that included peace building, reconciliation, and the social reconstruction of war-torn Chinese society. Despite its insistence to the contrary, the expansion of its mandate beyond emergency medical relief complicated its efforts to divorce its humanitarian endeavours from national or global politics.

Paradoxically, pacifist idealism was both the China Convoy's strength and its weakness. Although pacifism had different meanings for members of the Convoy, it provided a strong sense of collective identity that inspired members to carry on despite tangled political relationships or personal hardships. Successful cross-cultural brokerage depended on skillful staff at all levels, but the Convoy's advocacy of non-violence and its adherence to the principles of ethical compromise, mutual respect, and power sharing enhanced its negotiation of cross-cutting ties across the political divide. Ultimately, any humanitarian organization's negotiating capacity is determined by its ability to persuade and its relevance at a historical moment. In the absence of social trust and perceived mutual benefit as the civil war deepened, the process of cross-cultural negotiation broke down. As its numbers and finances dwindled, the FSU's humanitarian aid became less desirable and of little immediate value compared with its past efforts. Despite several attempts by the FSU to negotiate the continuation of its work on an impartial basis, and its dogged determination to continue its kala-azar work using locally trained personnel, it became an unwelcome interloper. Given Western aid to Chiang Kai-shek's regime, all Western groups were viewed as vehicles for transplanting Western culture into China and were challenged by the new Communist regime, which was determined to have its authority and legitimacy recognized on the world stage. From the Convoy's perspective, it sought to bear an independent witness to the birth of modern China that challenged the dominant Cold War American narrative. But the Convoy's pacifist views or motivation were not well understood among the Chinese people. From the Chinese perspective, the line between legitimate humanitarian action and illegitimate intervention had been crossed.

The China Convoy exposes one of the main myths of humanitarianism, namely, that there is a simple linear progression between good intentions and improved lives. As Spencer Coxe, who took charge of the AFSC China Desk in Philadelphia after his return, commented, "the most terrible thing of all is that ultimately the Unit is the casualty of the Cold War that we are all dedicated to oppose. Let us realize that pacifism usually ends in failure." In his opinion, this did not exonerate the FSU from responsibility for its record. He characterized the Unit's inability to survive as "a reflection of our own weakness."[17] Both the FAU and FSU viewed humanitarian space as "agency space," but in reality it is "a complex political, military and legal arena."[18] Humanitarian aid can never be uncoupled from the politics of its donor countries. Nor are humanitarian workers immune to their own cultural, social, or religious influences. The politics of humanitarian aid means that, at best, acting humanely, neutrally, and impartially provides a framework for the ethical conduct of humanitarian negotiations. The success of these also depends on a number of other factors: technical expertise, strong local ties, a degree of local acceptance and ownership, and flexibility to adapt. It is ironic that an organization that early on had recognized the need to take a community-based intersectoral approach to human security became a victim of the Cold War mentality. Focusing on knowledge transfer, training, and reduction of obstacles to local engagement in order to build community capacity and resilience across the relief/development divide constitutes the new gold standard of the humanitarian landscape. Managing the cleavages in transnational cooperation in today's kaleidoscopic global governance landscape continues to be a fundamental challenge of global civil society.

Pacifism continues to be a strong motivation for Quakers' civil engagement in global society. Whatever its shortcomings or strengths, the belief that recipients of humanitarian aid could distinguish the Quakers' distinctive pacifist mandate and impartiality from that of other American aid agencies or their government's foreign policy became deeply entrenched in the organizational culture of the American Friends Service Committee. In the decades to come, however, bearing witness to the human tragedy of war without compromising Quakers' tradition of apolitical engagement proved treacherous. The viability of an apolitical posture would be challenged during the Vietnam War, even as Quakers continued to deliver aid to both North and South Vietnam in defiance of US law. The AFSC's presence was decried in many circles as implying complicity with the American campaign to win the "hearts and minds" of the Vietnamese people.[19] While the ethics of outcome would remain a cardinal and controversial tenet of Quaker humanitarianism long after the Vietnam war, being a pacifist organization committed to social justice and reconciliation would present significant ethical dilemmas in navigating the turbulent politics of the Global South.[20] Sometimes it meant supporting groups whose goal was social justice but whose tactics endorsed violence. Those on the ground, as Convoy members before them, would continue to redefine the Friends' global engagement in a manner that other Quakers would find deeply disturbing.[21]

Equally important, the China Convoy's pacifist humanitarian practice supports those historians who see an overlap of human rights and humanitarianism before the end of the 1940s. Both the FAU and the FSU championed the protection of basic human dignity and the right to live free from violence well before it was codified in international law in the wake of the Second World War.

The China Convoy's experience foreshadowed a disturbing international trend: the militarization of humanitarian intervention. As Western states have continued to reaffirm their sovereignty over aid actors and policies, humanitarian "agency" space has been circumscribed. The China Convoy's history, however, punctures the widely held belief that there was a "golden age" when humanitarian actors had unrestricted access to vulnerable populations in need. Many of the problems humanitarian actors face today are familiar when compared with the past, and continue to be a consequence of the militarization of humanitarian engagement in conflict-affected areas. Humanitarian space remains the product of continuous transactions with local and international political and military forces, and is congruent with the organization's ambitions and political acumen and the interest of those wielding power. What the China Convoy's experience suggests, and the 2016 World Humanitarian Summit confirmed, is that humanitarian aid is not a substitute for political conflict resolution or a remedy for the failure to address the socio-economic determinants of human security. As the China Convoy members began to realize, economic development and humanitarian aid need to be better coordinated and geared to and led by the communities involved. Humanitarian aid appeared then, and continues to be perceived, as predominantly a Western vehicle representing Western values, interests, and behaviours to be distrusted. This perception of the humanitarian system persists, compromising individual non-governmental organizations that strive to fulfill their humanitarian imperative humanely, impartially, neutrally, and independently.

This book joins the scholarly conversations accompanying the recent expansion of transnational history to encompass a more far-reaching challenge to nation-centred historiography.[22] It continues to develop newer lines of inquiry that critically assess non-governmental activities across borders in the context of the twentieth century and considers the importance of the travelling of ideas, such as pacifism and social justice, across borders in the development of modern humanitarianism. It examines the lived experiences of travelling ideas and the reception, negotiation, and appropriation of pacifism and Western medical knowledge across cultural and linguistic borders.[23] It does not champion transnational history but seeks to open dialogues beyond history alone and suggest where new research interventions might profitably be directed.

Nurses working in non-governmental organizations were important transnational agents. This book shows that recentring global nursing history from the periphery of scholarly inquiry offers new perspectives that recast humanitarian nursing during and immediately following the Second World War. The diversity, greater autonomy, multidirectional learning, and constant negotiation of the humanitarian imperative experienced while nursing with the China Convoy refocuses our historical inquiry to consider how and by whom these cross-cutting humanitarian ties are negotiated in conflict zones. It considers individual trajectories marginalized within nation-centred historiography. Reconstructing women's wartime lives, discourse, and subjectivity provides a different analytical frame for examining the modern humanitarian architecture: one from the ground up. The Gadabout nurses' narratives provide intensely human complements to military and international relations accounts.

More specifically, the experiences of the China Convoy nurses invite a re-examination of postcolonial frames to interrogate humanitarianism in war-torn China from 1941 to 1951. Postcolonial scholars have persuasively challenged the "binary othering" that Eurocentric discourse invoked to perpetuate imperialism and racism in nursing work, and have convincingly critiqued the use of Western humanitarian medical aid to serve the self-interest of foreign powers. The cross-cultural humanitarian exchanges of neither Convoy nurses nor the wider Convoy are easily accommodated within this frame. Moving beyond postcolonial frames recognizes that Convoy nurses' tangled cross-cultural humanitarian exchanges were more complex and conflicted than previously acknowledged, peppered with tension among Western nurses, their Chinese colleagues, patients, and the physicians with whom they worked. Recovering Convoy nurses' narratives shows that their humanitarian nursing in China is better contextualized by a notion of constantly negotiated and contested professional space, rather than a cordon sanitaire where humanitarians' safety and right to deliver medical relief was sacrosanct. Convoy nurses did not embody their governments' foreign aspirations. Viewing Western Convoy nurses as agents of a top-down Western-driven humanitarian diplomacy fails to take account of the challenges, opportunities, or variations in their China odyssey. It obfuscates the complexity of the multiple identities that defined nurses' cross-cultural relationships as caregivers and purveyors of Western nursing knowledge and, in some cases, as committed pacifists. Moreover, viewing aid as a top-down process ignores the resistance to Western-based medicine in Chinese society. It underestimates Chinese nurses' agency and contribution to the Convoy's work and to the development of their national health system. It also fails to capture the significant ways in which Western nurses were changed by their China years. Transnational frames that grant historical agency to both sides of the cultural divide avoid recolonializing indigenous nurses and afford a more nuanced understanding of both the interconnectedness and different valency of humanitarian nursing's role in the development of health care nationally and globally.

This book demonstrates that nursing provides a multifaceted lens through which to view broader social attitudes towards race, gender, class, and nation and the value accorded care from a comparative perspective. Transnational scholarship, however, must continue to break down disciplinary boundaries to capture the liminal dimension of humanitarians' lived experiences and the humanitarian environment. The Gadabout nurses' experiences suggest that future studies of global nursing should consider the concept of hybridity within an intimate contact zone of patient care. Extending the contribution of Mary Louise Pratt to critical theory, the humanitarian nursing contact zone is a contested social space where different cultures and classes meet and grapple, often in the context of highly asymmetrical relations of power.[24] This frame admits the possibility of both cultural resistance and multidirectional learning and personal transformation when humanitarians confront unremitting suffering, and also better explains why some nurses became authentic knowers and more effective humanitarian diplomats.[25] This book makes clear that nursing was simultaneously being invented, appropriated, and translated within very different contact zones throughout China, and that some nurses were more effective interlocutors in that process. All China Convoy members, not just nurses, stressed the personal growth that accompanied their China years, and frequently referred to the Convoy as "my university."[26]

The concept of place should be extended to embrace liminality, originally an anthropological concept describing the in-between situations and conditions in the rites of passage as a category of cultural experience.[27] Liminality provides a different vantage point for viewing the transformation of the modern state, structures, and society. Lived experiences, as the Gadabouts attest, transform human beings and thereby contribute to the transmission and reformation of ideas and structures across borders with varying degrees of penetration. Liminality also more deftly captures the process by which China's and modern humanitarian systems transitioned through "in-between spaces," characterized by the dislocation of established structures and uncertainties about traditional cultural norms or future outcomes, and solidified into new normative structures and cultural behaviours. Until recently, however, international relations theorists have resisted incorporating liminality as an analytical lens. Transnational approaches that postulate the constancy of the "betwixt and between" space of humanitarian actors better contextualize the new normative global governance environment that emerged after 1945, characterized by increasing intrastate conflict.[28] If we take the position that today's individual humanitarian crises are not necessarily more complex than those the Gadabouts confronted, we can learn from past experiences.

Reframing studies of global nursing to move beyond a nation-centred approach towards a transnational frame foregrounds the complications of moving ideas, resources, and personnel when the right to receive and give aid impartially and neutrally had to be continuously negotiated. Making

humanitarian negotiations central to global nursing history inquiry illuminates the challenges of humanitarian nurses in high-risk conditions when
making life-and-death choices. In today's radicalized intrastate conflicts,
where there is continued political violence between armed groups representing the state and one or more non-state groups, humanitarian actors
such as the FAU/FSU must support the national government's obligation
under international law to meet its people's needs yet maintain some independence from those same authorities. At the same time, as the FSU experience demonstrates, those same principles must be applied to non-state
actors in order for humanitarian workers to operate safely and gain access
to those most in need of care. The preparation for humanitarian nursing,
indeed for all humanitarian staff, must move beyond mere technical competency and develop leadership and conflict resolution skills and disaster training appropriate to complex disasters and humanitarian crises.

But other challenges for collaborative scholarship, which supports the
view that women have experiences, knowledge, and perspectives crucial for
more effective global governance, remain. Feminist international relations
scholars continue to criticize their mainstream discipline for failing to admit
gender as a serious construct. The qualities associated with manliness have
traditionally been perceived as the basis for the exercise of leadership required
to preserve the national interest and a stable world order. Feminist international relations scholar Anne Tickner argues the necessity of making
women's global experiences visible to expose the limitations of gender as
conventionally constructed in the international relations field: "Drawing
attention to gender hierarchies that privilege men's knowledge and experiences permits us to see that these experiences about international politics
have formed most of our knowledge about international politics." Such reified
gender hierarchies perpetuate the marginalization of women's power in,
and their contribution to, global civil society. Contending that knowledge
must not simply be geared towards solving problems within existing power
structures but towards transforming such structures, Tickner contends that
it is "doubtful that we can achieve a more peaceful and just world ... while
these gender hierarchies remain in place."[29]

Convoy nurses and female physicians took their place in the male-
dominated humanitarian landscape and proved themselves to be risk takers,
skilled practitioners, cultural brokers, and humanitarian diplomats. To varying degrees, they began to develop a more nuanced understanding of the
limits of their own humanitarianism and, by association, of humanitarian

actions that failed to address the underlying determinants of human security. Choosing access over speaking out against human rights violations, and balancing cultural sensitivity, effectiveness, personal survival, and diplomatic acumen remain fundamental challenges for both humanitarian nursing and Quakers' global engagement today. This book attests that the voices of both male and female nurses need to be carefully listened to and critically recorded if we are to chart new directions in the history and practice of humanitarian nursing and a forward-looking human security agenda to ensure freedom from war and human rights that is inclusive and sustainable. If we are to improve their future effectiveness, satisfaction, and sustainability as front-line responders and empower their directive voice within the twenty-first-century global governance system, our scholarship needs to ground that engagement in a sound understanding of nurses' contested and complex historical role in the global humanitarian system. Future transitional scholarship, engaged across disciplines, offers innovative possibilities to restructure the decision-making circles tackling the problem of global security.

Appendix

WADE-GILES	PINYIN
Places	
Ch'angchih	Changzhi
Changte	Changde
Chengchow	Zhengzhou
Chengtu	Chengdu
Ch'ing Shun Ling	Qingshunling (Mountain)
Chungking	Chongqing
Chungmou	Zhongmou
Hangchow	Hangzhou
Hankow	Hankou
Hantan	Handan
Honan	Henan
Hsuchow	Xuzhou
Hupeh	Hubei
Hwang Ho	Huang He (Yellow River)
I Ho	Yi He (Yi River)
Kian	Ji'an
Kaifeng	Kaifeng
Kunming	Kunming
Kutsing	Qujing
Kweichow	Guizhou
Kweiyang	Guiyang
Liuchow	Liuzhou
Lungling	Dehong
Mohei	Mohei
Nanking	Nanjing
Paoshan	Baoshan

WADE-GILES	PINYIN
Places	
Peking	Beijing
Shantan	Shandan
Shanghai	Shanghai
Shihkiachwang	Shijiazhuang
Sian	Xi'an
Sinsiang	Xinxiang
Suchow	Suzhou
Szechwan	Sichuan
T'ai-hang Shan	Taihang Shan (a mountain range)
Tali	Tali
Tientsin	Tianjin
Tsinan	Jinan
Weihwei	Weihui
Wuchuan	Wuzhuang
Yenan	Yan'an
Yen Shan	Yanshan
Yangtze Kiang	Chang Jiang (Yangtze River)
Provinces	
Anhwei	Anhui
Honan	Henan
Hopei	Hebei
Kansu	Gansu
Kiangsi	Jiangxi
Kiangsu	Jiangsu
Shansi	Shanxi
Shantung	Shandong
Yunnan	Yunnan
Political party	
Nationalists	Guomindang

Abbreviations Used in Notes

Unit Letter 1942	file American Friends Service Committee (AFSC) Foreign Service (FS) 1942, China Friends Ambulance Unit (FAU) Reports – Unit Letters 1–38, 1 March 1942 – 24 December 1942, box General Files 1942, FS, FAU Reports # to Doukhobors, AFSC, AFSCA.
Unit Letter 1943	file Country – China FAU (Unit) Letters, 1943, box FS 1943, Country – China (Letters from J. Perry) to Country – China (FAU Reports to National Office), AFSC, AFSCA.
Unit Letter 1944	file Country – England FAU Un# Letters from 1944, box FS 1944, Country – China (FAU – Transport Reports) to Country –England [FAU – Newsletters #]), AFSC, AFSCA.
Newsletter 1945	file FAU Newsletters 1945, box FS 1945, Country – China (FAU Reports – Medical) to (Numbered KAB Letters from and to), AFSC, AFSCA.
Newsletter 1946	file Newsletters 1946, 5 January – 28 December, box FS 1946, Country – China (Numbered Letters to Shanghai to (FAU Newsletters), AFSC, AFSCA.
Newsletter 1947	file Country – China, FSU 1947 Chronicle, April 1947 –December 1947, box FS 1947, Country – China (FSU Minutes) to Country – Denmark, AFSC, AFSCA.
FSU Chronicle 1947	file Country – China, FSU 1947 Chronicle, April 1947 – December 1947, box FS 1947, Country – China (FSU Minutes) to Country – Denmark, AFSC, AFSCA.
FSU Chronicle 1948	file Country – China, Reports on Projects, box FS 1948, Country – China (China Letters to England) to Publicity, AFSC, AFSCA.
FSU Chronicle 1949	file FSU Chronicle, box FS 1949, Country – Austria (Reports from the Field) to Country – China (Letters Shanghai to Philadelphia), AFSC, AFSCA.
FSU Chronicle 1950	file Country – China 1950, Chronicle (Newsletters), box FS 1950, Country – China (Numbered HK Letters Philadelphia to Hong Kong), AFSC, AFSCA.

Others

AFSC	American Friends Service Committee
AFSCA	American Friends Service Committee Archives
ATL	Alexander Turnbull Library
CBCRC	Connie Bull Condick and Ron Condick Private Papers
CNRRA	Chinese National Relief and Rehabilitation Administration
CQYMA	Canadian Quaker Yearly Meeting Archives
DC	Douglas Clifford Private Papers
EA	Edwin Abbott Private Papers
FAU	Friends Ambulance Unit
FAUCC	Friends Ambulance Unit, China Convoy
FAUOHP	Friends Ambulance Unit Oral History Project
FHL	Friends House, London
FM	Frank Miles Private Papers
FS	Foreign Service
FSC	Friends Service Council
GF	General Files
IWM	Imperial War Museum
JD	Jack Dodds Private Papers
MCOHA	Midwest China Oral History and Archives Collection
MCOHAP	Midwest China Oral History and Archive Project
MR	Medical Reports
MS	Margaret Stanley Private Papers
NO	National Office
NQHA	National Quaker History Archive
PC	Pickering College
PDR	Patrick Rawlence Private Papers
RJP	Ralph Johnson Papers
SA	Sound Archives
SG	Shirley Gage Private Papers
UCA	United Church Archives
UCC	United Church of Canada
UCR	United China Relief
WQSC	Woodbrooke Quaker Study Centre

Notes

Introduction

Epigraph: Joan Kennedy Woodrow, personnel files, box 10, China Convoy Records, Friends Ambulance Unit (hereafter FAU) (1939–46), Friends House, London (hereafter FHL), National Quaker History Archive (hereafter NQHA), London.

1 The initiative evolved from cultural links forged by the FAU China Reunion Group with the Xi'an Municipal Administration for Cultural Heritage.

2 FAU China Convoy Reunion Group, "The Commemoration of Our Shared Memory Friends Ambulance Unit – China Exhibition." http://www.fauchinaconvoy.esy.es/?id=3.

3 The overall contribution of nursing remains eclipsed in the biography of Robert McClure, the iconic Canadian physician who directed the Convoy's medical operations. See Munroe Scott, *McClure: The China Years of Dr. Bob McClure: A Biography* (Don Mills, ON: Canec Publishing and Supply House, 1977). Apart from Tegla Davies's official history of the FAU, *Friends Ambulance Unit: The Story of the Friends Ambulance Unit in the Second World War* (London: Allen and Irwin, 1947), the majority of these autobiographical works depict the heroic tales of its medical transport drivers, with three exceptions: Andrew Hicks, *Jack Jones a True Friend to China: "The Lost Writings of a Historic Nobody"* (Hong Kong: Earnshaw Books, 2015); E.R. White, *South of the Clouds: Yunnan and the Salween Front, 1944: Memories of a British Nursing Sister* (London: China Society, 1985); and Teresa Hsu, with Sharana Rao and K.H. Eric Sim, *Love and Share: Memoirs of a Centenarian Teresa Hsu* (Singapore: Sharana Rao, 2011). More recent historical works that included nurses' stories but have limited focus are Susan Armstrong-Reid and David Murray, *Armies of Peace: Canada and the UNRRA Years* (Toronto: University of Toronto Press, 2008); Caitriona Cameron, *Go Anywhere, Do Anything: New Zealanders in the Friends Ambulance Unit, 1945–1951* (Wellington, NZ: Beechtree, 1996); and Lyn Smith, *Pacifists in Action: The Experience of the Friends Ambulance Unit in the Second World War* (York: William Sessions, 1998).

4 See Frederick W. Haberman, *Nobel Lectures, Peace 1926–1950* (Amsterdam: Elsevier, 1972).

5 Duncan Wood, "Talk by Duncan Wood, FAU China Convoy Reunion, York, 5 October 1996," in "Memoirs of Duncan Wood," copy in Lyn Smith FAU Collection, Imperial War Museum (hereafter IWM), London.

6 This perception is woven through Tony Reynolds's account, "Operation and Maintenance of a Road Transport System in West China, 1942–6," *Journal of the Hong Kong Branch of the Royal Asiatic Society* 16 (1976): 153.

7 Davies, *Friends Ambulance Unit.*

8 See Lyndon S. Back, "The Quaker Mission in Poland Relief, Reconstruction and Religion," *Quaker History* 101, 2 (2012): 1–23; Daniel Maul, "The Politics of Neutrality: The American Friends Service Committee and the Spanish Civil War, 1936–1939," *European Review of*

History 23, 1–2 (2016): 82–100; Ilana Feldman, "The Quaker Way: Ethical Labour and Humanitarian Relief," *American Ethnologist* 34, 4 (2007): 689–705; Nancy Gallagher, *Quakers in the Israeli-Palestine Conflict: The Dilemmas of NGO Humanitarian Activism* (Cairo: American University in Cairo Press, 2007); and Asaf Romirowsky and Alexander H. Joffe, "When Did the Quakers Stop Being Friends?" *The Tower,* December 2013, http://www.meforum.org/3693/quakers-friends-anti-israel.

9 See Arlene Keeling and Barbara Mann Wall, *Nurses and Disasters: Global, Historical Case Studies* (New York: Springer, 2015); Arlene Keeling and Barbara Mann Wall, *Nurses on the Front Line: When Disaster Strikes 1878–2010* (New York: Springer, 2011); Susan Armstrong-Reid, *Lyle Creelman: The Frontiers of Global Nursing* (Toronto: University of Toronto Press, 2014); Helen Sweet and Sue Hawkins, eds., *Colonial Caring: A History of Colonial and Post-colonial Nursing* (Manchester: Manchester University Press, 2015); Sonya Grypma, *China Interrupted: Japanese Internment and the Reshaping of a Canadian Mission Community* (Waterloo, ON: Wilfrid Laurier University Press, 2012).

10 M.R. Hunt, L. Schwartz, C. Sinding, and L. Elit. "The Ethics of Engaged Presence: A Framework for Health Professionals in Humanitarian Assistance and Developmental Work," *Developing World Bioethics* 14, 1 (2014): 47–55.

11 Cf. Sweet and Hawkins, *Colonial Caring,* 5–7.

12 Connie Bull Condick China Diary, 1 April 1944, Connie Bull Condick and Ron Condick Private Papers (hereafter CBCRC).

13 Cf. A. Tegla Davies, "Friends Ambulance Unit: The Far East," http://www.ourstory.info/library/4-ww2/Friends/fau07.html.

14 Ibid.

15 For further reading on the AFSC's work with the Civilian Public Service Corps see Steven White, "Quakers, Conscientious Objectors, the Friends Civilian Public Service Corporation and the World War Two," *Southern Friend* 14, 1 (1992): 6–18.

16 Among participants in these negotiations were the British Foreign Office, the British Red Cross Society, the British Fund for Relief of Distress in China, the British Relief Unit, the Friends Service Council, the Chinese Red Cross, the International Red Cross for Central China, the American Friends Service Committee, and the American Red Cross. See Gilbert White, 19 March 1945, file Country – China, Letters 1945, from KA 47 to 70, box Foreign Service (hereafter FS) 1945; Country – China, Letters: John Perry to FAU Newsletters, American Friends Service Committee (hereafter AFSC), American Friends Service Committee Archives (hereafter AFSCA).

17 David Brough, "The China Convoy: A Great Leveller," *The Friend: The Quaker Magazine,* 18 April 2013, https://thefriend.org/article/the-china-convoy-a-great-leveller/.

18 Christopher Sharman to John Rich and Tom Tanner, 6 December 1941, file General to England – Friends Service Council (hereafter FSC), box General Files (hereafter GF) 1941, FS, AFSC, AFSCA.

19 Ibid.

20 The former International Red Cross Committee.

21 *Observer,* 1 October 1968, cited in Helen Tangelder, "Reformed Reflections: Dr. Robert McClure New Moderator of the United Church (1969)," http://www.reformedreflections.ca/other-religions/uc-dr-robert-mcclure-moderator.html.

22 Armstrong-Reid and Murray, *Armies of Peace.*

23 See Chao Hsiang-ke and Lin Hsiao-ting, "Beyond the Carrot and Stick: The Political Economy of US Military Aid to China, 1945–1951," *Journal of Modern Chinese History* 5, 2 (2011): 199–216, http://dx.doi.org/10.1080/17535654.2011.627117.

24 Lieuwe Zijlstra, Andrej Zwitter, and Liesbet Heyse, "International Humanitarian Assistance: Legitimate Intervention or Illegitimate Interference?" in *Ethics and Crisis Management,*

ed. Lina Svedin (Charlotte, NC: Information Age Publishing, 2011), https://www.academia.edu/17397331/International_Humanitarian_Assistance_Legitimate_Intervention_or_Illegitimate_Interference.

25 See Maul, "The Politics of Neutrality," 93.

26 For a useful overview, see Humanitarian Policy Group, "Humanitarian Space: Concept, Definitions and Uses: Meeting Summary," Humanitarian Policy Group Overseas Development Institute, 20 October 2010, https://www.odi.org/sites/odi.org.uk/files/odi-assets/events-documents/4648.pdf.

27 See Sarah Collinson and Samir Elhawary, *Humanitarian Space: Trends and Issues,* HPG Policy Brief 46 (London: Humanitarian Policy Group, Overseas Development Institute, April 2012), http://www.odi.org/resources/docs/7644.pdf.

28 See, for example, Yoshiya Makita, "The Ambivalent Enterprise: Medical Activities of the Red Cross Society of Japan in the Northeastern Region of China during the Russo-Japanese War," in *Entangled Histories: The Transcultural Past of North East China,* ed. Dan Ben-Canaan and Frank Ines Prodohl (New York: Springer, 2014), 189–203. His study of the Japanese Red Cross medical initiatives in Northeast China demonstrated that the process of "othering" to legitimize imperial aspirations was not limited to Western nationals. Othering relies on a dyad that divides a population into "us," who belong, and "them," who do not. "Othering" – constructing negative identities often in binary opposition to Western ideals, values, and norms – creates a superior power over relationships that sustained imperial hierarchies predicated upon cultural superiority.

29 Sonya O. Rose, "Temperate Heroes: Concepts of Masculinity in Second World War Britain," in *Masculinities in Politics and War: Gendering Modern History,* ed. Stefan Dudink, Karen Hagemann, and Josh Tosh (Manchester: Manchester University Press, 2004), 189. Rose describes temperate masculinity as constructed to "combine 'good humour and kindliness with heroism and bravery'" (193). Expanding upon Rose, I explore whether the concept of temperate masculinity was relevant to the gendered perceptions of men's humanitarian work and experiences in nursing in wartime China portrayed within the Convoy's ranks.

30 See, for example, P. D'Antonio, J.C. Fairman, and J. Whelan, *Routledge Handbook on the Global History of Nursing* (New York: Taylor and Friend, 2013).

31 Several publications in particular have influenced this research project, such as J.F. Irwin, "Nurses without Borders: The History of Nursing as US International History," *Nursing History Review* 19, 1 (2011): 78–102; Angela Jackson, *"For Us It Was Heaven": The Passion, Grief and Fortitude of Patience Darton, from the Spanish Civil War to Mao's China* (Eastbourne, UK: Sussex Academic, 2012); Anne-Emanuelle Birn and Theodore M. Brown, eds., *Comrades in Health: US Health Internationalists Abroad and at Home* (New Brunswick, NJ: Rutgers University Press, 2013); Sweet and Hawkins, *Colonial Caring.*

32 Catherine Eschle, *Global Democracy, Social Movements and Feminism* (New York: Basic Books, 2000), quoted in Anne Sisson Runyan and V. Spike Peterson, *Global Gender Issues in the New Millennium* (New York: Westview, 2010), 236.

33 Jezewski defined *culture brokering* as "the act of bridging, linking or mediating between groups or persons of differing cultural backgrounds for the purpose of reducing conflict or producing change." Often, cultural brokers are capable of acting in both directions. See M.A. Jezewski and P. Sotnik, "Preface," in *Culture Brokering: Providing Culturally Competent Rehabilitation Services to Foreign-Born Persons,* ed. M.A. Jezewski and P. Sotnik (New York: Center for International Rehabilitation Research Information and Exchange, 2001), http://cirrie.buffalo.edu/culture/monographs/cb.php#introduction. The role covers more than being an interpreter, although this is an important attribute in cross-cultural situations where language is part of the role. Ibid.

34 Stephanie Chan, "Cross-Cultural Civility in Global Society: Transnational Cooperation in Chinese NGOs," *Global Net World* 8, 2 (2008): 232–52.

35 Ann J. Tickner, *Gender in International Relations: Feminist Perspectives on Achieving Global Security* (New York: Columbia University Press, 1992); Catherine Eschle, "Feminist Studies of Globalisation: Beyond Gender," *Global Society* 18, 2 (2004): 97–125.

36 The Geneva Conventions of 1949, which regulate the conduct of armed conflict and seek to limit its effects, and the Universal Declaration of Human Rights by the UN General Assembly in 1948, reinforcing the idea that humanitarian action should be based on rights rather than needs, were a watershed in the development of humanitarian law.

37 Valerie Amos, "Foreword," in *Coordination to Save Lives: History and Emerging Challenges,* ed. J. Meier, Interagency Standing Committee (New York: Office for the Coordination of Humanitarian Action, 2012).

38 On the value that history can provide in setting future directions for global governance of humanitarianism, see John Nicholas Borton, "Improving the Use of History by the International Humanitarian Sector," *European Review of History* 23, 1–2 (2016): 193–209, http://www.tandfonline.com/doi/full/10.1080/13507486.2015.1121973.

39 E. Davey, "An Introduction to the History of the Humanitarian System: Western Origins and Foundations," IHPG Working Paper (London: Overseas Development Institute, 2013). For further information, see United Nations Regional Information Centre for Europe, "The Responsibility to Protect – on a Case by Case Basis," http://www.unric.org/en/responsibility-to-protect/26988-the-responsibly-to-protect-on-a-case-by-case-basis.

40 D. Chandler, "The Road to Military Humanitarianism: How the Human Rights NGOs Shaped a New Humanitarian Agenda," *Human Rights Quarterly* 23, 3 (2001): 678–700. Direct action is justified on the grounds of serving the greater good, protecting human rights, or promoting peace.

41 Keith David Watenpaugh, *Bread from Stones: The Middle East and the Making of Modern Humanitarianism* (Oakland: University of California Press, 2015). Watenpaugh's provocative book added fuel to the scholarly debate focusing on the overlap between the development of human rights and humanitarianism. He views modern humanitarianism as a distinctive form, phase, and "ideology of organized compassion." It was, he argues, a "phenomenon of late colonialism" at the end of the interwar period, imbricated by race, ethnicity, and nation (4, 179–80). He contends that modern humanitarianism diverged from its predecessor by adopting a largely secular approach "to addressing the root causes of human suffering" (44), and through its adoption of social scientific methods and representative forms across its transnational practice to legitimize its institutional integrity. Disagreeing with scholars who find a greater intersection between the history of human rights and humanitarianism, he postulates that "the reason of humanitarianism pivoted not on the rights of victims of war or genocide, but on the humanity of those providing and those receiving it." It was, he asserts, only because of the disenchantment with humanitarian setbacks that the human rights system crystallized in the 1940s (180).

42 The term is used by Maul in "The Politics of Neutrality," 87.

43 By "one estimate the number of registered NGOs more than doubled between 2001 and 2011, jumping from just over 200,000 to approximately 450,000. Financial support from international partners has become an important source of funding for China's growing number of NGOs" and led to a recent crackdown on their operations by the Chinese government. See Asia Pacific Foundation of Canada, "China's New Order: The Regulation of Foreign Organizations," APF Canada Blog, 24 May 2016, https://www.asiapacific.ca/blog/chinas-new-order-regulation-foreign-organizations.

44 Scholars must be attentive to the ways in which their own vantage point and values shape their historical interpretation; they must also be alert to ethical and methodological

challenges in conducting a particular research project. See Ellen Fleischmann, Sonya Grypma, M. Marten, and Inger Marie Okkenhug, eds., *Transnational and Historical Perspectives on Global Health Welfare and Humanitarianism* (Kristiansand, Norway: Portal Books, 2013), ch. 4; Sonya Grypma, "When We Were (Almost) Chinese: Identity and the Internment of Missionary Nurses in China, 1941–1945," *Histoire sociale/Social History* 43, 86 (2010): 315–44; G. Boschma, S. Grypma, and F. Melchior, "Reflections on Researcher Subjectivity in Nursing History," in *Capturing Nursing History: A Guide to Historical Research*, ed. Sandra Lewenson and Eleanor Hermann (New York: Springer, 2008), 99–121.

45 See Joan Tumblety, *Memory and History: Understanding Memory as Source and Subject* (Abingdon, UK: Routledge, 2013).

46 For a discussion of redemptive narratives, see Grypma, *China Interrupted*, 76.

47 For a useful perspective on "the methodologies used to read different sources 'against the grain' of reality to uncover and give voice to different nurses' experiences deserve greater attention." See the works of life-writing critics such as Sidonie Smith and Julia Watson and their analysis of autobiographies, memoirs, and biographies. Their work cogently challenged the gendered and elitist nature of the grand narrative. Together with other literary theorists and critics of autobiography, they sought to map a more nuanced understanding of the making of the self in society. Their latest collaboration, *Reading Autobiography: A Guide for Interpreting Life Narratives* (Minneapolis: University of Minnesota Press, 2010), delineates the differences between autobiography, memoir, biography, and the more inclusive "life writing" and "life narrative," as well as the six foundational concepts for situating the complexity of autobiographical subjectivity: memory, experience, identity, space, embodiment, and agency. As a historian seeking to contextualize and situate humanitarian nursing's contested place within the global governance landscape, I use agency as an analytical concept in a different way from authors such as Smith and Watson. Despite all the constraints that class and gender place upon their life choices, nurses exercised agency to advance their lives personally and professionally. I am interested in how humanitarian work gave meaning to women's lives as nurses and to their private lives, and how they carved out personal and professional space despite a chaotic, unfamiliar, and sometimes hostile environment to create a sense of home and belonging. Since this perspective shaped my book, I found that Smith and Watson's account of agency did not easily accommodate the gradations of free will that I saw evidenced in the Gadabouts' professional and private lives.

48 For a discussion of the challenges presented by oral history as methodology, see Thomas P. Socknat, "The Canadian Contribution to the China Convoy," *Quaker History* 69, 2 (Autumn 1980): 69–90.

49 Naomi Rogers, "The Most Admired Woman in the World: Forgetting and Remembering in the History of Nursing," *Nursing History Review* 23 (2015): 30.

Introduction to Part 1

1 The FAU had sent an ambulance convoy to the Russo-Finnish front, but the withdrawal of the Allied forces left little immediate prospect for further ambulance work; the first opportunity for work overseas came from China.

2 See Jacqueline Bruzio, "Historical Survey of the AFSC Efforts in China, 1917–2005," 2. Moreover, women's contributions, especially those of the Chinese nurses, are often embedded in male narratives. Uncatalogued AFSC document; copy available at AFSCA.

3 Ibid., 1.

4 Edward J. Drea and Hans Van de Ven, "An Overview of Major Military Campaigns during the Sino-Japanese War, 1937–1945," in *The Battle for China: Essays on the Military History*

of the Sino-Japanese War of 1937–1945, ed. Mark Peattie, Edward Drea, and Hans Van de Ven (Stanford, CA: Stanford University Press, 2013), 34.

5 S.C.M. Paine, *The Wars for Asia, 1911–1949* (Cambridge: Cambridge University Press, 2012), 137.

6 Headquartered in New York, the United China Relief was composed of six American organizations interested in raising funds and coordinating their relief for China: the American Bureau for Medical Aid, the Associated Boards for Christian Colleges, the Associated Boards for Christian Colleges in China, the China Emergency Relief Committee, the Church Committee for China Relief, and the China Aid Council.

7 Leonard Tomkinson, 11 December 1942, file AFSC FS China – FAU Letters and Cables, box GF 1942, FS, Country – China, FAU Reports # to Doukhobors, AFSC, AFSCA.

8 Thomas Tanner to Dear Friends, 6 October 1941, file AFSC FS China – FAU, box GF 1941, FS, General to England – FSC 1941, AFSC, AFSCA.

9 Sydney D. Bailey, handwritten memo, 13 July 1943, file International FAU Misc 1943, box FS Coms. and Orgs. United China Relief to Country – China 1943, United Church of Canada Archives (hereafter UCA).

10 Leonard Tomkinson, 11 December 1942.

11 Henry Louderbough to Dear Mamsie, 20 December 1941, file AFSC, 1941, Country – China Individuals: Henry Louderbough Personal Letters, etc., box GF 1941, FS, General to England – FSC, AFSC, AFSCA.

12 W.H. Auden and Christopher Isherwood, *Journey to a War* (New York: Random House, 1939), 77.

13 Cf. Christopher Sharman to Clarence Pickett, 12 May 1941, file General to England – FSC, box GF 1941, FS, AFSC, AFSCA.

14 Quoted in L.A. Kauffmann, "The Theology of Consensus," *Jacobin,* 27 May 2015, https://www.jacobinmag.com/2015/05/consensus-occupy-wall-street-general-assembly/.

15 Elizabeth Molina-Markham, "Finding the 'Sense of the Meeting': Decision Making through Silence among Quakers," *Western Journal of Communication* 78, 2 (2014): 155.

16 Report 7, 16 March 1942, file AFSC FS China – FAU Reports, Numbered, box GF 1942, FS, Country – China, FAU Reports # to Doukhobors, AFSC, AFSCA.

17 Bob McClure to Clarence E. Pickett and Christopher Sharman, 21 August 1941, file General to England – FSC, box GF 1941, FS, AFSC, AFSCA.

18 John Rich to Leonard Tomkinson, 11 December 1942, file AFSC China – FAU Letters and Cables, box GF 1942, Country – China, FAU Reports # to Doukhobors, AFSC, AFSCA.

19 Davies, *Friends Ambulance Unit.*

20 Douglas Turner, interview with Lyn E. Smith, 24 June 1986, catalogue no. 9338, Sound Archives (SA), IWM.

21 Brough, "The China Convoy: A Great Leveller."

22 Formerly called the International Red Cross Committee for Central China (IRCCC), for whom McClure had worked in the past.

23 Wood, "Memoirs of Duncan Wood," app. 3, 70.

24 Henry Louderbough to Dear M, 21 December 1941, file AFSC, FS 1941, Country – China Individuals: Henry Louderbough Personal Letters, etc., box GF 1941, Foreign Service General to England – FSC, AFSC, AFSCA.

25 Ibid., 20 December 1941.

26 Robert McClure to Dr. Hume, n.d., file AFSC, FS 1941 China, box GF 1941, Foreign Service General to England – FSC, AFSC, AFSCA.

27 Memo, 18 November 1941, file FS 1941 Country – China, box GF 1941, FSC to England – FSC, AFSC, AFSCA.

28 Tom Tanner to Robert McClure, 5 December 1941, file FS, China FAU 1941, box GF 1941, General to England – FSC, AFSC, AFSCA.
29 Tom Tanner to Brandon Cadbury, 19 November 1941, file FS, China FAU 1941, box GF 1941, General to England – FSC, AFSC, AFSCA.
30 Davies, *Friends Ambulance Unit.*
31 Leonard Tomkinson, "With the China Convoy of the FAU," n.d., file AFSC FS China – Friends Ambulance Unit, Letters and Cables, box GF 1942, FS, Country – China (FAU report to Doukhobors), AFSC, AFSCA.
32 Leonard Tomkinson to Clarence Pickett, 21 November 1942, file AFSC FS China – FAU Letters and Cables, box GF 1942, FS, Country – China, FAU Reports # to Doukhobors, AFSC, AFSCA.
33 Sydney D. Bailey, "Draft for China Pamphlet," 30, file Country China – FAU Letters # 1946, box FS 1946, Country – China (Committee and Organizations to Country China FAU), AFSC, AFSCA.
34 John Rich to his wife, 30 April 1943, file Country – China 1943, FAU Letters from John Rich un #, box GF 1941, FS, AFSC, AFSCA.
35 Wood, "Memoirs of Duncan Wood," app. 3: "Quakerism, Pacifism and Wartime Service," 30, John Duncan Wood Private Papers (hereafter JDW). See John Duncan Wood, interview with Lyn E. Smith, 7 August 1986, catalogue no. 9371, SA, IWM.
36 Paine, *Wars for Asia,* 127.
37 Ibid., 131.
38 Ibid., 133.
39 Ibid., 150–51.
40 Cf. ibid., 133–34.
41 Drea and Van de Ven, "Overview of Major Military Campaigns during the Sino-Japanese War," 39.
42 Paine, *Wars for Asia,* 168.
43 Marvin Williamsen, "The Military Dimension, 1937–1941," in *China's Bitter Victory: War with Japan, 1937–1945,* ed. James C. Hsiung and Steven I. Levine (New York: Routledge, 2015), 148.

Chapter 1: Trial by Fire

Epigraph: Davies, *Friends Ambulance Unit.*
1 Sydney D. Bailey, "Draft for China Pamphlet," 41.
2 "Work and Plans of FAU China Convoy," 20 May 1943, file AFSC FS China – FAU 1942 Reports, General, box GF 1942, FS, Country – China, FAU Reports # to Doukhobors, AFSC, AFSCA.
3 H.T. Laycock, "Experiences in a Military Hospital in Free China," *British Medical Journal* (27 February 1943): 262–63, http://pubmedcentralcanada.ca/pmcc/articles/PMC2282315/pdf/brmedj03979-0021.pdf.
4 Scott, *McClure,* 309.
5 Robert McClure, "Memo on the Work of Mobile Surgical Medical Teams," 26 January 1943, file Country – China, FAU Medical Papers from China 1943, box FS 1943, Country – China (Letters from J. Perry) to Country – China (FAU – Reports to National Office [hereafter NO]), AFSC, AFSCA.
6 Alarmed at the prospect of losing the vital Burma Road, the Chinese government offered the British several divisions to help fight the Japanese.
7 Peter Tennant, Report on the Medical Work, n.d., 1942, file AFSC FS China – FAU 1942 Reports, General, box GF 1942, FS, Country – China, FAU Reports # to Doukhobors, AFSC, AFSCA.

8 The son of American Baptist missionaries, Gordon Seagrave was born in Rangoon and received his medical training at Denison University in Granville, Ohio, and Johns Hopkins University in Baltimore. After completing an internship at Union Memorial Hospital in Baltimore, he and his wife settled in Namkham in the Shan State of northeastern Burma in 1922, where they ran a hospital. After war broke out in Burma, Seagrave and his unit were assigned by the British to offer mobile medical support for the Chinese 6th Army, operating in the Shan State and the Karen State in eastern Burma. After Stilwell arrived, Seagrave's unit was placed under American command and subsequently ordered to move just behind the front lines at Pyinmana. It was then that Seagrave was also informed that a volunteer group called the Friends Ambulance Unit would join them.

9 Peter Tennant, Report on the Medical Work, n.d., 1942.

10 Davies, *Friends Ambulance Unit*.

11 Smith, *Pacifists in Action*, 177.

12 Report 8, 22 April 1942, file AFSC FS China – FAU Reports, Numbered, box GF 1942, FS, Country – China, FAU Reports # to Doukhobors, AFSC, AFSCA.

13 Devizes Peace Group, "Exit from Burma: A Conscientious Objector's Story," BBC, 12 November 2005, http://www.bbc.co.uk/history/ww2peopleswar/stories/71/a6913271. shtml.

14 Alan K. Lathrop, "Dateline: Burma," *Dartmouth Medicine*, http://dartmed.dartmouth.edu/ spring04/html/dateline_burma.shtml.

15 Devizes Peace Group, "Exit from Burma."

16 Lathrop, "Dateline: Burma."

17 Dwight Edwards, "Diary of Involuntary Traveller," 7–8, file Personnel Files – Personnel Movements FHL, box 8, FAU, China Convoy (hereafter FAUCC), Friends House, London (hereafter FHL), National Quaker History Archive (hereafter NQHA).

18 Gordon S. Seagrave, *Burma Surgeon* (London: Victor Gollancz, 1944), 189.

19 Devizes Peace Group, "Exit from Burma."

20 Seagrave, *Burma Surgeon*, 292.

21 Medical Report for the Second Quarter, July/September 1942, file AFSC FS China – FAU 1942 Reports, General, box GF 1942, FS, Country – China, FAU Reports # to Doukhobors, AFSC, AFSCA.

22 Dr. Laycock, "The Friends Ambulance Unit in North Assam, 1942," file AFSC FS China – FAU 1942 Reports, General, box GF 1942, FS, Country – China, FAU Reports # to Doukhobors, AFSC, AFSCA.

23 FAU, Medical Report for the Second Quarter 1942, 19 October 1943, file AFSC FS China – FAU 1942 Reports, General, box GF 1942, FS, Country – China, FAU Reports # to Doukhobors, AFSC, AFSCA.

24 Dr. Laycock, "The Friends Ambulance Unit in North Assam, 1942."

25 FAU, Medical Report for the Second Quarter 1942, 19 October 1943.

26 Peter Tennant, Report on the Medical Work, n.d., 1942.

27 Copy of letter, Joseph F. Stilwell to Gordon Keith, 18 January 1943, file American Friends Service Committee, box 19 American Friends Service Committee (DG 002), section 5: Later Accessions, accession 06A-019, UCA; FAU (China) 06A-019 Correspondence, 1943.

28 Davies, *Friends Ambulance Unit*, 269.

29 Compare with David Brough, "The China Convoy: What Was the Right Thing to Do?" *The Friend: The Quaker Magazine*, 9 May 2013, https://thefriend.org/article/the-china-convoy -what-was-the-right-thing-to-do/.

30 Robert McClure to Robert W. Barnett, Program of FAU for 1942, 7 May 1942, file AFSC FS China – FAU 1942 Reports, General, box GF 1942, FS, Country – China, FAU Report # to Doukhobors, AFSC, AFSCA.

31 Robert McClure, 1 June 1942, file AFSC FS China – FAU 1942 Reports, General, box GF 1942, FS, Country – China, FAU Reports # to Doukhobors, AFSC, AFSCA.

32 Robert McClure to Dr. Bachman, 6 May 1942, file AFSCA FS China – FAU 1942, Letter and Cables, box GF 1942, FS, Country – China, FAU Reports # to Doukhobors, AFSC, AFSCA.

33 Report of the Year's Work 1942–43, 1.

34 Robert McClure, 1 June 1942.

35 George William Parsons, interview with Lyn E. Smith, 27 March 1987, catalogue no. 9789, SA, IWM.

36 Report 10, 19 June 1942, file AFSC FS China – FAU Reports, Numbered, box GF 1942, FS, Country – China, FAU Reports # to Doukhobors, AFSC, AFSCA.

37 Leonard Tomkinson to John F. Rich and Michael Cadbury, "Descriptive Reports on Condition and Work from an FAU Medical Team," 1 December 1944, file Country – China, FAU Medical Papers from China 1943, box FS 1943, Country – China (Letters from J. Perry) to Country – China (FAU – Reports to NO), AFSC, AFSCA.

38 *Unit Letter* 23, 22 August 1942.

39 Nelson Fuson, Summary of John Rich's Information from China thru Letter no. 18, 5 July 1943; also cable of 4 August 1943, file Country – China Reports (General, including CPS men), box FS 1942, Country – China, AFSC, AFSCA.

40 John Rich, Dear Ken and Duncan, 5 July 1943, file China – John Rich Correspondence 1943, box FS 1943, FS, Country – China, AFSC, AFSCA.

41 Report 22, 8 July 1943, file Country – China 1943, FAU Reports, Numbered, box FS 1943, FS, Country – China (FAU Numbered Reports) to Country – Egypt, AFSC, AFSCA.

42 John Rich, 3 September 1943, file China – FAU Letters from 1943, to John [Rich], box FS 1943, Country – China, AFSC, AFSCA.

43 Ken Bennett to John Rich, 28 June 1943, file China – John Rich Correspondence 1943, box GF 1943, FS, Country – China, AFSC, AFSCA.

44 Nelson Fuson, Summary of John Rich's Information from China thru Letter no. 18, 5 July 1943; also cable of 4 August 1943.

45 *Unit Letter* 36, 28 November 1942.

46 Report 10, 19 June 1942.

47 Leonard Tomkinson to John F. Rich and Michael Cadbury, "Descriptive Reports on Condition and Work from an FAU Medical Team," 1 December 1944.

48 See Peter Tennant, Friends Ambulance Unit Report #14, file AFSC FS China – FAU Reports, Numbered, box GF 1942, FS, Country – China, FAU Reports # to Doukhobors, AFSC, AFSCA.

49 John Rich, 26 June 1943, file China – John Rich Correspondence 1943, box GF 1943, FS, Country – China, AFSC, AFSCA.

50 *Unit Letter* 27, 19 September 1942.

51 Duncan Wood to Jane Wong, 9 March 1944, file Chinese Volunteers, box 19, FAUCC, FHL, NQHA.

52 Report 11, 10 September 1942, file AFSC FS China – FAU Reports, Numbered, box GF 1942, FS, Country – China, FAU Reports # to Doukhobors, AFSC, AFSCA.

53 Robert McClure, 1 June 1942.

54 *Unit Letter* 38, 28 July 1942.

55 Report 10, 19 June 1942.

56 Duncan Wood to Yang Shao Nan, 5 October 1943, file Chinese Volunteers, box 19, FAUCC, FHL, NYQA.

57 *Newsletter* 151, 24 March 1945.

Chapter 2: A Marriage of Convenience
Epigraph: Robert McClure, MST2 Baoshan, 28 July 1942. *Unit Letter* 22, 16 August 1942.

1 Art Barr to Dear Michael, 29 September 1943, file Country – China, FAU Medical Papers from China 1943, box FS 1943, Country – China (Letters from J. Perry) to Country – China (FAU – Reports to NO), AFSC, AFSCA.
2 See *Unit Letter* 25, 2 September 1942; *Unit Letter* 26, 12 September 1942.
3 Scott, *McClure*, 323.
4 "Work of the Mobile Surgical Teams in China April to November, 1942," file AFSC FS China – FAU 1942 Reports, General, box GF 1942, FS, Country – China, FAU Reports # to Doukhobors, AFSC, AFSCA.
5 FAU Report, December 1942, file AFSC FS China – FAU 1942 Reports, General, box GF 1942, FS, Country – China, FAU Reports # to Doukhobors, AFSC, AFSCA.
6 Compare with *Independent*, "Lives Remembered: Michael Harris," 23 October 2011, http://www.independent.co.uk/news/obituaries/lives-rememberedmichael-harris-1699434.html.
7 *Unit Letter* 27, 19 September 1942.
8 Scott, *McClure*, 343.
9 Robert McClure to A.E. Armstrong, 15 January 1945, file McClure, box 5, FAUCC, FHL, NQHA.
10 Henry Louderbough, "Report on Medical & Surgical Work of the 2nd MST," n.d., file AFSC FS China – FAU 1942 Reports, General, box GF 1942, FS, Country – China, FAU Reports # to Doukhobors, AFSC, AFSCA.
11 Leonard Tomkinson to Clarence Pickett, 21 September 1942, file AFSC FS China – FAU Letters and Cables, box GF 1942, FS, Country – China, FAU Reports # to Doukhobors, AFSC, AFSCA. Compare with John Rich to Leonard Tomkinson, 11 December 1942.
12 John Rich to Clarence [Pickett], James and Edgar, 20 May 1943, file Country – China 1943, FAU Letters from John Rich, box FS 1943, Country – China (Letters from J. Perry) to Country – China (FAU – Reports to NO), AFSC, AFSCA.
13 Report 21, 8 June 1943, file Country – China 1943, FAU Reports, Numbered, box GF 1943, FS, Country – China (FAU Numbered Reports) to Country – Egypt, AFSC, AFSCA.
14 John Rich to Clarence Pickett, Elmore Jackson, C. Reed Cary, and James Vail, 2 February 1943, file China – FAU Personnel 1943, box GF 1943, FS, Country – China, AFSC, AFSCA.
15 Henry Louderbough to Dear Mamsie, 20 December 1941.
16 Art Barr to Dear Folks, 6 October 1942, file AFSC FS China – FAU Letters and Cables, box GF 1942, FS, Country – China, FAU Reports # to Doukhobors, AFSC, AFSCA.
17 AFSC, "Reporting on the Activities of the Friends Ambulance in China, March 1943," file AFSC FS China – FAU Letters and Cables, box GF 1942, FS, Country – China, FAU Reports # to Doukhobors, AFSC, AFSCA.
18 Henry Louderbough to Dear Mamsie, 4 October 1942, file AFSC FS China – FAU Letters and Cables, box GF 1942, FS, Country – China, FAU Reports # to Doukhobors, AFSC, AFSCA.
19 Ernest Evans to his parents, n.d., copy, file Country – China 1943, FAU Personal Letters from Members, box FS 1943, Country – China (Letters from J. Perry) to Country – China (FAU – Reports to NO), AFSC, AFSCA.
20 AFSC, "Reporting on the Activities of the Friends Ambulance in China, March 1943."
21 Arthur Barr to Dear Folks, 6 October 1942.
22 FAU, "Report on the Use of the British Grant for the Third Quarter October to December 1942," file AFSC FS China – FAU 1942 Reports, General, box GF 1942, FS, Country – China, FAU Reports # to Doukhobors, AFSC, AFSCA.

23 John Rich to John Judkyn, 21 May 1943, file Country – China 1943, FAU Letters from John Rich, box FS 1943, Country – China (Letters from J. Perry) to Country – China (FAU – Reports to NO), AFSC, AFSCA.

24 Robert McClure to A.E. Armstrong, 15 January 1945.

25 Report 18, n.d., file AFSC FS China – FAU Reports, Numbered, box GF 1942, FS, Country – China, FAU Reports # to Doukhobors, AFSC, AFSCA.

26 Allen Longshore to his parents (excerpt), 27 February 1944, file Country – China, FAU Letters from American Members Un#, box FS 1944, FS, Country – China (A) to Country – China (FAU), AFSC, AFSCA.

27 Nelson Fuson, Summary of Correspondence from John Rich from China thru Letter no. 18, 5 July; also cable of 4 August 1943. The file contains scathing letters from several members of MST1 about Evans's behaviour, lack of surgical skill, and negativity. All recommended against his being appointed team leader in the near future.

28 John Rich to Clarence [Pickett], James and Edgar, 20 May 1943.

29 Letters from Ernest Evans to his parents, received October 1943, 18, file Country – China 1943, FAU Personal Letters from Members, box FS 1943, Country – China (Letters from J. Perry) to Country – China (FAU – Reports to NO), AFSC, AFSCA.

30 Ibid., 15.

31 Ibid., 19.

32 Ibid., 17.

33 "Extracts from the August 1943 Report," file Country – China, FAU Medical Papers from China 1943, Medical Reports (hereafter MR), box FS 1943, Country – China (Letters from J. Perry) to Country – China (FAU – Reports to NO), AFSC, AFSCA.

34 "Report of the Year's Work, 1942–43," file AFSC FS China – FAU 1942 Reports, General, box GF, 1942, FS, Country – China, FAU Reports, # to Doukhobors, AFSC, AFSCA.

35 Letters from Ernest Evans to his parents, received October 1943, 14–15.

36 Ibid.

37 Japanese Red Cross physicians experienced similar difficulties. See Makita, "The Ambivalent Enterprise," 202.

38 Robert McClure to Brandon (Cadbury) Re: Future of Medical Teams, n.d., file Chinese Red Cross, box 13, FAUCC, FHL, NQHA.

39 Robert McClure to Michael Harris, 26 November 1943, file Chinese Red Cross, box 13, FAUCC, FHL, NQHA.

40 Robert McClure to John Rich, 4 October 1943, file China – John Rich Correspondence 1943, box GF 1943, FS, Country – China, AFSC, AFSCA.

41 Robert McClure to Michael Harris, 26 November 1943.

42 William Rahill to Passmore Elkinton, 25 February 1944, file Country – China, FAU Letters from American Members Un#, box GF 1944, FS, Country – China (A) to Country – China (FAU), AFSC, AFSCA.

43 "Report on Medical Work for the Year 1944," file Country – China, FAU MR 1944, FAU, China Convoy, box FS 1944, Country – China (FAU – Letters from & to FAU – Supplies), AFSC, AFSCA.

44 *Newsletter* 171, 11 August 1945.

45 Patrick Rawlence, unpublished memoir, 5, Patrick Rawlence Private Papers (hereafter PDR).

46 *Unit Letter* 133, 11 November 1944.

47 *Unit Letter* 131, 28 October 1944.

48 "General Medical Report for the Month of December 1944," 30 December 1944, file MR, box 5, FAUCC, FHL, NQHA.

49 Patrick Rawlence, unpublished memoir, 5–6.

50 "General Medical Report for the Month of December 1944," 30 December 1944.

51 *Newsletter* 148, 3 March 1945.

52 Edwin Abbott, 26 July 1945, letters to his future wife, Viv, Edwin Abbott Private Papers (hereafter EA).

53 Patrick Rawlence, unpublished memoir, 7.

54 Ibid., 6.

55 Ibid., 12.

56 Edwin Abbott to Viv, 9 July 1945, EA.

57 Ibid., 24 August 1945.

58 Patrick Rawlence, unpublished memoir, 6.

59 Edwin Abbott to Viv, 10 September 1945, EA.

60 Robert McClure to Whom It May Concern, 6 October 1945, file Jane Wong, box 10, FAUCC, FHL, NQHA.

61 *Newsletter* 184, 17 November 1945.

62 Spencer Coxe to David Johnson, 13 November 1947, file FSU, China (Letters from China to London) 1947, box FS 1947, Country – China (FSU Minutes) to Country – Denmark, AFSC, AFSCA.

63 David Johnson to Spencer Coxe, 3 December 1947, file FS China (Letters from China to London) 1947, box FS 1947, Country – China (FSU Minutes) to Country – Denmark, AFSC, AFSCA.

64 Spencer Coxe to Jane Wong, 27 May 1947, file Jane Wong, box 10, FAUCC, FHL, NQHA.

65 Ibid., 23 January 1948.

66 *Unit Letter* 131, 28 October 1944.

67 *Newsletter* 150, 17 March 1945.

68 "General Medical Report through the Month of March 1945," 30 April 1945, file MR, box 5, FAUCC, FHL, NQHA. Compare with *Newsletter* 157, 5 May 1945.

69 "Medical Report for the Month of November 1944," file Country – China (FAU – Letters from) to (FAU – Supplies), Country – China (FAU MR 1944) box FS 1944, Country – China, AFSC, AFSCA.

70 *Newsletter* 140, 6 January 1945.

71 Ibid.

72 "General Medical Report through the Month of March 1945," 30 April 1945; *Newsletter* 150, 17 March 1945.

73 Ibid. See also *Newsletter* 157, 5 May 1945.

74 *Newsletter* 168, 21 July 1945.

75 Michael Harris, 20 September 1943, file Chinese Red Cross, box 13, FAUCC, FHL, NQHA.

76 Ibid.

77 Colin Bell to Dr. P.Z. King, medical director Chinese National Relief and Rehabilitation Administration (hereafter CNRRA), 21 March 1946, file Sheila Iu, box 9, FAUCC, FHL, NQHA.

Chapter 3: The Salween Campaign
Epigraph: Friends Ambulance Unit Chronicle, 7 October 1944, FHL, NQHA.

1 For a more detailed description of the campaign, see Drea and Van de Ven, "Overview of Major Military Campaigns during the Sino-Japanese War," 44–46.

2 Report of the Medical Director, 7 June 1943, file Country – China, FAU Medical Papers from China, box FS 1943, Country – China (Letters from J. Perry) to Country – China (FAU – Reports to NO), AFSC, AFSCA.

3 Leonard Tomkinson, the British Friends Service Council worker who had been asked to be its liaison officer because of his long experience of China, was invited to become the Convoy's chairman.

4   Leonard Tomkinson to Dear Michael and Tegla, 3 September 1943, file Country – China, FAU Letters to and from, box FS 1943, Country – China (Letters from J. Perry) to Country – China (FAU – Reports to NO), AFSC, AFSCA.
5   Jane Wong to Duncan Wood, 20 December 1943, file Personnel Files: Jane Wong, box 10, FAUCC, FHL, NQHA.
6   Chiang Kai-shek launched the New Life Movement on 19 February 1934. For a more positive reassessment of the unfolding and contribution of the NLM, see Federica Ferlanti, "The New Life Movement in Jiangxi Province, 1934–1938," *Modern Asian Studies* 44, 5 (2010): 961–1000.
7   *Newsletter* 176, 19 September 1945.
8   Unknown, Dear Tegla and Michael, 23 November 1943, file Country – China 1943, FAU Reports, Numbered, Report 25, box FS 1943, FS, Country – China (FAU Numbered Reports) to Country – Egypt, AFSC, AFSCA.
9   For a description of the tumultuous beginnings of the Army Nursing School, see "China's Nurses Carry On," *American Journal of Nursing* 44, 7 (July 1944): 642–44.
10   John Perry to Dear Mamsie, 30 December 1943, file Country – China 1944, FAU, Perry, John (Letters), box FS 1944, Country – China (FAU Letters from & to), AFSC, AFSCA. Although this letter was written in 1943, it is included in the box according to the date received by AFSC.
11   Ibid., 19 January 1944.
12   Ibid., 6 February 1944.
13   Ibid., 13 February 1944.
14   Ibid., 17 February 1944.
15   Ibid., 7 February 1944.
16   Ibid., 8 February 1944.
17   Ibid., 11 February 1944.
18   Ibid., 19 February 1944.
19   Arthur Barr, "Report of Medical Team 3," file Country – China, 1943 FAU Medical Papers from China, box FS 1943, Country – China (Letters from J. Perry) to Country – China (FAU – Reports to NO), AFSC, AFSCA.
20   "Report of the Year's Work, 1942–43," 2.
21   Letter 13, 5 December 1943, copies of letters from Allen Longshore to his parents, file Country – China, 1943 FAU Medical Papers from China, box FS Country – China 1943, AFSC, AFSCA.
22   "Reporting the Activities of the Friends Ambulance Unit in China," October 1943, file Country – China, FAU Reports to NO, box FS 1943, Country – China (Letters from J. Perry) to Country – China (FAU – Reports to NO), AFSC, AFSCA.
23   Allen Longshore to Dear Folks, 5 March 1944, file Country – China 1944, FAU Letters from American Members Un#, box FS 1944, Country – China to County (A) – China (FAU), AFSC, AFSCA.
24   Allen Longshore to Dear Folks, 7 November 1943, file Country – China 1943, FAU Personal Letters from Members, box FS 1943 Country – China (Letters from J. Perry) to Country – China (FAU – Reports to NO), AFSC, AFSCA.
25   *Unit Letter* 103, April 1944.
26   *Unit Letter* 116, 1 July 1944.
27   *Newsletter* 176, 15 September 1945.
28   Robert McClure to Edward Cunningham, 29 November 1944, file Medical Files, Robert McClure 1945, box 5, FAUCC, FHL, NQHA.

29 Scott, *McClure*, 323.
30 John Wilks had begun his studies at Guy's Medical School in 1936 and qualified in 1942. He held house posts at Guy's before joining the China Convoy.
31 *Newsletter* 176, 15 September 1945.
32 *Unit Letter* 134, 25 November 1944.
33 Ibid.
34 Ibid.
35 *Unit Letter* 122, 18 August 1944. Compare with Michael Harris, "Medical Report through July 1944 (Military Teams Only)," 1 September 1944, file MR, box 5, FAUCC, FHL, NQHA.
36 *Unit Letter* 134, 25 November 1944. Compare with Michael Harris, ibid.
37 *Unit Letter* 122, 18, August 1944.
38 *Unit Letter* 134, 25 November 1944.
39 Margaret So to Duncan Wood and Michael Harris, 7 November 1944, file Margaret So, box 10, FAUCC, FHL, NQHA.
40 Duncan Wood to Margaret So, 7 November 1944, file Margaret So, box 10, FAUCC, FHL, NQHA.
41 Duncan Wood to Whom It May Concern, 2 December 1944, file Margaret So, box 10, FAUCC, FHL, NQHA.
42 "Medical Report," 9 November 1944. Compare also with file "Medical Report through October 1944 (Military Teams Only)," box 5, FAUCC, FHL, NQHA.
43 *Newsletter* 157, 5 May 1945.
44 *Newsletter* 153, 19 May 1945.
45 *Newsletter* 159, 7 April 1945.
46 *Newsletter* 153, 19 May 1945.
47 Theo Willis to Bob McClure, 12 January 1945, file MR 1945, Robert B. McClure, box 6, FAUCC, FHL, NQHA.
48 Jack Goss to Colin Bell, "Notes on Interview with Doris Wu 4 January 1945," 5 January 1945, file Personnel Files: Wu, Doris, box 10, FAUCC, FHL, NQHA.
49 John Perry to Dear Mamsie, 7 June 1945, file Country – China 1945, FAU, Perry, John (Letters) 1945, box FS 1945, Country – China (FAU Reports – Medical) to (Numbered KAB Letters from and to), AFSC, AFSCA.
50 Ibid., 17 June 1945. (Ibid., 17 June 1945).
51 Ibid., 3 July 1945.
52 Jack Dodds to Dear Mother, Dad and all, 8 July 1945, Jack Dodds Private Papers (hereafter JD).
53 John Perry to Dear Mamsie, 14 July 1945, file Country – China 1945, Perry, John (Letters) 1945, box FS 1945, Country – China (FAU Reports – Medical) to (Numbered KAB Letters from and to), AFSC, AFSCA.
54 Ibid.
55 Ibid., 18 August 1945.
56 Ibid., 29 August 1945.
57 Ibid.
58 John Perry, Nantan Project, n.d., file Country – China 1945, FAU Reports (Medical & Orders), box FS 1945, Country – China (FAU Reports – Medical) to (Numbered KAB Letters from and to), AFSC, AFSCA.
59 *Newsletter* 179, 12 September 1945.
60 Compare with Jack Dodds to Dear Mother, Dad and all, 13 July 1945, 27 July 1945.
61 John Perry to Dear Mamsie, 14 July 1945.

62 A. Perry, FAU Book: Some Comments, FAU 4.7, SA, IWM.

63 "General Medical Report through the Month of January 1945," 7 February 1945, file MR, box 5, FAUCC, FHL, NQHA.

64 Timothy Hayworth, "Hwa Mei Hospital, Memorandum of Discussion Held 21 January 1947," file Hospitals, box 15, FAUCC, FHL, NQHA.

65 Scott, *McClure*, 386.

66 Robert McClure, "Miscellany: Miss Li," *Canadian Medical Association Journal* 53, 3 (September 1945): 295.

67 Ibid., 296.

68 Robert McClure to George Armstrong, 5 February 1945, file MR, box 5, FAUCC, FHL, NQHA.

69 Ibid., 15 January 1945.

70 Copy of Duncan Wood, "Talk by Duncan Wood, FAU China Convoy Reunion, York, 5 October 1996," in "Memoirs of Duncan Wood," Lyn Smith FAU Collection, IWM.

71 Jackson Progin, "Reflections on Repatriation," *Friends Ambulance Unit Chronicle*, 3 March 1945, FHL, NQHA.

72 Duncan Wood, "Further Thoughts on China," *Friends Ambulance Unit Chronicle*, 2 June 1945, FHL, NQHA.

73 Cf. Stephanie Chan, "Cross-Cultural Civility in Global Civil Society: Transnational Cooperation in Chinese NGOs," *Global Net World* 8, 2 (2008): 232–52.

74 Email correspondence with Chris Bonsall, 21 April 2014.

75 Colin Bell to Whom It May Concern, 27 February 1945, file Personnel Files: Nellie Wee, box 9, FAUCC, FHL, NQHA.

76 Teresa Hsu's account of her educational background in convent school in her letters of application to British nursing schools differs from her self-published memoir, *Love and Share*. In her redemptive memoir, she claims that a combination of abject poverty and gender discrimination prevented her from obtaining any formal education during her childhood. While the memoir likely embellished her dire circumstances growing up, her belief that education was key to women's autonomy and health rings true, given her later life of service to those in need in Paraguay, Cambodia, Malaysia, and Singapore. She was the founder of several non-profit charities – Heart to Heart Service and the Home for the Aged Sick, one of the first homes for the aged sick in Singapore.

77 Colin Bell to Ken Bennett, 16 December 1945, file Personnel Files: Teresa Hsu, box 9, FAUCC, FHL, NQHA.

Chapter 4: "China Needs Good Men, and Still Better Women"

Epigraph: Colin Bell to Eric Johnson, and Wil Jenkins, 14 December, file 1945, Letters FAU KA 100–164, box FS 1945, Country – China (FAU – Reports Medical) to (Numbered KAB Letters from and to), AFSCA, AFSC.

1 Robert McClure, 18 July 1944, copy of airgraph, file Country – China 1944, FAU McClure, Robert, box FS 1944, Country – China (FAU – Letters from) to (FAU – Supplies), AFSC, AFSCA.

2 Duncan Wood to John Rich, 26 June 1943, file China – John Rich Correspondence 1943, box FS 1943, FS, Country – China, AFSC, AFSCA.

3 Nelson Fuson, Summary of John Rich's Information from China thru Letter no. 18, 5 July 1943; also cable of 4 August 1943, file Country – China Reports (General including CPS men), box FS 1942, Country – China, AFSC, AFSCA.

4 Gilbert White, "Minutes of China Convoy Staff Meeting, November 1944 Which Have a Bearing on Personnel Policies," minute 17, file Country – China 1944, FAU Inter-office Memos, box FS 1944, Country – China (A) to Country – China (FAU), AFSC, AFSCA.

5 Robert McClure to Dear Michael (Cadbury), 9 January 1945, file MR, box 5, FAUCC, FHL, NQHA.
6 *FAU Chronicle* 69, 3 March 1945, FHL, NQHA.
7 Elaine Ethel Conyers Bell, interview with Lyn E. Smith, 2 November 1993, catalogue no. 13499, SA, IWM.
8 Margaret Matheson Briggs, interview with Lyn E. Smith, 29 August 1990, catalogue no. 11531, SA, IWM.
9 Ibid.
10 Evelyn Rita Dangerfield White, interview with Lyn E. Smith, 22 January 1988, catalogue no. 10142, SA, IWM.
11 Email correspondence with Sasha Denton White, 25 February 2016.
12 P.J. Hume, personnel officer, "Bull, Constance Margaret, Case no. L.W. 12, sheet No. 2, Line No. 4, Further Evidence Obtained at Hearing" (copy), CBCRC.
13 Copy of Connie Bull's Application to Local Tribunal by a Person Provisionally Registered in the Register as a Conscientious Objectors, 1 April 1942, CBCRC.
14 Elaine Ethel Conyers Bell, interview with Lyn E. Smith, 2 November 1993.
15 Ron Condick to Connie Bull, June 1943, from Kutsing [Qujing], CBCRC.
16 Evelyn Rita Dangerfield White, interview with Lyn E. Smith.
17 In a 1944 article exploring the Chinese concept of face, Hsien Chin Hu distinguished two criteria: "*mien-tzu,* a reputation for getting on with life, through success and ostentation," and "*lien,*" which is "respect of the group for a man with a good moral reputation ... it represents the confidence of society in the integrity of ego's moral character, the loss of which makes it impossible for him to function properly within the community. *Lien* is both a social sanction for enforcing moral standards and an internalized sanction." Hsien Chin Hu, "The Chinese Concept of 'Face,'" *American Anthropologist* 46 (1944): 45.
18 Evelyn Rita Dangerfield White, interview with Lyn E. Smith.
19 *Unit Letter* 110, 19 July 1944.
20 Ibid.
21 Report 11, 16 September 1942, file AFSC FS China – FAU Reports, Numbered, box GF 1942, Country – China, FAU Reports # to Doukhobors, AFSC, AFSCA.
22 See, for example, *Unit Letter* 37, 5 November 1942.
23 Rita Dangerfield White, Diary, 19 April 1944, Rita Dangerfield White Private Papers (hereafter RDWD).
24 Evelyn Rita Dangerfield White, interview with Lyn E. Smith.
25 Rita Dangerfield White, Diary, 3 May 1944.
26 *Unit Letter* 110, 19 July 1944.
27 Rita Dangerfield White, Diary, 18 May 1944.
28 Allen Longshore to Dear Folks, 29 May 1944, file Country – China, FAU Letters from American Members Un#, box FS 1944, FS, Country – China (A) to Country – China (FAU), AFSC, AFSCA.
29 Evelyn Rita Dangerfield White, interview with Lyn E. Smith. See also Lyn Denton-White, "Nursing in China," Bemerton Local History Society, BBC – WW2 People's War, http://www.bbc.co.uk/history/ww2peopleswar/stories/65/a4255265.shtml.
30 Sydney D. Bailey, "Draft for China Pamphlet," 30.
31 Ibid.
32 Evelyn Rita Dangerfield White, interview with Lyn E. Smith. See also Denton-White, "Nursing in China."
33 Connie Bull Condick, China Diary, 1 April 1944.
34 Margaret Briggs Matheson, interview with Lyn E. Smith.
35 Peter Tennant, Friends Ambulance Unit Report #14.

Chapter 5: Baoshan

Epigraph: Connie Bull Condick China Diary, 12 October 1944.

1 Gas gangrene, also known as "clostridial myonecrosis," is a form of tissue death caused by infection of muscle tissue with gas-producing *Clostridium perfringens* bacteria. It is a medical emergency. The term "myonecrosis" refers to necrotic damage specific to muscle tissue.

2 John Perry to Dearest Wonderful Mamsie, 2 June 1944, file Country – China 1944, FAU, Perry, John (Letters), box FS 1944, Country – China, FAU Letters to and from, AFSC, AFSCA.

3 Ibid., 29 May 1944.

4 Ibid., 22 September 1944.

5 Ibid., 31 May 1944.

6 Ibid.

7 Ibid., 2 June 1944.

8 Ibid., 23 September 1944.

9 Connie Bull Condick China Diary, 10 June 1944.

10 John Perry to Dearest Mamsie, 8 September 1944, file Country – China 1944, FAU, Perry, John (Letters), box FS 1944, Country – China, FAU Letters to and from, AFSC, AFSCA.

11 Evelyn Rita Dangerfield White, interview with Lyn E. Smith.

12 Denton-White, "Nursing in China."

13 Evelyn Rita Dangerfield White, interview with Lyn E. Smith.

14 Rita Dangerfield White, Diary, 24 June 1944.

15 McClure to Michael Harris, 31 July 1944, file Chinese Red Cross, box 13, FAUCC, FHL, NQHA.

16 Connie Bull Condick, China Diary, 3 August 1944. The diary entry ends mid-sentence, and several of the following pages are torn out.

17 *Unit Letter* 115, 24 June 1944.

18 *Unit Letter* 131, 1 July 1944.

19 John Perry to Dear Mamsie, 6 August 1944, file Country – China 1944, FAU, Perry, John (Letters), box FS 1944, Country – China, FAU Letters, AFSC, AFSCA.

20 Ibid., 8 September 1944.

21 Ibid.

22 *Unit Letter* 135, 2 December 1944.

23 *Unit Letter* 137, 16 December 1944.

24 Ibid.

25 Margaret Briggs Matheson, interview with Lyn E. Smith.

26 Clement White, an account of his time with FAU, untitled and n.d., file Country – China 1944, FAU Letters from American Members Un#, box FS 1944, FS, Country – China (A) to Country – China (FAU), AFSC, AFSCA.

27 Ibid.

28 *Unit Letter* 125, 2 September 1944.

29 Rita Dangerfield White, Diary, 24 June 1944.

30 Ibid.

31 Connie Bull Condick China Diary, 10 June 1944.

32 John Perry to Dear Mamsie, 24 September 1944, file Country – China 1944, FAU, Perry, John (Letters), box FS 1944, Country – China, FAU Letters, AFSC, AFSCA.

33 Allen Longshore to Dear Folks, 7 May 1944, file Country – China, FAU Letters from American Members Un#, box FS 1944, FS, Country – China (A) to Country – China (FAU), AFSC, AFSCA.

34 *Unit Letter* 106, 22 April 1944.

35 Margaret Briggs Matheson, interview with Lyn E. Smith.

36 Connie Bull Condick China Diary, 19 May 1944.

37 Ibid., 24 May 1944.

38 John Perry to Dear Mamsie, 8 June 1944, file Country – China 1944, FAU, Perry, John (Letters), box FS 1944, Country – China, FAU Letters, AFSC, AFSCA.

39 Connie Bull Condick China Diary, 10 June 1944.

40 Ibid.

41 Ibid., 17 October 1945.

42 Ibid., 8 January 1945.

43 Ibid., 10 February 1945.

44 Ibid., 19 March 1945.

45 *Newsletter* 182, 3 November 1945.

46 Ibid.

47 I am grateful to Frances Hurd, Connie's daughter, for helping me to understand several difficult periods of her mother's life. Connie had confided in Frances not long before her death some of the painful memories of her childhood and China. Ron never knew how unhappy his wife was until he discovered her diary after her death. It is unclear who tore out the missing pages of her diary.

48 White, *South of the Clouds*, 13.

49 Ibid., 14.

50 Denton-White, "Nursing in China."

51 *Newsletter* 143, 27 January 1945.

52 Scott, *McClure*, 394.

53 Margaret Briggs Matheson, interview with Lyn E. Smith.

54 Duncan Wood to Colin Bell, 3 May 1945, file Country – China, Letters London to China, box FS 1945, Country – China (FAU Reports – Medical) to (Numbered KAB Letters from and to), AFSC, AFSCA.

55 I am indebted to Sasha Denton-White for helping me clarify Margaret Briggs's references to Rita's American fiancé. Email correspondence, 25 February 2016.

56 Evelyn Rita Dangerfield White, interview with Lyn E. Smith.

57 The Burma Star was a campaign medal normally awarded for service in the Second World War to British Commonwealth forces between 11 December 1941 and 2 September 1945, but it was also awarded for specific service in China.

58 *Newsletter* 177, 29 September 1945.

59 *Newsletter* 178, 6 October 1945.

60 *Newsletter* 187, 8 December 1945; *Newsletter* 185, 24 November 1945.

61 Cf. Scott, *McClure*, 392.

62 Margaret Briggs to Ken [Bennett], 4 February 1945, Country China 1945, FAU Reports – Medical and Orders, box FS 1945, Country – China (FAU Reports Medical) to (Numbered KAB Letters from and to), AFSC, AFSCA.

63 Scott, *McClure*, 372.

64 Neil Johnson to Joan Oldman, 21 February 1946, Letters from Neil Johnson to Joan Oldman, MS – Papers – 11840–16, Ralph Johnson Papers (hereafter RJP), Alexander Turnbull Library (hereafter ATL), Wellington.

65 Eschle, *Global Democracy, Social Movements and Feminism*, 236.

66 *Newsletter* 161, 2 June 1945.

67 Ibid.

Introduction to Part 2

1 John Perry, "Rehabilitation in Tengchung," n.d., file Country – China 1945, FAU Reports (Medical & Orders), box FS 1945, Country – China (FAU Reports – Medical) to (Numbered KAB Letters from and to), AFSC, AFSCA.

2 Michael Barnett, *Empire of Humanity: A History of Humanitarianism* (Ithaca, NY: Cornell University Press, 2011), 120.

3 For a more detailed discussion of the origins of UNRRA and its potential as a template for future international collaboration, see Armstrong-Reid and Murray, *Armies of Peace,* 17–40.

4 Ben Shephard, "'Becoming Planning Minded': The Theory and Practice of Relief 1940–1945," *Journal of Contemporary History* 43, 3 (2008): 406, quoted in Barnett, *Empire of Humanity,* 110.

5 George Woodbridge, *UNRRA: The History of the United Nations Relief and Rehabilitation Administration* (New York: Columbia University Press, 1950), 2: 214.

6 Armstrong-Reid and Murray, *Armies of Peace,* 290.

7 Ibid., 288.

8 Spencer Coxe, "The UNRRA Program in China and the Friends Ambulance Unit (China Convoy) and the Friends Service Unit, China, 22 March 1948," file Country – China, Report UNRRA Program in China, box FS 1948, Country – China (Receiving Home for Children) to Country – Denmark, AFSC, AFSCA.

9 Daniel G. Cohen, "Between Relief and Politics: Refugee Humanitarianism in Occupied Germany, 1945–46," *Journal of Contemporary History* 43, 3 (2008): 439, quoted in Barnett, *Empire of Humanity,* 111.

10 Unknown to Eric Johnson, n.d., file Country – China, FAU Future Program, box FS 1945, Country – China to Country – China (FAU), AFSC, AFSCA.

11 For a detailed account of the Convoy's symbiotic relationship with UNRRA/CNRRA, see Coxe, "The UNRRA Program in China and the Friends Ambulance Unit (China Convoy) and the Friends Service Unit, China, 22 March 1948."

12 Scott, *McClure,* 161. For a more in-depth analysis of the Chinese-American relationship during the Chinese civil war, 1946–49, see Chao and Lin, "Beyond the Carrot and Stick."

13 The view of Chiang Kai-shek has softened in the recent historiography; historians have challenged the prevailing view of him as a failure for having lost mainland China to Mao's People's Liberation Army. See Sarah Paine's *Wars for Asia, 1911–1949* and Jay Taylor's groundbreaking complex study *The Generalissimo: Chiang Kai-shek and the Struggle for Modern China* (Cambridge, MA: Belknap Press, 2009).

14 Cf. Council Report for the China Convoy, 15 May 1946, file "Country – China," "Letters 1946, from KA 100 to 154," box FS 1946, "Country – China, Letters: John Perry to FAU News Letters," AFSC, AFSCA.

15 Bronson Clark, letter to *Newsletter,* 23 October 1946, file Country – China, FAU, Letters from 1946, box FS 1946, Country – China (Committees and Organizations) to Country – China (FAU – L), AFSC, AFSCA.

16 Ibid.

17 Cf. a short explanation of the Henan scheme by Eric Johnson, FSC secretary, at the request of Taber Jenkins and included as a postscript in his letter home. Copy of Letter #17, April 1946, file Country – China, FAU, Letters from 1946, box FS 1946, Country – China (Committees and Organizations) to Country – China (FAU – L), AFSC, AFSCA.

18 See the riveting account by Andrews Hicks, *Jack Jones a True Friend of China.*

19 For an engaging account of New Zealanders' medical and reconciliation work in Hankou, see Cameron, *Go Anywhere, Do Anything.*

Chapter 6: The Road to Henan

Epigraph: John Perry, "Rehabilitation in Tengchung."

1 "General Medical Report, 1 April 1945 to 19 May 1945," file Country – China 1945, FAU Reports (Medical & Orders), box FS 1945, Country – China (FAU Reports – Medical) to (Numbered KAB Letters from and to), AFSC, AFSCA.

2 Friends Ambulance Unit: China Convoy, "Report on Medical Work for the Period November 1944 to September 1945," file Country – China 1945, FAU Reports (Medical & Orders), box FS 1945, Country – China (FAU Reports – Medical) to (Numbered KAB Letters from and to), AFSC, AFSCA.

3 Scott, *McClure,* 374.

4 Ibid., 387.

5 Socknat, "The Canadian Contribution to the China Convoy."

6 Travis Jones and Hilarie Jones (daughter), correspondence with Susan Armstrong-Reid, 16 August 2005.

7 Harriet Alexander and Hilarie Jones (daughter), telephone interview with Susan Armstrong-Reid, 26 July 2005.

8 Socknat, "The Canadian Contribution to the China Convoy," 70.

9 "Walter James Alexander Tells of His Life," n.d., Walter James Alexander Private Papers.

10 Harriet Alexander and Hilarie Jones, telephone interview.

11 Harriet Brown file, Personnel Files: British, American, Canadian, 1943–1947, box 8, FAUCC, FHL, NHQA.

12 Ibid.

13 *Canadian Friends Service Committee Newsletter,* 7 April 1945, FAU, Canadian Quaker Yearly Meeting Archives (hereafter CQYMA), Pickering College (hereafter PC).

14 Harriet J. Brown, circular letter, 15 August 1945, FAU, CQYMA, PC.

15 Harriet Alexander and Hilarie Jones, telephone interview.

16 Harriet J. Brown, circular letter, 15 August 1945.

17 Courtney Archer, interview with Caitriona Cameron, 7 July 1988, Friends Ambulance Unit Oral History Project (hereafter FAUOHP), ATL.

18 Harriet J. Brown, circular letter, 15 August 1945.

19 Ibid.

20 Ibid.

21 John Perry to Dear Mamsie, 2 September 1945, file Country – China 1945, FAU, Letters, Perry, John, box FS 1945, Country – China (FAU Reports – Medical) to (Numbered KAB Letters from and to), AFSCA, AFSC.

22 I am indebted to Graham Milne for furnishing me with a copy of his account of this incident, titled "Two Women."

23 Milne, "Two Women."

24 Harriet J. Brown, circular letter, 10 November 1945, FAU, CQYMA, PC.

25 Milne, "Two Women."

26 J.D. McMurtry to Fred [Haslam], 31 October 1945, CQYMA, PC.

27 Harriet J. Brown, circular letter, 10 November 1945.

28 *Newsletter* 181, 27 October 1945.

29 Harriet J. Brown, circular letter, 10 November 1945.

30 John Perry to Dear Mamsie, 9 September 1945, file Country – China 1945, FAU, Perry, John (Letters), box FS 1945, Country – China (FAU Reports – Medical) to (Numbered KAB Letters from and to), AFSCA, AFSC.

31 Jack Dodds to Dear Folks, 18 November 1945, JD.

32 Jack Dodds to Dear Mother, Dad, and all, 8 July 1945.

33 Harriet J. Brown, circular letter, 10 November 1945.

34 General Medical Report, May 1946, file Country – China FAU Medical Reports and Orders, box FS 1946, Country – China (Numbered Letters to Shanghai to FAU – Newsletters), AFSC, AFSCA.

35 Griffith Levering to Ed Peacock, 17 September 1946, file Country – China, FAU, Letters Series KA from 155, box FS 1946, Country – China (Committee and Organizations) to Country – China (FAU), AFSC, AFSCA.

36 See also Griffith Levering, 30 August 1946, file Country – China, FAU, Letters Series KA from 155, box FS 1946, Country – China (Committee and Organizations) to Country – China (FAU), AFSC, AFSCA.
37 Council Report for the China Convoy, 15 May 1946.
38 Harriet Alexander and Hilarie Jones, telephone interview.
39 Harriet J. Brown, circular letter, June 1946, FAU, CQYMA, PC.
40 Ibid.
41 Walter Alexander, circular letter, 5 August 1945, CQYMA, PC. In fact, the language of her circular letter echoed Alexander's private letters home.
42 Cf. Council Report for the China Convoy, 15 May 1946.
43 Travis Jones and Hilarie Jones, correspondence with Armstrong-Reid, 16 August 2005.
44 *Newsletter* 142, 20 January 1945.
45 *Newsletter* 141, 15 January 1945.
46 Theo Willis to Doris Woodward, 11 April 1945, copy found in file Personnel Files: Wu, Doris, box 10, FAUCC, FHL, NQHA.
47 Ibid.
48 *Newsletter* 150, 17 March 1945.
49 *Newsletter* 157, 5 May 1945.
50 *Unit Letter* 143, 27 January 1943.
51 *Newsletter* 172, 18 August 1945.
52 Perry, "Rehabilitation in Tengchung."
53 *Newsletter* 167, 15 July 1945.
54 *Newsletter* 172, 18 August 1945.
55 *Newsletter* 173, 6 October 1945.
56 Edwin Abbott to Dear Viv, 29 December 1945, EA.
57 *Newsletter* 195, 1 February 1946.
58 *Newsletter* 205, 27 April 1946.
59 Walter Alexander to Isabel Showler, 30 October 1945, file 200, box 12, fond 502, FA186, series 4/3 China (Honan) Mission 1912–1952, United Church of Canada (hereafter UCC), Board of Overseas Missions, UCA.
60 Edwin Abbott to Dear Viv, 11 December 1945, EA.
61 Perry, "Rehabilitation in Tengchung."
62 Constance Shen to the president, Wellesley College, 7 January 1946, file Personnel Files: Constance Shen, box 10, FAUCC, FHL, NQHA.
63 Colin Bell to Whom It May Concern, n.d., file Personnel Files: Constance Shen, box 10, FAUCC, FHL, NQHA.
64 Edwin Abbott to Dear Viv, 11 December 1945, EA.
65 Edwin Abbott to Dear Viv, 13 February 1946, EA.
66 Edwin Abbott to Dear Viv, 2 March 1946, EA.
67 Edwin Abbott to Dear Viv, 26 January 1945, EA.
68 Edwin Abbott to Dear Viv, 21 February 1946, EA.
69 *Newsletter* 210, 1 June 1946.
70 *Newsletter* 205, 27 April 1946.
71 *Newsletter* 213, 22 June 1946.
72 *Newsletter* 228, 20 September 1946.
73 Bob McClure to Dick Ruddell, 24 September 1948, file Country – China, Letters from China to Philadelphia, box FS 1948, Country – China (Communist negotiations) to (Unnumbered Letters to), AFSC, AFSCA.
74 Ibid.

75 Ken Grant to Spencer Coxe, 28 June 1948, file Personal Files: Doris Woodward, box 10, FAUCC, FHL, NQHA.
76 Council Meeting Minutes, 13 July 1948, xviii, file Country – China, Minutes – Council Section, box FS 1948, Country – China (China Letters to England) to Publicity, AFSC, AFSCA.
77 Colin Bell to Elizabeth Hsu, 25 February 1946, file Personnel Files: Hsu, Elizabeth, box 9, FAUCC, FHL, NQHA.
78 Juliet (Chiu) to Dear Dennis [Frone], 28, file Personnel Files: Chiu, Juliet, box 9, FAUCC, FHL, NQHA.
79 John Perry was instrumental in arranging a full scholarship for Constance to do a preparatory year at Walnut Hill School for the Arts in Massachusetts before entering Wellesley College on a four-year scholarship.
80 Elizabeth's parents arranged a fellowship to Westhampton College at the University of Richmond in Virginia, where she received a BS in biochemistry. She then received a scholarship to the University of Michigan, where she obtained her MS in microbiology, graduating Phi Beta Kappa. "Elizabeth Lee," *Ann Arbor News,* 18–20 January 2013, http://obits.mlive.com/obituaries/annarbor/obituary.aspx?pid=162443490.
81 Robert McClure to Art Barr, 9 September 1945, file Country – China, 1945 FAU Reports (Miscellaneous), box FS China Letters 1945, Country – China to China (FAU), AFSC, AFSCA.
82 Brandon Cadbury to Victor Hayward, regional associate director UNRRA Kwangsi Regional Office, 31 January 1946, file UNRRA/CNRRA HQ Chungking/Chengchow-Kweiyang/Hankow/Kaifeng 1945–47, box 14, FAUCC, FHL, NQHA.
83 John Perry, Liuchow [Liuzhou] Report, n.d., file Country – China 1945, FAU Reports (Medical & Orders), box FS 1945, Country – China (FAU Reports – Medical) to (Numbered KAB letters from and to), AFSC, AFSCA.

Chapter 7: Henan

1 Taber Jenkins to R.J. Jenkins, 18 May 1946, file Country – China, FAU Letters Un# from 1946, box FS 1946, Country – China (Committees and Organizations) to Country – China (FAU – L), AFSCA, AFSCA.
2 Scott, *McClure,* 384.
3 Tony Gibson, FAU Relief Department, Report for March 1946, file Honan: IRC Project Files, box 17, FAUCC, FHL, NQHA.
4 Margaret Stanley, "A Year in Yenan," unpublished, vi, Margaret Stanley Private Papers (hereafter MS).
5 Edith [Elizabeth] Hughes, interview with Lyn E. Smith, 11 November 1986, catalogue no. 9437, SA, IWM.
6 Colin Bell to Kenneth A. Bennett, 24 September 1945, file Country – China (Letters to London), box FS 1945, Country – China to Country – Dominican Republic, AFSC, AFSCA.
7 Ibid.
8 Ken Bennett to Colin Bell, 11 October 1945, file Country – China, (Letters to China), box FS 1945, Country – China to Country – Dominican Republic, AFSC, AFSCA.
9 Margaret Stanley, interview with Jane Baker Koons, 15 and 17 April 1977. Original tapes are held in Margaret Stanley's Private Papers. Transcripts are available from Midwest China Oral History and Archive Project (hereafter MCOHAP), Midwest China Oral History and Archives Collection (hereafter MCOHA).
10 CV and biographical background sheet, n.d., file Personnel Files: Joan B. Kennedy Woodrow, box 10, FAUCC, FHL, NQHA.
11 Ibid.

12 Memo, "Joan Kennedy," 21 September 1946, file Personnel Files: Joan B. Kennedy Woodrow, box 10, FAUCC, FHL, NQHA.

13 Cf. Victor W. Turner, "'Betwixt and Between': The Liminal Period in the Rites of Passage," in *Proceedings of the American Ethnological Society*, ed. M. Banton (Seattle: American Ethnological Society, 1964).

14 Elizabeth Hughes, interview with Margaret Stanley, 31 May 1977, Burlington, Ontario. Original tapes are available in Margaret Stanley's Private Papers; transcript available: Hughes, Elizabeth, "Midwest China Oral History Interviews" (1977), *China Oral Histories*, Book 64, http://digitalcommons.luthersem.edu/china_histories/64.

15 Margaret Stanley, interview with Jane Baker Koons, 15 and 17 April 1977.

16 Margaret Stanley, Diary, 1: 53, MS.

17 Margaret Stanley, interview with Jane Baker Koons, 15 and 17 April 1977.

18 Scott, *McClure*, 393.

19 Bunny and Heath Thompson, "Report for FS on Kwang Sheng I Yuan," file Changte Hospital, 1946, box 12, FAUCC, FHL, NQHA.

20 New Zealander nurse/physiotherapist Bunny Thompson, quoted in Cameron, *Go Anywhere, Do Anything*, 130.

21 Bunny and Heath Thompson, "Report for FS on Kwang Sheng I Yuan."

22 Lewis Hoskins to Eric, Etta, and Ed, 22 May 1946, file Country – China, FAU, Letters Un# from 1946, box FS 1946, Country – China (Committees and Organizations) to Country – China (FAU – L), AFSC, AFSCA.

23 American Members of FAU China Convoy and Their Assignments as of 15 July 1946, file Country – China, Personnel August to December 1946, box FS 1946, Country China (Individuals) to Country – Denmark, AFSC, AFSCA.

24 Margaret Stanley, Diary, 1: 53.

25 Park Woodrow to Lewis Hoskins, 5 September 1946, file Changte 1946, box 12, FAUCC, FHL, NQHA.

26 Stanley, "A Year in Yenan," 2.

27 Memo to Jack Norton, 4 September 1946, file Hwei Min Hospital, 1946–47, box 19, FAUCC, FHL, NHQA.

28 Stanley, "A Year in Yenan," 24.

29 Ibid., 25.

30 Margaret Stanley, Diary, 1: 58.

31 Margaret Stanley, interview with Jane Baker Koons, 15 and 17 April 1977.

32 Walter Alexander to Bimbo Stokes, 15 July 1946, file Weihwei: Chengchow HQ to Hwei Min Hospital, Weihwei: 1946–47, box 19, FAUCC, FHL, NQHA.

33 Walter Alexander, Hwei Min Hospital, Monthly Report for July 1946, file 200, box 12, fond 502, FA186, series 4/3 China (Honan) Mission 1912–52, UCC Board of Overseas Missions, UCA.

34 China scholar Sonya Grypma identified Tuan as Dr. Duan Mei-Qing. I have used the spelling found in FAU documents. See S. Grypma, *Healing Henan: Canadian Nurses at the North China Mission, 1888–1947* (Vancouver: UBC Press, 2008).

35 Walter Alexander, "Confidential Hwei Min Hospital, Weihwei, Honan," Monthly Report for July 1946, file Weihwei: Chengchow HQ to Weimin, box 19, FAUCC, FHL, NQHA.

36 Ibid.

37 Scott, *McClure*, 392.

38 Ibid. See also Grypma's *Healing Henan*, 149–51.

39 George K. King to Robert McClure, 16 May 1946, file Weihwei: Chengchow HQ to Weimin Hospital, 1946–47, box 19, FAUCC, FHL, NQHA; George K. King to Kenneth Cross, 7 May 1946, file Weihwei: Chengchow HQ to Weimin Hospital, 1946–47, box 19, FAUCC,

FHL, NQHA. The hospital board had wanted to standardize hospital salary levels with other Henan hospitals, but within a three-month period, Dr. Tuan purportedly raised his own salary by 600 percent. Tuan was demanding $200,000 (Chinese currency) per month.

40 Robert McClure to George K. King, 13 May 1946, file Weihwei: Chengchow HQ to Weimin Hospital, 1946–47, box 19, FAUCC, FHL, NQHA.

41 George K. King to Kenneth Cross, 7 May 1946.

42 Memo: Weihwei General, 13 May 1946, file Weihwei: Chengchow HQ to Weimin Hospital, 1946–47, box 19, FAUCC, FHL, NQHA; see also Chris Barber to Griff Levering, Glyn Hughes, and Bob McClure, 20 June 1946, Weihwei General Hospital, file Weihwei: Chengchow HQ to Weimin Hospital, 1946–47, box 19, FAUCC, FHL, NQHA.

43 Walter Alexander to Bimbo (Kathleen Stokes), 16 August 1946, file Weihwei: Chengchow HQ to Weimin Hospital, 1946–47, box 19, FAUCC, FHL, NQHA.

44 Liu Tse was a graduate nurse who had received additional clinical training, especially in surgery, from the physician-in-chief, R.G. Struthers, at the Hwei Min Hospital, Weihwei, before the Japanese occupation. He had passed the state exams during the war and was given a state certificate as a doctor during the Sino-Japanese War.

45 Walter Alexander to Bimbo [Stokes], 27 July 1946, file Weihwei: Chengchow HQ to Weimin Hospital, 1946–47, box 19, FAUCC, FHL, NQHA.

46 Walter Alexander, Hwei Min Hospital – Monthly Report for July [1946], file Medical Reports, Hwei Min Hospital, Weihwei, box 5, FAUCC, FHL, NQHA.

47 Aydee, "Life at Weihwei," *Newsletter* 215, 6 July 1946.

48 Walter Alexander, Hwei Min Hospital – Monthly Report for July [1946].

49 Walter Alexander to Kathleen Stokes, 5 September 1946, file Weihwei: Chengchow HQ to Weimin Hospital, 1946–47, box 19, FAUCC, FHL, NQHA.

50 Walter Alexander to Kathleen Bimbo [Stokes], 15 August 1946, file Weihwei: Chengchow HQ to Weimin Hospital, 1946–47, box 19, FAUCC, FHL, NQHA.

51 Walter Alexander to Bimbo [Stokes], 27 July 1946.

52 See Henry Stokes to Lewis Hoskins and Walter Alexander, 22 June 1946, file Changte Hospital, 19 November 1946, box 12, FAUCC, FHL, NQHA; Memo: "To All Concerned," 22 June 1946, file Chungking-Honan Project, 1945–46, box 16, FAUCC, FHL, NQHA. This memo also identified Margaret Stanley as head nurse.

53 Margaret Stanley, Diary, 1: 63.

54 Henry [Stokes], 30 June 1946, file Weihwei, box 5, FAUC, FHL, NQHA.

55 Cf. Henry Stokes to Margaret Stanley, 5 September 1946, file Changte Hospital, 19 November 1946, subject files continued, box 12, FAUCC, FHL, NQHA.

56 Ibid.

57 Al [Dobson] to Henry Stokes, 30 June 1946; Memo to Jack Norton, business manager, 4 September 1946, file Weihwei, box 5, FAUCC, FHL, NQHA.

58 Margaret Stanley, Diary, 1: 63.

59 Ibid., 1: 83.

60 Margaret Stanley to Henry and Bimbo [Stokes], 9 September 1946, file Weihwei, box 5, FAUCC, FHL, NQHA.

61 Margaret Stanley, Diary, 1: 83–84.

62 Jack Norton to K. Sangrea Stokes, 24 September 1946, file Huei Min Hospital, box 19, FAUCC, FHL, NQHA.

63 Margaret Stanley, Diary, 1: 81.

64 Ibid., 1: 83.

65 Ibid., 1: 94.

66 Kenneth Cross, section leader, 3 November 1946, file Weihwei, box 5, FAUCC, FHL, NQHA.

67 Margaret Stanley, Diary, 1: 95.

68   Ibid., 1: 103.
69   Tagore's main principles – that the universe is a manifestation of God, that there is no unbridgeable gulf between our world and God's, and that God is the one who can provide the greatest love and joy – resonated with the Quakers' own belief system.
70   Margaret Stanley, Diary, 1: 103–4.
71   Ibid., 1: 103.
72   Ibid., 1: 106.
73   Elizabeth Hughes, interview with Margaret Stanley, 31 May 1977.
74   Stanley, "A Year in Yenan," 30.
75   Elizabeth Hughes, interview with Margaret Stanley, 31 May 1977.
76   Margaret Stanley, Diary, 1: 103.
77   Cf. Elizabeth Hughes, interview with Margaret Stanley, 31 May 1977.
78   Stanley, "A Year in Yenan," 20.
79   Ibid., 28.
80   Elizabeth Hughes, interview with Margaret Stanley, 31 May 1977.
81   Margaret Stanley, Diary, 1: 88.

Chapter 8: "Early Team"

Epigraph: Bronson Clark, "Behind the Communist Lines, Chengchow, Honan," 25 September 1946, file Country – China, FAU, 1946, Letter Series (KA from 155 to), box FS 1946, Country – China (Committees and Organizations) to Country – China (FAU [L]), AFSC, AFSCA.

1   Bronson Clark, "Talk to the Chengchow Section and the Yenan Medical Team on the Eve of Their Departure, 1 December 1946," file Country – China, Reports (Medical & Orders), box FS 1946, Country – China (Numbered Letters to Shanghai) to FAU Newsletter, AFSC, AFSCA.
2   Ibid.
3   See Armstrong-Reid and Murray, *Armies of Peace,* 308–9.
4   Bronson Clark, "Talk to the Chengchow Section and the Yenan Medical Team on the Eve of Their Departure, 1 December 1946."
5   See, for example, Elizabeth Hughes, interview with Margaret Stanley, 31 May 1977.
6   Cf. Douglas Clifford, interview with Margaret Stanley, 6 June 1977, Burlington, Ontario. The original tapes are found in Margaret Stanley's Private Papers. A transcript is now available at *China Oral Histories,* Book 16, http://digitalcommons.luthersem.edu/china_histories/16.
7   Elizabeth Hughes, interview with Margaret Stanley, 31 May 1977.
8   Douglas Clifford completed his basic medical training at the University of Otago Medical School in 1943 and was granted a bachelor of surgery degree in 1944.
9   Douglas Clifford, interview with Margaret Stanley, 6 June 1977.
10   For a description of Peter Early's earlier work with the FAU, see A. Tegla Davies, "Friends Ambulance Unit: Civilian Relief in Europe," http://ourstory.info/library/4-ww2/Friends/fau11.html.
11   Frank Miles, "A Quaker's War," in *World War II Remembered,* ed. Clinton C. Gardner et al. (Hanover, NH: Kendal at Hanover Residents Association, 2012), 193.
12   Frank Miles, interview with Margaret Stanley. The original tapes are found in Margaret Stanley's Private Papers. A transcript is now available at: "Midwest China Oral History Interviews" (1977), *China Oral Histories,* Book 52, http://digitalcommons.luthersem.edu/china_histories/52.
13   Jack Dodds, interview with Margaret Stanley. The original tapes are found in Margaret Stanley's Private Papers. A transcript is now available at: "Midwest China Oral History

Interviews" (1977), *China Oral Histories,* Book 23, http://digitalcommons.luthersem.edu/china_histories/23.

14 Douglas Clifford, interview with Margaret Stanley, 6 June 1977.
15 Frank Miles to Dear Folks, 12 July 1947, Frank Miles Private Papers (hereafter FM).
16 Jack Dodds, interview with Margaret Stanley.
17 Stanley, "A Year in Yenan," 15.
18 Margaret Stanley, Diary, 1: 133–34.
19 Edith [Elizabeth] Hughes, interview with Lyn E. Smith, 11 November 1986.
20 Jack Dodds, interview with Margaret Stanley.
21 Douglas Clifford to Dear Mum and Alan, 15 January 1947, Douglas Clifford Private Papers (hereafter DC).
22 Edith [Elizabeth] Hughes, interview with Lyn E. Smith, 11 November 1986.
23 Stanley, "A Year in Yenan," 15.
24 Margaret Stanley, "Working West and East of the Yellow River," *Eastern Horizon* 17, 5 (1977): 40–43.
25 Ibid., 41.
26 Douglas Clifford to Dear Mum and Alan, 10 July 1947, DC.
27 Douglas Clifford to Dear Mum and Alan, 15 January 1947.
28 Jack Dodds to Dear Mom Dad, and All, 6 January 1947, JD.
29 Neil Johnson to Dear Joan, letter 114, n.d., Letters from Neil Johnson, nos. 90–119, RJP, ATL.
30 Bronson Clark to Spencer Coxe and Company, 28 March 1947, file Country – China, FSU, Letters from Series #AF 1947, box FS 1947, Country – China (Committees and Organizations – United Service to China) to (FSU – Numbered Letters to Shanghai), AFSC, AFSCA.
31 Spencer Coxe to Bronson Clark, 19 April 1947, file Country – China, FSU Letters from Series #AF 1947, box FS 1947, Country – China (Committees and Organizations – United Service to China) to (FSU – Numbered Letters to Shanghai), AFSC, AFSCA.
32 Frank Miles, telephone conversation with Susan Armstrong-Reid, August 2012.
33 I am indebted to Peter Woodrow for sharing his mother's life story with me. Telephone conversation, 9 September 2016.
34 Medical Team 19, First Annual Report, 16 January 1948, file Country – China, Report on Projects, box FS 1948, Country – China (China Letters to England) to Publicity, AFSC, AFSCA.
35 Elizabeth Hughes, interview with Margaret Stanley, 31 May 1977.
36 Medical Team 19, First Annual Report.
37 Ibid.
38 Margaret Stanley, "Two Experiences of an American Public Health Nurse in China a Quarter of a Century Apart," *American Journal of Public Health Nursing* 63, 2 (1973): 112.
39 Medical Team 19, First Annual Report.
40 Margaret Stanley, interview with Jane Baker Koons, 15 and 17 April 1977; Margaret Stanley, "Gunfire, Shepherd's Flute and an American Nurse," *Eastern Horizon* 16 (March 1977): 36.
41 Margaret Stanley, interview with Jane Baker Koons, 15 and 17 April 1977.
42 Medical Team 19, First Annual Report.
43 Margaret Stanley, "Mobile Hospital Unit in China," *American Journal of Nursing* 48, 6 (1948): 6.
44 Ibid.
45 Margaret Stanley, interview with Jane Baker Koons, 15 and 17 April 1977.
46 Ibid., 53.

47 Margaret Stanley Tesdell, "Hospital Beds: North China Style," *American Journal of Nursing* 50, 2 (February 1950): 113.

48 Ibid.

49 Ibid., 112.

50 Elizabeth Hughes, interview with Margaret Stanley, 31 May 1977.

51 Jack Norton to David Johnstone, 7 October 1947, file FS, China (Letters from China to London), box FS 1947 Country – China (FSU Minutes) to Country – Denmark, AFSC, AFSCA.

52 Transcript of a radio interview given by Eric and Elizabeth Hughes on 9 December 1948. I am indebted to David Brough for sharing this document with me.

53 Medical Team 19, First Annual Report.

54 Stanley, "A Year in Yenan," 57.

55 Margaret Stanley, Diary, 1: 147.

56 Ibid., 1: 155.

57 Ibid., 1: 165.

58 Ibid., 1: 155.

59 Stanley, "A Year in Yenan," 93; Margaret Stanley, "Barefoot Doctors and the Los Angeles Nursery," *Eastern Horizon* 16, 6 (June 1977): 39.

60 Medical Team 19, First Annual Report.

61 Stanley, "Working West and East of the Yellow River," 43.

62 Margaret Stanley, Diary, 1: 167.

63 Stanley, "A Year in Yenan," 67.

64 Stanley, "Working West and East of the Yellow River," 40.

65 Margaret Stanley, Diary, 1: 138.

66 Margaret Stanley, interview with Jane Baker Koons, 15 and 17 April 1977.

67 Margaret Stanley, "A Slow Journey Home," *Eastern Horizon* 16, 7 (July 1977): 40.

68 Stanley, "A Year in Yenan," 201.

69 Medical Team 19 in Shansi Province, copy of Margaret Stanley's report, *FSU Chronicle* 57, 8 May 1948, file Country – China, Reports on Projects, box FS 1948, Country – China (China Letters to England) to Publicity, AFSC, AFSCA.

70 Margaret Stanley, Diary, vol. 2, 27 April 1947.

71 Ibid., 20 March 1947, 18 March 1947.

72 Ibid., 18 March 1947.

73 Stanley, "A Year in Yenan," 212.

74 Frank Miles, Journal, 3 February 1948, FM.

75 Frank Miles to Dear Folks, 2 May 1948, FM.

76 Margaret Stanley, Diary, vol. 2, 25 April 1948.

77 Frank Miles, Journal, 21 April 1948.

78 Ibid., 16 April 1948.

79 Ibid., 26 April 1948.

80 Margaret Stanley, Diary, vol. 2, 8 May 1948.

81 Ibid., 16 May 1947.

82 Frank Miles, Journal, 20 May 1948. Compare with ibid., 24 January 1948.

83 Margaret Stanley, Diary, vol. 2, 27 May 1947.

84 Stanley, "A Year in Yenan," 230.

85 "Situational identities refer to role, relationship, race, work, and symbolic identifies that are adaptive self-images and highly situationally dependent. The identities are changeable – dependent on the configuration of the interaction of goals, individual wants and needs, roles, statuses, and activities in the situation." Stella Ting-Toomey, *Communicating across Cultures* (New York: Guilford Press, 1999), 36.

86 Stanley, "A Year in Yenan," 228.

87 Margaret Stanley, Diary, vol. 2, 28 May 1947.

88 Ibid., 6 June 1947.

89 Stanley, "A Year in Yenan," 233.

90 Ibid., 234.

91 Ibid., 238.

92 Elizabeth Hughes, interview with Margaret Stanley, 31 May 1977.

93 I am indebted to Lee Tesdell and Rebecca Tesdell for sharing, during our many phone conversations and visits over the past five years, their views on how their mother's passion for China and its people figured throughout Margaret Stanley's life.

94 Jackson Progin, "Reflections on Repatriation," *FAU Chronicle*, 3 March 1945.

95 Margaret Stanley, interview with Jane Baker Koons, 15 and 17 April 1977.

96 Stanley, "A Year in Yenan," 68.

97 Margaret Stanley, interview with Jane Baker Koons, 15 and 17 April 1977.

98 Ibid.

99 Stanley, "A Year in Yenan," 8.

100 Ibid., 68.

101 For a more extensive discussion of the schism between the "work" and "faith" concerning the religious purpose of the China Convoy, see Socknat, "The Canadian Contribution to the China Convoy," 69–90.

102 Stanley, "A Year in Yenan," 85.

103 Ibid., 24.

104 Margaret Stanley to Mrs. Clifford, 1 September 1948, DC.

105 Douglas Clifford to Bronson Clark and David Johnson, 14 January 1948, file Country – China, Reports on Projects, Medical Team 19, box, FS 1948, Country – China (China Letters to England) to Publicity, AFSC, AFSCA.

Introduction to Part 3

Epigraph: FSU Chronicle 1, 5 April 1947.

1 *FSU Chronicle* 3, 19 April 1947.

2 *Newsletter* 17, 26 July 1946.

3 The doctrine of "helping people to help themselves" was applied in Europe as well. "The Right to Responsibility," *Quaker World Service*, March 1949, WQSC.

4 William A. Ritz, "The Failure of the China White Paper," *Constructing the Past* 11, 1 (2009), http://digitalcommons.iwu.edu/constructing/vol11/iss⅛.

5 Lyman P. Van Slyke, in the introduction to US Department of State, *China White Paper* (Palo Alto, CA: Stanford University Press, 1967). Ritz also supports this viewpoint, noting that "previous sporadic expressions of anti-Americanism on the mainland became a nationwide campaign vilifying the United States." Ritz, ibid., 81.

6 *FSU Chronicle* 3, 19 April 1947.

7 *FSU Chronicle* 9, 21 May 1947.

8 *FSU Chronicle* 11, 12 June 1948 (the year typed in should have been 1947).

9 *Newsletter* 246, 15 February 1947.

10 *FSU Chronicle* 18, 2 August 1947.

11 *FSU Chronicle* 20, 16 August 1947.

12 *FSU Chronicle* 1, 5 April 1947.

13 *FSU Chronicle* 9, 21 May 1947.

14 Ibid.

15 *FSU Chronicle* 12, 21 June 1947.

16 *FSU Chronicle* 8, 24 May 1947.

17 *FSU Chronicle* 6, 10 May 1947. See also *FSU Chronicle* 7, 17 May 1947.

18 *FSU Chronicle* 7, 17 May 1947.

19 The FSU operated five projects in Communist areas: (1) MT19 in Yan'an; (2) the loan of a horticulturalist to an agricultural experiment station in Hsinchi, Hopei (Hebei); (3) the MT22 kala-azar team in western Shangtung (Shandong); (4) MT24, an emergency team dispatched to the Communist-controlled battle area of Hschow (Xuzhou); and (5) MT 21, the village rehabilitation and medical project at Chungmou (Zhongmou) that shifted several times between Guomindang and Communist control. As a balancer, MT20, a new malaria team in southwestern China had been approved, and in 1949 a spearhead team, MT23, was sent forward to Nanjing to deal with the refugee, civilian, and military casualties when it too changed hands. The final FSU project, MT25 at Chungking (Chongqing) opened as the Communists "liberated" the city in 1949.

20 E. Tuckman, "Rural Health Problems in China," *Lancet* 255, 6603 (18 March 1950): 477–524.

21 Ibid., 524. See also E. Tuckman, "Off the Beaten Track – Some Experiences in China," *Medical Press*, 20 January 1954. I am indebted to Sarah Tuckman for sharing this document.

22 *FSU Chronicle* 65, 3 July 1948.

23 Staff Meeting Documents, Shanghai, October 1948, FSU, file Country – China (Letters Shanghai to Philadelphia 1949), box FS 1949, Country – Austria to Country – China (Letters Shanghai to Philadelphia), AFSC, AFSCA.

24 Spencer Coxe, China Desk, to Dear Friends, 15 June 1949, FSU, file Country – China (Letters Shanghai to Philadelphia 1949) box FS 1949, Country – Austria to Country – China (Letters Shanghai to Philadelphia), AFSC, AFSCA.

25 *FSU Chronicle* 98, 2 and 7 August 1949.

26 Frank Miles to Spencer Coxe, 4 June 1949, FSU, file Country – China (Letters to Philadelphia RM#), box FS 1949, Country – Austria to Country – China (Letters Shanghai to Philadelphia), AFSC, AFSCA.

27 Frank Miles to Spencer Coxe, Douglas Turner, 20 September 1949, FSU, file Country – China (Letters to Philadelphia RM#), box FS 1949, Country – Austria to Country – China (Letters Shanghai to Philadelphia), AFSC, AFSCA.

28 *FSU Chronicle* 98, 2 and 7 August 1949.

29 *FSU Chronicle* 97, 6 August 1949.

30 Chris Evans (chairman) to London, Chungmou, Hongkong, Chungking, 1949, FSU, file Country – China (Letters Shanghai to Philadelphia 1949), box FS 1949, Country – Austria to Country – China (Letters Shanghai to Philadelphia), AFSC, AFSCA.

31 *FSU Chronicle* 89, 29 January 1949.

32 Chris Evans to Spencer Coxe, 21 December 1947, FSU, file Country – China (Letters Shanghai to Philadelphia 1949), box FS 1949, Country – Austria to Country – China (Letters Shanghai to Philadelphia), AFSC, AFSCA.

33 Memorandum, Friends Service Unit (China) to FSU (China Sub-Committee FSU) China Standing Committee, 31 January 1951. I am indebted to Caitriona Cameron for sharing this document with me.

34 *FSU Chronicle* 22, 30 August 1947.

35 Jack Jones to Spencer [Coxe], 3 October 1949, file Country – China (Letters Chungking to Philadelphia), box FS 1949, Country – China (Individuals – Hubert Wang) to Personnel Repatriation, AFSC, AFSCA.

Chapter 9: Nursing beyond the Trenches, 1947–50

Epigraph: Friends Service Council, *Annual Report 1948,* WQSC.

1 FSC, *Annual Report 1949,* FSC, Woodbrooke Quaker Study Centre (WQSC).

2 Hicks, *Jack Jones,* 11–12.

3 Lewis Hoskins to Dear Colin [Bell], Bronson [Clark], and David [Johnstone], 30 October 1947, file Country – China, FSU, Letters from Unit # 1947, box FS 1947, Country – China (Committees and Organizations – United Service to China) to (FSU Numbered Letters to Shanghai), AFSC, AFSCA.

4 *FSU Chronicle* 56, 1 May 1948.

5 *FSU Chronicle* 57, 8 May 1948.

6 *FSU Chronicle* 63, 19 June 1948.

7 Spencer Coxe to Bronson Clark, 24 May 1947, file Country – China, FSU, Letters from Series AD, 1947, box FS 1947, Country – China (Committees and Organizations – United Service to China) to (FSU Numbered letters to Shanghai), AFSCA, AFSC.

8 Francis Star to Dear Friends, 1 January 1946, FAUCC, CQYMA, PC, Starr.

9 I am indebted to Andrew Hick, who carried out a telephone interview with Timothy Tyndall on my behalf to gain a better understanding of Jean Liu's role in the China Convoy; correspondence by email, Andrew Hicks to Susan Armstrong-Reid, 1 September 2016.

10 Mark Shaw to Mardy, 22 March 1947, Mark and Mardy Shaw Private Papers (hereafter MMS).

11 Ibid.

12 Timothy Tyndall, "Almost 70 Years On: A Retrospect by Timothy Tyndall," 17 May 2014, http://fauchinaconvoy.xyz/images/sampledata/docs/FAU%20China%20Convoy%20 Reunion%20Meeting%20Tim%20Tyndall.pdf.

13 Ibid.

14 *FSU Chronicle* 63, 19 June 1948.

15 *FSU Chronicle* 64, 26 June 1948.

16 Ibid.

17 Ibid.

18 *FSU Chronicle* 68, 24 July 1948.

19 *FSU Chronicle* 70, 7 August 1948.

20 Unknown to Spencer Coxe, 1 February 1949, FSU, file Country – China (Letters to Philadelphia RM#), box FS 1949, Country – Austria to Country – China (Letters Shanghai to Philadelphia), AFSC, AFSCA.

21 Untitled personnel data sheet, 4 March 1945, Liu, Lung-chien, file Chinese Volunteers, box 19, FAUCC, FHL, NQHA.

22 Francis Starr to Dear Star Elmer, 20 October 1946, Francis Starr Private Papers (uncatalogued), CQYMA, PC.

23 "History, Background and Present Condition of FSU Projects as Listed in Article 7 Section A," file China 1949, Reports Miscellaneous, box FS 1949, Country – China (Individuals – Hubert Wang) to Personnel Repatriation, AFSC, AFSCA.

24 Frank Miles to Spencer Coxe and Douglas Turner, 12 March 1949, FSU, file Country – China (Letters Shanghai to Philadelphia 1949), box FS 1949, Country – Austria to Country – China (Letters Shanghai to Philadelphia), AFSC, AFSCA.

25 Alex Dobson to Dear Friends, 31 August 1945, FAUCC, CQYMA, PC.

26 Alex Dobson to Dear Friends and Companions, 18 February 1947, FAUCC, CQYMA, PC.

27 Cf. Socknat, "Canadian Contribution to the China Convoy."

28 Jack Dodds to Mother, Dad and et al., 12 September 1946, JD.

29 Alex Dobson to Dear Friends and Companions, 18 February 1947.

30 Smith, *Pacifists in Action,* 210.

31 See John Anthony (Tony) Gibson, interview with Lyn E. Smith, 28 August 1991, catalogue no. 12267, SA, IWM.

32 Tyndall, "Almost 70 Years On."

33 *FSU Chronicle* 55, 24 April 1948.

34 Cf. Christine Ayoub, *Memories of the Quaker Past: Stories of Thirty-Seven Senior Quakers* (Bloomington, IN: Xlibris, 2014), 72–73.
35 Frank Miles to Spencer Coxe, 19 March 1949, FSU, file Country – China (Letters UN # from), box FS 1949, Country – China (Letters Philadelphia to Shanghai) to Individual An Min Wang, AFSC, AFSCA.
36 Spencer Coxe to unknown, 2 March 1948, FSU, file Country – China (Letters from London to China LS 1948), box FS 1948, Country – China (Communist Negotiations) to (Unnumbered Letters to), AFSC, AFSCA.
37 London to Lewis Hoskins, 15 April 1948, FSU, file Country – China (Letters from London to China LS 1948), box FS 1948, Country – China (Communist Negotiations) to (Numbered Letters to), AFSC, AFSCA.
38 *FSU Chronicle* 69, 31 July 1948.
39 Spencer Coxe to David Johnstone, 5 October 1948, FSU, file Country – China (Letters from China to Philadelphia), box FS 1948, Country – China (Communist Negotiations) to (Unnumbered Letters to), AFSC, AFSCA.
40 Frank Miles to Spencer Coxe, 19 March 1949.
41 I am indebted to Craig Shaw, who shared these excerpts from his mother's letters, written 18–28 June 1948 and 17–19 August 1948.
42 Spencer Coxe to David Johnstone, 5 October 1948.
43 Frank Miles to Spencer Coxe, 19 March 1949.
44 Ibid.
45 Unknown to Spencer Coxe and David Johnstone, 24 November 1948, FSU, file Country – China (Letters from China to Philadelphia), box FS 1948, Country – China (Communist Negotiations) to (Unnumbered Letters to), AFSC, AFSCA.
46 Lewis Hoskins to Shirley Gage, 16 November 1948, FM.
47 I am indebted to Shirley Gage's daughter for sharing the details of her mother's life that were not contained in official records. Orion Hyson, telephone interview by Susan Armstrong-Reid, 14 November 2016.
48 *FSU Chronicle* 93, 19 March 1949.
49 *FSU Chronicle* 88, 8 January 1949.
50 Frank Miles to Spencer Coxe, 19 March 1949.
51 Shirley Gage to Eldridge Campbell, 17 November 1948, Shirley Gage Private Papers (hereafter SG).
52 Gladys Saint, Report of Investigation Hsuchow [Xuzhou] Area, January 1949, FSU, file China 1949, Miscellaneous Reports, box FS 1949, Country – China (Personnel Training) to Country – Denmark, AFSC, AFSCA.
53 Ibid.
54 Ibid.
55 Ibid.
56 Ibid.
57 Ibid.
58 Rupert Stanley to Dick Ruddell, 2 September 1948, FSU, file Country – China (Letters YF Series Philadelphia – China), box FS 1948, Country – China (Communist Negotiations) to (Unnumbered Letters to), AFSC, AFSCA.
59 Shirley Gage to Eldridge Campbell, 15 February 1949, SG.
60 Medical Report of MT24, n.d., FSU, file Country – China, Projects MT24, MR, box FS 1949, Country – China (Personnel Training) to Country – Denmark, AFSC, AFSCA.
61 Staff Meeting Documents, Chungking, 1949, Report of the Chairman, Projects, FSU, file Country – China, Minutes Miscellaneous, box FS 1949, Country – China (Letters Philadelphia to Shanghai) to Individual An Min Wang, AFSC, AFSCA.

62 Medical Report of MT24, n.d.

63 Ibid.

64 Ibid.

65 Ibid.

66 "History, Background and Present Condition of FSU Projects."

67 Frank Miles to Spencer Coxe, 8 November 1949, FSU, file, Country – China (Letters Confidential 1949), box FS 1949, Country – China (Individuals – Hubert Wang) to Personnel Repatriation, AFSC, AFSCA.

68 Shirley Gage to Eldridge Campbell, 23 November 1949, SG.

69 Ibid.

70 Orion Hyson, telephone interview by Susan Armstrong-Reid, 14 November 2016.

71 Frank Miles to Spencer Coxe and Douglas Turner, 9 March 1949, FSU, file Country – China (Letters Shanghai to Philadelphia 1949), box FS 1949, Country – Austria to Country – China (Letters Shanghai to Philadelphia), AFSC, AFSCA.

72 Frank Miles to Spencer Coxe and Douglas Turner, 4 June 1949, FSU, file Country – China (Letters Shanghai to Philadelphia 1949), box FS 1949, Country – Austria to Country – China (Letters Shanghai to Philadelphia), AFSC, AFSCA.

73 Spencer Coxe, China Desk, to Dear Friends, 15 June 1949, FSU, file FSU Chronicle, box FS 1949, Country – Austria (Reports from the Field) to Country – China (Letters Shanghai to Philadelphia), AFSC, AFSCA. For two months, the *FSU Chronicle* failed to publish, and the AFSC published *Overseas Chronicle* to keep former members informed about events in China.

74 "The FSU in China," *Friend,* 8 September 1950, 675.

75 Frank Miles to Spencer Coxe, 9 September 1949.

76 Ibid.

77 Frank Miles to Spencer Coxe and Douglas Turner, 20 September 1949.

78 *FSU Chronicle* 112, 18 March 1950.

79 Frank Miles to Spencer Coxe, 8 November 1949.

80 Mary Jones left in August 1950.

81 *FSU Chronicle* 124, 19 November 1950.

82 Fred Haslam to Spencer Coxe, 16 November 1948, FSU, file Country – China (Letters, Philadelphia – Toronto), box FS 1948, Country – China (Communist Negotiations) to (Numbered letters to), AFSC, AFSCA; Fred Haslam to Spencer Coxe, 3 November 1948, FSU, file Country – China (Letters, Philadelphia – Toronto), box FS 1948, Country – China (Communist Negotiations) to (Numbered Letters to), AFSC, AFSCA; D. Johnson, Memo: Confidential, Friends Service Unit Preliminary Interview Notes, 14 September 1948, FSU, file Country – China (Letters from London to Philadelphia), box FS 1948, Country China (Communist Negotiations) to (Unnumbered Letters to), AFSC, AFSCA.

83 Since File was not a fully qualified nurse, her application initially faced resistance in Philadelphia. CFS believed that she merited "careful consideration," as she "has what I consider very good motivation" and "exceptional experience in areas having similar conditions to China." No further details were provided.

84 Frank Miles to Spencer Coxe, 9 September 1949, FSU, file Country – China (Letters Confidential 1949), box FS 1949, Country – China (Individuals – Hubert Wang) to Personnel Repatriation, AFSC, AFSCA.

85 For a more detailed account of how UNICEF was unprepared for the volte-face of the Communist regime, see Perry O. Hanson, "UNICEF in China, 1947–1951," UNICEF History Project, Ripton, Vermont, 20 August 1984, http://www.cf-hst.net/unicef-temp/CF-hst/cf-hst-073-unicef-in-china-p-hanson.pdf.

86 Ibid., 58.

87 Ibid., 71.

88 Phyllida Thornton and Edna Hadfield arrived there on 22 October. Roy Mason, regarded as a loner, remained in Nanjing, dividing his time between the hospital and university, as well as teaching English to the university students. Thornton left the Unit in early November 1949. Secondments that kept personnel occupied without incurring financial costs until new opportunities opened up were arranged. Elizabeth File and Edna Hadfield were seconded to Church World Service (CWS) in Shanghai. In April 1950, Elizabeth wound up her work with the CWS and began working full-time in the FSU Shanghai office, where she met her future husband, Jack Gerson. She left Shanghai in September 1950 to begin the long journey home via Tihang, as it was not possible embark from Shanghai. The US government backed the Guomindang's blockade of the port and threatened to revoke the permits of American shipowners who ran the blockade. Hadfield enjoyed working in several Christian orphanages sponsored by the CWS.

89 Spencer Coxe to Douglas Turner, 25 November 1949, FSU, file Country – China (Letters Philadelphia to London) box FS 1949, Country – China (Individuals – Hubert Wang) to Personnel Repatriation, AFSC, AFSCA.

90 *Overseas Chronicle* 2, 8 November 1949, FSU, file FSU Chronicle, box FS 1949, Country – Austria (Reports from the Field) to Country – China (Letters Shanghai to Philadelphia), AFSC, AFSCA.

91 Douglas [Turner] to Frank Miles or Betty Ringeisen, 5 May 1949, FSU, file Country – China (Letters London to Shanghai), box FS 1949, Country – China (Individuals – Hubert Wang) to Personnel Repatriation, AFSC, AFSCA.

92 Jack Jones to Mark Shaw, Frank Miles, Doug Turner, Spencer Coxe, 24 November 1949, FSU, file Country – China (Letters Chungking to Philadelphia), box FS 1949, Country – China (Individuals – Hubert Wang) to Personnel Repatriation, AFSC, AFSCA.

93 Ibid.

94 Jack Jones to Mark Shaw, 15 November 1949, quoted in Hicks, *Jack Jones,* 211.

95 Ibid., 214.

96 Frank Miles to Spencer Coxe, 31 January 1949, FSU, file Country – China (Letters to Philadelphia RM#), box FS 1949, Country – Austria to Country – China (Letters Shanghai to Philadelphia), AFSC, AFSCA.

97 Andrew Hicks, "My Quest for John Peter," *China Eye* 43 (Autumn 2014): 12–14.

98 I am indebted to Andrew Hicks for sharing with me this document from the Reuman's Private Papers. Dorothy Reuman, Chungking, to O.G. Reuman, 11 December 1949, in Bob and Dorothy Reuman, "Letters from China."

99 Jack Jones, Report to 1949 Staff Meeting, North Bank Clinic Chungking (MT25), FSU, file Country – China, Project Clinic (South Bank Clinic Chungking) MT25, box FS 1950, Country – China (Maps) to (Supplies and Famine Relief), AFSC, AFSCA.

100 Ibid.

101 Dorothy Reuman, Chungking, to O.G. Reuman, 11 December 1949, in Bob and Dorothy Reuman, "Letters from China." I am indebted to Andrew Hicks for sharing this document with me: Transcription of part of a three-page typed letter written by Dorothy Reuman, 11 December 1949, from the FAU depot at Ssu Kung Li Pan, Chungking, to Revd. OG Reuman, 270 South Chestnut Street, Ravenna, Ohio.

102 Ibid.

103 Jack Jones, Report to 1949 Staff Meeting.

104 Bob Reuman, quoted in Hicks, *Jack Jones,* 318. (Note: Andrew Hicks does not use references.)

105 Jack Reynolds, *Daughters of an Ancient Race* (Hong Kong: Heinemann Educational Books [Asia], 1974), 9.

106 Hicks, *Jack Jones,* 269.
107 *FSU Chronicle* 119, 17 June 1950.
108 Jack Jones, Report to 1949 Staff Meeting.
109 See also Daniel Maul, "American Quakers, the Emergence of International Humanitarianism, and the Foundation of the American Friends Service Committee, 1890–1920," in *Dilemmas of Humanitarian Aid in the Twentieth Century,* ed. Johannes Paulmann (Oxford: Oxford University Press, 2016).
110 Frank Miles to Spencer Coxe and Douglas Turner, 12 March 1949.

Conclusion: Nurses without Weapons, 1941–51
Epigraph: Smith, *Pacifists in Action,* 188.

1 Cf. Joan Wallace Scott, *Gender and the Politics of History: Gender and Culture* (New York: New York University Press, 1988), 6.
2 Armstrong-Reid and Murray, *Armies of Peace,* Appendix C, "UNRRA salary scales"; Appendix D, "Military salaries."
3 Margaret Stanley, "Universality of Nursing," *American Journal of Nursing* 47, 4 (1947): 256.
4 Margaret Stanley, interview with Jane Baker Koons, 15 and 17 April 1977.
5 Diane Hamilton, "Constructing the Mind of Nursing," *Nursing History Review* 2 (1994): 14.
6 See, for example, M. Bjerneld, G. Lindmark, P. Diskett, and M.J. Garrett, "Perceptions of Work in Humanitarian Assistance: Interviews with Returning Swedish Health Professionals," *Disaster Management and Response* 2, 4 (2004): 101–8; M. Bjerneld, G. Lindmark, L.N. McSpadden, and M.J. Garrett, "Motivations, Concerns, and Expectations of Scandinavian Health Professions Volunteering for Humanitarian Assignments," *Disaster Management and Response* 4, 2 (2006): 49–58. This qualitative study examined health professionals' motivation for volunteering within the framework of Hertzberg's theory of motivations and Maslow's hierarchy of needs.
7 Sonya Grypma and Cheng Zhen noted this trend in the early development of modern nursing in China. See "The Development of Modern Nursing in China," in *Medical Transitions in Twentieth-Century China,* ed. Bridie Andrews and Mary Brown Bullock (Bloomington: Indiana University Press, 2014), 297.
8 Convoy rhetoric reflects the discourse characterizing nurses prevalent throughout the First and Second World Wars. See Charlotte Dale, "The Social Exploits and Behaviour of Nurses during the Anglo-Boer War," in Sweet and Hawkins, *Colonial Caring,* 64.
9 For an analysis of the idea of compassion as virtue in nursing, see Hamilton, "Constructing the Mind of Nursing," 3–28.
10 Margaret Stanley, interview with Jane Baker Koons, 15 and 17 April 1977.
11 Compare with Douglas Clifford, interview with Margaret Stanley, 6 June 1977. Douglas Clifford's uneasiness with the limitations surgeons faced in China resonates throughout his meticulous case-by-case reconstruction of his work in this interview.
12 I am indebted to Don Davis for drawing the following document to my attention: Minutes of the Board of Directors Meeting, 17 April 1946, held at Hannah Clothier Hill's Home, Swarthmore, PA.
13 Historians have explored how medicine has extended national power and interests, but have only recently begun to address this lacuna in the history of nursing. For a succinct literature review, see Helen Sweet and Sue Hawkins, "Introduction: Contextualizing Colonial and Post-colonial Nursing," in Sweet and Hawkins, *Colonial Caring,* 1–17.
14 I was struck, for example, by the differences in the Gadabouts' articulation of their professional identities compared with those of US Army Corps nurses or missionary nurses portrayed by Winifred C. Connerton, "Working towards Health, Christianity and Dem-

ocracy: American Colonial and Missionary Nurses in Puerto Rico, 1900–30," in Sweet and Hawkins, *Colonial Caring*, 126–44.

15 Stanley, "A Year in Yenan," 252.

16 See Claire Magone, Michaël Neuman, and Fabrice Weissman, eds., *Humanitarian Negotiations Revealed: The MSF Experience* (London: Hurst, 2011).

17 Spencer Coxe to Dear Unit, 29 August 1950, reprinted in *FSU Chronicle* 122, 9 September 1950.

18 Sarah Collinson and Samir Elhawary, *Humanitarian Space: A Review of Trends and Issues*, HPG Report 32 (London: Humanitarian Policy Group, Overseas Development Institute, April 2012), 1. https://www.odi.org/sites/odi.org.uk/files/odi-assets/publications-opinion -files/7643.pdf.

19 See Mary Hershberger, *Traveling to Vietnam: American Peace Activists and the War* (Syracuse, NY: Syracuse University Press, 1998).

20 Within transnational studies, the Global South is commonly used to refer to what used to be called the Third World, developing countries or less-developed regions.

21 Compare with Dick Erstad, Memorandum: American Friends Service Committee to the Board of Directors: L.A. Program All-Staff Conference Consensus Statement, 16 January 1979. In the wake of Latin American political struggles for economic and political reform, the All-Staff Conference struggled to identify a vision that reconciled Quakers' "identification with the oppressed and commitment to non-violence" and their concern with "ends and means." The statement issued a significant challenge to the Peace Testimony: it proposed continuing to provide support, through non-violent methods, to groups dedicated to the goals of equality and justice, even when the group adopted violent as well as non-violent methods. I am again indebted to Don Davis, the archivist at the American Friends Service Committee, for drawing my attention to this document.

22 Compare with Simon Macdonald, "Transnational History: A Review of Past and Present Scholarship," https://www.ucl.ac.uk/centre-transnational-history/objectives/simon_ macdonald_tns_review.

23 Compare with the Matthew Evangelista, "Transnational Organizations and the Cold War," in *The Cambridge History of the Cold War*, ed. Mervyn P. Leffler and Odd Arne Westad (Cambridge: Cambridge University Press, 2010), and Sarah B. Snyder, *Human Rights Activism and the End of the Cold War: A Transnational History of the Helsinki Process* (Cambridge: Cambridge University Press, 2011).

24 See M.L. Pratt's discussion of the contact zone in *Imperial Eyes: Travel Writing and Transculturation* (New York: Routledge, 1992); and H. Bhabha's discussion of hybridity in *Location of Culture* (London: Routledge, 1994).

25 Eschle, *Global Democracy, Social Movements and Feminism*, 236.

26 Lyn Smith, "Quakers in Uniform: The Friends Ambulance Unit," in *Challenge to Mars: Essays on Pacifism from 1918 to 1945*, ed. Peter Brock and Thomas Socknat (Toronto: University of Toronto Press, 1999), 253.

27 Compare with P. D'Antonio, "Thinking about Place: Researching and Reading the Global History of Nursing," *Texto and Contexto Enfermagem* 18, 4 (2009): 766–72.

28 See Maria Mälksoo, "The Challenge of Liminality for International Relations Theory," *Review of International Studies* 38, 2 (April 2012): 481–94.

29 J. Ann Tickner, *Gender in International Relations: Feminist Perspectives on Achieving Global Security* (New York: Columbia University Press, 1992), iv. Tickner's work falls within a more expansionist concept of security that advocates the accumulation of power and military strength. Her concept is more closely associated with social justice and human security. Compare also with J. Ann Tickner, *A Feminist Voyage through International Relations* (Oxford: Oxford University Press, 2014). The book captures the core arguments

and debates in feminist international relations (IR) to produce unique insights into the masculinism of IR theory. Never satisfied to simply add women to the international narrative, Tickner interrogates how the gendered hierarchies in institutions and practices operate to signify power. More recently, her scholarship has expanded the category of otherness beyond gender alone, to encompass religion, fundamentalism, race, and postcolonialism.

Bibliography

Archival Sources

Alexander Turnbull Library, Wellington, New Zealand

Mary Greig Campbell Papers

Friends Service Unit, China Convoy Oral Histories
Courtney Archer
George Lindsay Crozier
Owen and Wilfred Jackson
John Francis Johnson
Reginald Ewart Lawry
W. Roy Lucas
Graham Anderson Milne
Bernice and Heath Thompson

Johnson Family: Correspondence between Neil Johnson and Joan Oldman

Photographs relating to the work of the Friends Ambulance Unit in China

American Friends Service Committee Archives, Philadelphia
China Convoy Records
Annual Report of the Friends Ambulance Unit
Canadian Friends Service Committee
Friends Ambulance Unit Chronicle
Friends Ambulance Unit Great Britain
Friends Ambulance Unit Post-war Service

Canadian Quaker Yearly Meeting Archives, Pickering College, Pickering, Ontario
Canadian Friends Service Committee
The Canadian Friend
Circular letters

The China Convoy Private Papers
Harriet Brown Alexander
Walter Alexander
Al Dobson
Jack Dodds
Albert Dorland
Delf Fransham

Gordon Keith
J. Douglas McMurtry
Francis Starr

Oral Histories
Wilfred Howarth, volumes 1 and 2 (1986)

Haverford College, Haverford, Pennsylvania

Magill Library Special Collections
Howard Haines Brinton and Anna Shipley Cox Brinton Papers
William Warder Cadbury Papers

Imperial War Museum Archives, London
Sound Collection
Christopher B. Barber
Michael H. Cadbury
Elaine Ethel (Bell) Conyers
Spencer Coxe
George Lindsay Crozier
John Anthony Gibson
Michael Rendell Harris
Lewis Maloney Hoskins
Wilfred Howarth
Lu Hsiung
Elizabeth Hughes
Margaret (Briggs) Matheson
George William Parsons
Patrick Rawlence
William Antony Reynolds
Margaret Stanley
Douglas Gordon Turner
Evelyn Rita Dangerfield White
John Duncan Wood

Library and Archives Canada, Ottawa
Department of External Affairs
Department of National Defence

Library of the Religious Society of Friends in Britain, Friends House, London
Annual and Quarterly Reports
Post War Service Reports
Papers of Former Unit Members (unpublished)
Friends Ambulance Unit, China Convoy Fonds

Midwest China Oral History and Archives Collection, St. Paul, Minnesota
Douglas Clifford
Jack Dodds
Elizabeth Hughes
Margaret Stanley

Presbyterian Church Archives, Knox College, Dunedin, New Zealand
  Graham A. Milne Fonds, South China Mission

Private Papers
  Edwin V. Abbott
  Walter and Harriet (Brown) Alexander
  Douglas Clifford
  Connie Bull Condick and Ron Condick
  Al Dobson
  Jack Dodds
  Shirley Elliott Gage
  Gordon Keith
  J. Douglas McMurtry
  Frank Miles
  Kathleen Green Savan
  Mark and Mardy Shaw
  Margaret Stanley
  Francis Starr
  Elizabeth Rita Dangerfield White

United Church of Canada Records
  Katherine Hockin Records
  Robert Baird McClure Fonds

Western University Archives, London
  Hugh MacKenzie Papers

Oral Interviews and Correspondence
  Edwin Abbott
  Harriet Brown Alexander and Hilarie Jones (daughter)
  Chris Bonsall
  Douglas Clifford
  Cathy Miles Grant
  Andrew Hicks
  Francis Hurd
  Orion Hyson
  Rebecca Miles
  Craig Shaw
  Erica Tesdell
  Lee Tesdell
  Sasha Denton White
  Peter Woodrow

Secondary Sources
Allen, A. Stewart. "Modern Medicine in China: Its Development and Its Difficulties." *Canadian Medical Association Journal* 56, 2 (February 1947): 211–13.
Armstrong-Reid, Susan. *Lyle Creelman: The Frontiers of Global Nursing.* Toronto: University of Toronto Press, 2014.
–. "Soldiers of Peace in the China Convoy: Edward Abbott and Francis Starr." *Canadian Quaker Journal* 72 (2008): 44–67.

Armstrong-Reid, Susan, and David Murray. *Armies of Peace: Canada and the UNRRA Years.* Toronto: University of Toronto Press, 2008.

Asia Pacific Foundation of Canada. "China's New Order: The Regulation of Foreign Organizations." APF Canada Blog, 24 May 2016. https://www.asiapacific.ca/blog/chinas-new -order-regulation-foreign-organizations.

Auden, W.H., and Christopher Isherwood. *Journey to a War.* New York: Random House, 1939.

Awmack, J.W. *In China with the Friends Ambulance Unit, 1945–1946.* Victoria: author, n.d.

Ayoub, Christine. *Memories of the Quaker Past: Stories of Thirty-Seven Senior Quakers.* Bloomington, IN: Xlibris, 2014.

Back, Lyndon S. "The Quaker Mission in Poland Relief, Reconstruction and Religion." *Quaker History* 101, 2 (2012): 1–23.

Barnett, Michael. *Empire of Humanity: A History of Humanitarianism.* Ithaca, NY: Cornell University Press, 2011.

Bhabha, H. *Location of Culture.* London: Routledge, 1994.

Birn, Anne-Emanuelle, and Theodore M. Brown, eds. *Comrades in Health: US Health Internationalists Abroad and at Home.* New Brunswick, NJ: Rutgers University Press, 2013.

Bjerneld, M., G. Lindmark, P. Diskett, and M.J. Garrett. "Perceptions of Work in Humanitarian Assistance: Interviews with Returning Swedish Health Professionals." *Disaster Management and Response* 2, 4 (2004): 101–8.

Bjerneld, M., G. Lindmark, L.N. McSpadden, and M.J. Garrett. "Motivations, Concerns, and Expectations of Scandinavian Health Professions Volunteering for Humanitarian Assignments." *Disaster Management and Response* 4, 2 (2006): 49–58.

Borton, John Nicholas. "Improving the Use of History by the International Humanitarian Sector." *European Review of History* 23, 1–2 (2016): 193–209. http://www.tandfonline.com/doi/full/10.1080/13507486.2015.1121973.

G. Boschma, S. Grypma, and F. Melchior. "Reflections on Researcher Subjectivity in Nursing History." In *Capturing Nursing History: A Guide to Historical Research,* ed. Sandra Lewenson and Eleanor Hermann, 99–121. New York: Springer, 2008.

Brock, Peter, and Thomas P. Socknat. *Challenge to Mars: Essays on Pacifism from 1918 to 1945.* Toronto: University of Toronto Press, 1999.

Brough, David. "The China Convoy: A Great Leveller." *The Friend: The Quaker Magazine,* 18 April 2013. https://thefriend.org/article/the-china-convoy-a-great-leveller/.

–. "The China Convoy: What Was the Right Thing to Do?" *The Friend: The Quaker Magazine,* 9 May 2013. https://thefriend.org/article/the-china-convoy-what-was-the -right-thing-to-do/.

Cameron, Caitriona. *Go Anywhere, Do Anything: New Zealanders in the Friends Ambulance Unit in China, 1945–1951.* Wellington, NZ: Beechtree, 1996.

Chan, Stephanie. "Cross-Cultural Civility in Global Society: Transnational Cooperation in Chinese NGOs." *Global Net World* 8, 2 (2008): 232–52.

Chandler, D. "The Road to Military Humanitarianism: How the Human Rights NGOs Shaped a New Humanitarian Agenda." *Human Rights Quarterly* 23, 3 (2001): 678–700.

Chao Hsiang-ke and Lin Hsiao-ting. "Beyond the Carrot and Stick: The Political Economy of US Military Aid to China, 1945–1951." *Journal of Modern Chinese History* 5, 2 (2011): 199–216. http://dx.doi.org/10.1080/17535654.2011.627117.

"China's Nurses Carry On." *American Journal of Nursing* 44, 7 (July 1944): 642–44.

Clifford, Douglas. "Midwest China Oral History and Archives Collection" (1977). *China Oral Histories,* Book 16. http://digitalcommons.luthersem.edu/china_histories/16.

Cohen, Daniel G. "Between Relief and Politics: Refugee Humanitarianism in Occupied Germany, 1945–46." *Journal of Contemporary History* 43, 3 (2008): 437–49.

Collinson, S., and Samir Elhawary. Humanitarian Space: A Review of Trends and Issues. HPG Report 32. London: Humanitarian Policy Group, Overseas Development Institute, April 2012. https://www.odi.org/sites/odi.org.uk/files/odi-assets/publications-opinion-files/7643.pdf.

–. *Humanitarian Space: Trends and Issues*. HPG Policy Brief 46. London: Humanitarian Policy Group, Overseas Development Institute, April 2012. http://www.odi.org/resources/docs/7644.pdf.

Coxe, Spencer. "Quakers and Communists in China." *Far Eastern Survey* 18, 13 (June 1949): 152–55.

Cruikshank, Kathleen. "Education, History and the Art of Biography." *American Journal of Education* 107, 3 (1999): 231–39.

D'Antonio, P. "Thinking about Place: Researching and Reading the Global History of Nursing." *Texto and Contexto Enfermagem* 18, 4 (2009): 766–72.

D'Antonio, P., J.C. Fairman, and J. Whelan. *Routledge Handbook on the Global History of Nursing*. New York: Taylor and Friend, 2013.

Davey, E. "An Introduction to the History of the Humanitarian System: Western Origins and Foundations." IHPG Working Paper. London: Overseas Development Institute, 2013.

Davies, A. Tegla. "Friends Ambulance Unit." http://www.ourstory.info/library/4-ww2/Friends/fauTC.html.

–. *Friends Ambulance Unit: The Story of the Friends Ambulance Unit in the Second World War*. London: Allen and Unwin, 1947.

Denton-White, Lyn. "Nursing in China." Bemerton Local History Society, BBC – WW2 People's War. http://www.bbc.co.uk/history/ww2peopleswar/stories/65/a4255265.shtml.

Devizes Peace Group. "Exit from Burma: A Conscientious Objector's Story." BBC, 12 November 2005. http://www.bbc.co.uk/history/ww2peopleswar/stories/71/a6913271.shtml.

Drea, Edward J., and Hans Van de Ven. "An Overview of Major Military Campaigns during the Sino-Japanese War, 1937–1945." In *The Battle for China: Essays on the Military History of the Sino-Japanese War of 1937–1945*, ed. Mark Peattie, Edward Drea, and Hans Van de Ven, 27–47. Stanford, CA: Stanford University Press, 2013.

Easton-Thompson, Isobel. *Yellow River Mules and Mountains: A New Zealand Nurse in China, 1947–1950*. Pleasanton, CA: Eagle Pearly, 2010.

"Elizabeth Lee." *Ann Arbor News*, 18–20 January 2013. http://obits.mlive.com/obituaries/annarbor/obituary.aspx?pid=162443490.

Eller, Cynthia. "Oral History as Moral Discourse: Conscientious Objectors and the Second World War." *Oral History Review* 18, 1 (Spring 1990): 45–75.

Eschle, Catherine. *Global Democracy, Social Movements and Feminism.* New York: Basic Books, 2000.

Evangelista, Matthew. "Transnational Organizations and the Cold War." In *The Cambridge History of the Cold War,* ed. Mervyn P. Leffler and Odd Arne Westad. Cambridge: Cambridge University Press, 2010.

Feldman, Ilana. "The Quaker Way: Ethical Labour and Humanitarian Relief." *American Ethnologist* 34, 4 (2007): 689–705.

Ferlanti, Federica. "The New Life Movement in Jiangxi Province, 1934–1938." *Modern Asian Studies* 44, 5 (2010): 961–1,000.

Fleischmann, Ellen, Sonya Grypma, M. Marten, and Inger Marie Okkenhug, eds. *Transnational and Historical Perspectives on Global Health Welfare and Humanitarianism*. Kristiansand, Norway: Portal Books, 2013.

Friends Ambulance Unit (China). *FAU China Convoy: A Year in Honan*. Shanghai: FAU, 1947.

Gallagher, Nancy. *Quakers in the Israeli-Palestine Conflict: The Dilemmas of NGO Humanitarian Activism*. Cairo: American University in Cairo Press, 2007.

Gardner, Clinton C., et al. *World War II Remembered*. Hanover, NH: Kendal at Hanover Residents Association, 2012.

Grypma, S. *China Interrupted: Japanese Internment and the Reshaping of a Canadian Mission Community*. Waterloo, ON: Wilfrid Laurier University Press, 2012.

–. *Healing Henan: Canadian Nurses at the North China Mission, 1888–1947*. Vancouver: UBC Press, 2008.

–. "When We Were (Almost) Chinese: Identity and the Internment of Missionary Nurses in China, 1941–1945." *Histoire sociale/Social History* 43, 86 (2010): 315–44.

–. "Withdrawal from Weihui: China Missions and the Silence of Missionary Nursing, 1888–1947." *Nursing Inquiry* 14, 4 (December 2007): 306–19.

Grypma, Sonya, and Cheng Zhen. "The Development of Modern Nursing in China." In *Medical Transitions in Twentieth-Century China*, ed. Bridie Andrews and Mary Brown Bullock, 297–317. Bloomington: Indiana University Press, 2014.

Haberman, Frederick. *Nobel Lectures, Peace 1926–1950*. Amsterdam: Elsevier, 1972.

Hamilton, Diane. "Constructing the Mind of Nursing." *Nursing History Review* 2 (1994): 3–28.

Hanson, Perry O. "UNICEF in China, 1947–1951." UNICEF History Project, Ripton, Vermont, 20 August 1984. http://www.cf-hst.net/unicef-temp/CF-hst/cf-hst-073-unicef -in-china-p-hanson.pdf.

Haslam, Fred. *A Record of Experiences with Canadian Friends (Quakers) and the Canadian Ecumenical Movement, 1921–1967*. Birmingham, UK: Woodbrooke College, 1968.

Hershberger, Mary. *Traveling to Vietnam: American Peace Activists and the War*. Syracuse, NY: Syracuse University Press, 1998.

Hicks, Andrew. *Jack Jones a True Friend to China: "The Lost Writings of a Historic Nobody."* Hong Kong: Earnshaw Books, 2015.

–. "My Quest for John Peter." *China Eye* 43 (Autumn 2014): 12–14.

Hsiung, James C., and Steven I. Levine, eds. *China's Bitter Victory: War with Japan, 1937–1945*. New York: Routledge, 2015.

Hsu, Teresa, with Sharana Rao and K.H. Eric Sim. *Love and Share: Memoirs of a Centenarian Teresa Hsu*. Singapore: Sharana Rao, 2011.

Hu, Hsien Chin. "The Chinese Concept of 'Face.'" *American Anthropologist* 46 (1944): 45–64.

Hughes, Elizabeth. "Midwest China Oral History Interviews" (1977). *China Oral Histories*, Book 64. http://digitalcommons.luthersem.edu/china_histories/64.

Hunt, M.R., L. Schwartz, C. Sinding, and L. Elit. "The Ethics of Engaged Presence: A Framework for Health Professionals in Humanitarian Assistance and Developmental Work." *Developing World Bioethics* 14, 1 (2014): 47–55.

Independent. "Lives Remembered: Michael Harris." 23 October 2011. http://www. independent.co.uk/news/obituaries/lives-remembered-michael-harris-1699434.html.

Irwin, J.F. "Nurses without Borders: The History of Nursing as US International History." *Nursing History Review* 19, 1 (2011): 78–102.

Jackson, Angela. *"For Us It Was Heaven": The Passion, Grief and Fortitude of Patience Darton, from the Spanish Civil War to Mao's China*. Eastbourne, UK: Sussex Academic, 2012.

Jezewski, M.A., and P. Sotnik, eds. *Culture Brokering: Providing Culturally Competent Rehabilitation Services to Foreign-Born Persons*. New York: Center for International

Rehabilitation Research Information and Exchange, 2001. http://cirrie.buffalo.edu/culture/monographs/cb.php#introduction.

Kauffmann, L.A. "The Theology of Consensus." *Jacobin,* 27 May 2015. https://www.jacobinmag.com/2015/05/consensus-occupy-wall-street-general-assembly/.

Keeling, Arlene, and Barbara Mann Wall. *Nurses and Disasters: Global, Historical Case Studies.* New York: Springer, 2015.

–. *Nurses on the Front Line: When Disaster Strikes 1878–2010.* New York: Springer, 2011.

Lathrop, Alan K. "Dateline: Burma." *Dartmouth Medicine.* http://dartmed.dartmouth.edu/spring04/html/dateline_burma.shtml.

Laycock, Handley T. "Experiences in a Military Hospital in Free China." *British Medical Journal* (27 February 1942): 262–63. http://pubmedcentralcanada.ca/pmcc/articles/PMC2282315/pdf/brmedj03979-0021.pdf.

–. "With the Friends Ambulance Unit in China." *British Medical Journal* (4 March 1944): 333. https://www.ncbi.nlm.nih.gov/pmc/articles/PMC2283684/pdf/brmedj03928-0021.pdf.

Llewellyn, B. *The Friends of the China Road.* London: Friends Home Service Committee, 1946.

–. *I Left My Roots in China.* London: George Allen and Unwin, 1953.

Macdonald, Simon. "Transnational History: A Review of Past and Present Scholarship." https://www.ucl.ac.uk/centre-transnational-history/objectives/simon_macdonald_tns_review.

Magone, Claire, Michaël Neuman, and Fabrice Weissman. *Humanitarian Negotiations Revealed: The MSF Experience.* London: C. Hurst, 2011.

Makita, Yoshiya. "The Ambivalent Enterprise: Medical Activities of the Red Cross Society of Japan in the Northeastern Region of China during the Russo-Japanese War." In *Entangled Histories: The Transcultural Past of North East China,* ed. Dan Ben-Canaan and Frank Ines Prodohl, 189–203. New York: Springer, 2014.

Mälksoo, Maria. "The Challenge of Liminality for International Relations Theory." *Review of International Studies* 38, 2 (April 2012): 481–94.

Maul, Daniel. "American Quakers, the Emergence of International Humanitarianism, and the Foundation of the American Friends Service Committee, 1890–1920." In *Dilemmas of Humanitarian Aid in the Twentieth Century,* ed. Johannes Paulmann. Oxford: Oxford University Press, 2016.

–. "The Politics of Neutrality: The American Friends Service Committee and the Spanish Civil War, 1936–1939." *European Review of History* 23, 1–2 (2016): 82–100.

McCall, Leslie. "The Complexity of Intersectionality." *Signs* 30, 3 (Spring 2005): 1771–1800.

McClure, Robert B. "The Chinese Doctor." *Canadian Medical Journal* 50, 6 (June 1944): 543–46.

–. "Miss Li." *Canadian Medical Association Journal* 53, 3 (September 1945): 295–96.

Miles, Frank. "Midwest China Oral History Interviews" (1977). China Oral Histories, Book 52. http://digitalcommons.luthersem.edu/china_histories/52.

Molina-Markham, Elizabeth. "Finding the 'Sense of the Meeting': Decision Making through Silence among Quakers." *Western Journal of Communication* 78, 2 (2014): 155–74.

Morris, David Elwyn. *China Changed My Mind.* London: Cassell, 1948.

–. "Quakers in China." *The Spectator,* 21 October 1948.

Murphey, Rhoads. *A China Convoy Anthology.* Chungking: FAU, 1945.

–. *Fifty Years of China to Me: Personal Recollections of 1942–1992.* Ann Arbor, MI: Association for Asian Studies, 1994.

Narain, Seema. "Gender in International Relations: Feminist Perspectives of J. Ann Tickner." *Indian Journal of Gender Studies* 21, 2 (June 2014):179–97.

Paine, S.C.M. *The Wars for Asia, 1911–1949.* Cambridge: Cambridge University Press, 2012.

Pratt, M.L. *Imperial Eyes: Travel Writing and Transculturation.* New York: Routledge, 1992.

Reynolds, Jack. *Daughters of an Ancient Race.* Hong Kong: Heinemann Educational Books (Asia), 1974.

Reynolds, Tony. "Operation and Maintenance of a Road Transport System in West China, 1942–6." *Journal of the Hong Kong Branch of the Royal Asiatic Society* 16 (1976): 136–61.

Reynolds, W.A. "A Journey to Yan'an." *Journal of the Hong Kong Branch of the Royal Asiatic Society* 17 (1977): 43–54.

Ritz, William A. "The Failure of the China White Paper." *Constructing the Past* 11, 1 (2009). http://digitalcommons.iwu.edu/constructing/vol11/iss⅙.

Rogers, Naomi. "The Most Admired Woman in the World: Forgetting and Remembering in the History of Nursing." *Nursing History Review* 23 (2015): 28–55.

Romirowsky, Asaf, and Alexander H. Joffe. "When Did the Quakers Stop Being Friends?" *The Tower,* December 2013. http://www.meforum.org/3693/quakers-friends-anti-israel.

Rose, Sonya O. "Temperate Heroes: Concepts of Masculinity in Second World War Britain." In *Masculinities in Politics and War: Gendering Modern History,* ed. Stefan Dudink, Karen Hagemann, and Josh Tosh, 177–95. Manchester: Manchester University Press, 2004.

Schenectady Gazette. "Dr. Gage Now Army Capt.; Hopes to Serve in Korea." 1 October 1951. http://fultonhistory.com/newspaper%208/Schenectady%20NY%20Gazette/Schenectady%20NY%20Gazette%201951%20Grayscale/Schenectady%20NY%20Gazette%201951%20Grayscale%20-%202721.pdf.

Scott, Joan Wallace. *Gender and the Politics of History: Gender and Culture.* New York: New York University Press, 1988.

Scott, Munroe. *McClure: The China Years of Dr. Bob McClure: A Biography.* Don Mills, ON: Canec Publishing and Supply House, 1977.

Seagrave, Gordon S. *Burma Surgeon.* London: Victor Gollancz, 1944.

Simpson, J.E.R. *Letters from China: Quaker Relief Work in Bandit Country, 1944–46.* Cambridge: Ross Evans, 2001.

Sisson Runyan, Anne, and V. Spike Peterson. *Global Gender Issues in the New Millennium.* New York: Westview, 2010.

Smith, Lyn. *Pacifists in Action: The Experience of the Friends Ambulance Unit in the Second World War.* York: William Sessions, 1998.

–. "Quakers in Uniform: The Friends Ambulance Unit. " In *Challenge to Mars: Essays on Pacifism from 1918 to 1945,* ed. Peter Brock and Thomas Socknat, 243–55. Toronto: University of Toronto Press, 1999.

Snyder, Sarah B. *Human Rights Activism and the End of the Cold War: A Transnational History of the Helsinki Process.* Cambridge: Cambridge University Press, 2011.

Socknat, Thomas P. "The Canadian Contribution to the China Convoy." *Quaker History* 69, 2 (Autumn 1980): 69–90.

Solheim, K. "Patterns of Community Relationships: Nurses, Non-Governmental Organisations and Internally Displaced Persons." *International Nursing Review* 52 (2005): 60–67.

Stanley, Margaret. "Barefoot Doctors and the Los Angeles Nursery." *Eastern Horizon* 16, 6 (June 1977): 39–41.

–. *Foreigners in Areas of China under Communist Jurisdiction before 1949: Biographical Notes and Comprehensive Bibliography of the Yenan Hui.* Lawrence: Centre for East Asian Studies, University of Kansas, 1987.

–. "Gunfire, Shepherd's Flute and an American Nurse." *Eastern Horizon* 16 (March 1977): 36–37.

–. "Mobile Hospital Unit in China." *American Journal of Nursing* 48, 6 (1948): 6, 8.

–. "A Slow Journey Home." *Eastern Horizon* 16, 7 (July 1977): 40–43.

–. "Two Experiences of an American Public Health Nurse in China a Quarter of Century Apart." *American Journal of Public Health Nursing* 63, 2 (1973): 111–16.

–. "Universality of Nursing." *American Journal of Nursing* 47, 4 (1947): 256.

–. "Visiting Health Teams in the People's Republic of China." *Journal of Nurse- Midwivery* 18, 2 (Summer 1973): 14–18.

–. "What Was It Like in Yenan?" *Eastern Horizon* 16 (March 1977): 42–47.

–. "Working West and East of the Yellow River." *Eastern Horizon* 17, 5 (1977): 40–43.

Stewart-Winter, Timothy. "Not a Soldier, Not a Slacker: Conscientious Objectors and Male Citizenship." *Gender and History* 19, 3 (November 2007): 519–42.

Sweet, Helen, and Sue Hawkins, eds., *Colonial Caring: A History of Colonial and Post-colonial Nursing.* Manchester: Manchester University Press, 2015.

Tangelder, Helen. "Reformed Reflections: Dr. Robert McClure New Moderator of the United Church (1969)." http://www.reformedreflections.ca/other-religions/uc-dr-robert-mcclure-moderator.html.

Taylor, Jay. *The Generalissimo: Chiang Kai-shek and the Struggle for Modern China.* Cambridge, MA: Belknap Press, 2009.

Tesdell, Margaret Stanley. "Hospital Beds: North China Style." *American Journal of Nursing* 50, 2 (February 1950): 112–13.

Tickner, Ann J. *A Feminist Voyage through International Relations.* Oxford: Oxford University Press, 2014.

–. *Gender in International Relations: Feminist Perspectives on Achieving Global Security.* New York: Columbia University Press, 1992.

Ting-Toomey, Stella. *Communicating across Cultures.* New York: Guilford Press, 1999.

Trent, Bill. "Dr Robert McClure: Missionary-Surgeon Extraordinaire." *Canadian Medical Association Journal* 132 (February 1985): 431–41.

Tuckman, E. "Rural Health Problems in China." *Lancet* 255, 6603 (18 March 1950): 477–524.

Tumblety, Joan. *Memory and History: Understanding Memory as Source and Subject.* Abingdon, UK: Routledge, 2013.

Turner, Victor W. "'Betwixt and Between': The Liminal Period in the Rites of Passage." In *Proceedings of the American Ethnological Society,* ed. M. Banton, 4–20. Seattle: American Ethnological Society, 1964.

Watenpaugh, Keith David. *Bread from Stones: The Middle East and the Making of Modern Humanitarianism.* Oakland: University of California Press, 2015.

White, Evelyn R. *South of the Clouds: Yunnan and the Salween Front, 1944: Memories of a British Nursing Sister.* London: China Society, 1985.

White, Steven. "Quakers, Conscientious Objectors, the Friends Civilian Public Service Corps and the World War Two." *Southern Friend* 14, 1 (1992): 5–21.

Williamsen, Marvin. "The Military Dimension, 1937–1941." In *China's Bitter Victory: War with Japan, 1937–1945,* ed. James C. Hsiung and Steven I. Levine, 135–56. New York: Routledge, 2015.

Woodbridge, George. *UNRRA: The History of the United Nations Relief and Rehabilitation Administration.* 3 vols. New York: Columbia University Press, 1950.

Zijlstra, Lieuwe, Andrej Zwitter, and Liesbet Heyse. "International Humanitarian Assistance: Legitimate Intervention or Illegitimate Interference?" In *Ethics and Crisis Management,* ed. Lina Svedin, 57–74. Charlotte, NC: Information Age Publishing, 2011. https://www.academia.edu/17397331/International_Humanitarian_Assistance_Legitimate_Intervention_or_Illegitimate_Interference.

Index

Abbott, Edwin, 62, 63–64, 147–48
acclimatization: Brown and, 139; Bull and, 112; Chinese colleagues and, 84; Chinese nurses and, 257; factors shaping, 116–17; magnitude of, 53; McClure as underestimating, 52; Perry on, 102; Western nurses and, 143. *See also* British nurses, unpreparedness of
acculturation: agency/assimilation/accommodation and, 192; British nurses and, 96, 223; Chinese nurses and, 53; Chinese nurses' role in, 50; factors shaping, 116–17; individual differences in, 192–93, 223, 257–58; of MT24 recruits, 235; of nurses *vs.* physicians, 255. *See also entries beginning* cross-cultural
Alexander, Walter: beliefs, 144; joining the Bruderhof, 144, 259; and Keinshui nursing school, 142; later life, 259; marriage to Brown, 138, 142; repatriation, 142, 143, 163; at Weihui hospital, 162, 163; on Woodward, 147
ambulance service: abandonment of ambulance work, 30; Burma Road too narrow for, 31; McClure's new definition as transportation of supplies *vs.* wounded, 46–47; redundancy of work, 54; "rogue" Convoy drivers in Burma, 42–43; sale of ambulances, 30; shift of focus to civilian medical work/rehabilitation of medical facilities, 35–36
American Friends Board of Foreign Missions: and Friends Centre in Shanghai, 27; UCR and, 28

American Friends Service Committee (AFSC): and BFSC reconvention of FAU, 8–9; and conscientious objectors, 9; establishment of, 27; exploration of opportunities for China project, 27; and Foreign Office grant-in-aid to British Fund for the Relief of Distress in China, 28; formation of, 9; and FSU, 9; and FSU funding, 205; and impartial humanitarian aid, 264; inauguration of FSU, 201; and McClure, 30; Nobel Prize awarded to, 5–6; and pacifist humanitarian aid, 263–64; and recruits' pacifist views, 90; redefinition of wartime mandate, 27; schisms with FAU, 27; Second World War and, 9; Vietnam War and, 264; on Western nurses in China, 48
American Red Cross, 56; China Convoy providing transport for, 31; supplies for Yan'an, 172
Amos, Baroness, 17
assimilation. *See* acculturation
"authentic knowers," 16, 116, 118, 267

Baoshan: 71st Army Hospital, Baoshan, 54; mission hospital, 99; MST2 at, 41–42, 54; MT5 at, 79, 100, 106–7, 145
Barr, Arthur (Art): on army officials as cooperative, 66; on brotherhood of man, 53; on China as test of Christian service concept, 53; on Chinese nurses, 74; convalescence in Kunming from typhus, 74; on fully trained nurses, 90; in Liuzhou, 140; on MST2 troubles, 55; with MT3, 73; with MT6, 60; with MT7, 65; on Wei Shen